STEPS FORWARDS IN DIAGNOSING AND CONTROLLING INFLUENZA

Edited by **Manal Mohammad Baddour**

Steps Forwards in Diagnosing and Controlling Influenza
http://dx.doi.org/10.5772/61910
Edited by Manal Mohammad Baddour

Contributors

Yasemin Budama Kilinc, Rabia Cakir Koc, Andrey Dmitrievich Protasov, Mikhail Kostinov, Alexander Zhestkov, Mikhail Shteiner, Svetlana Kazharova, Yuriy Tezikov, Igor Lipatov, Chen Wang, Chengshui Liao, Wufan Zhang, Deyuan Li, Puyan Chen, Atsushi Yasuda, Motoyuki Esaki, Kristi Moore Dorsey, Zoltan Penzes, Vilmos Palya, Darrell Kapczynski, Yannick Gardin, Anna Maria Iorio, Barbara Camilloni, Emilia Nunzi, Michela Basileo, Tsunetaka Ohta, Majid Laassri, Ewan P Plant, Tatiana Zagorodnyaya, Elvira Rodionova, Alin Voskanian-Kordi, Vahan Simonyan, Zhiping Ye, Ronghui Wang, Yanbin Li, Ted Ross, Terianne Wong, Jill Manske, Hanna Radecka

Published by InTech

Janeza Trdine 9, 51000 Rijeka, Croatia

Publishing Process Manager Dajana Pemac

Technical Editor SPi Global

Cover InTech Design team

First published October, 2016

Printed in Croatia

Additional hard copies can be obtained from orders@intechopen.com

Steps Forwards in Diagnosing and Controlling Influenza, Edited by Manal Mohammad Baddour

p. cm.

Print ISBN 978-953-51-2732-1

Online ISBN 978-953-51-2733-8

For EU product safety concerns:
IN TECH d.o.o., Prolaz Marije Krucifikse Kozulić 3, 51000 Rijeka, Croatia,
info@intechopen.com or visit our website at intechopen.com.

Meet the editor

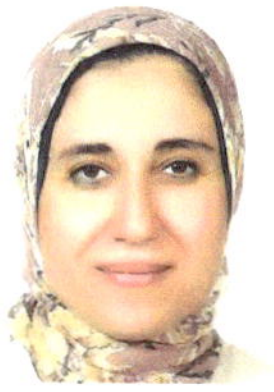

Manal Mohammad Baddour is a Professor of Medical Microbiology and Immunology, Faculty of Medicine, Alexandria University, Egypt. She serves as a Clinical Microbiologist and Microbiology Consultant in the Alexandria University Hospital as well as in several private sector hospitals. She has been Principal Investigator or Coinvestigator of 18 research projects from various academic granting agencies. She has supervised 4 PhD and 13 master's degree theses. She has reviewed manuscripts for 18 international journals. She has served as Editor and Associate Editor on the board of several international journals. She has published 32 microbiology articles mostly in renowned journals and has authored 2 internationally published books with an h-index of 9. She has also edited an open-access book. She shares in many conferences and workshops related to microbiology and infection control.

Contents

Preface

Continuous sporadic transmission of avian influenza H5N1 and swine influenza H1N1 to large numbers of humans has prompted concerns that conditions are suitable for emergence of a pandemic influenza virus.

There have been five influenza pandemics during the past 100 years, and each has been caused by the emergence of a novel virus. Adaptability of influenza virus to various host species and evasion of natural immunity make this ubiquitous pathogen particularly difficult to eradicate. We are always prone to influenza pandemics and their consequences. Influenza epidemics and pandemics have an enormous toll on human health and economy. Estimates of potential global mortality related to pandemic avian influenza are as high as 62 million deaths.

Rapid and accurate diagnosis is a key factor in order to timely instate therapeutic and control measures. Current diagnostic techniques are not as rapid and as sensitive/specific as we would like them to be, and their application demands high-quality laboratories. Biosensors are attractive alternatives. They are self-contained integrated analytical instruments, which are capable of providing specific quantitative or semiquantitative analytical information applying a biological recognition element, which is in direct spatial contact with a transducer element. Main parameters describing the quality of biosensors are selectivity, sensitivity, reproducibility, and time of response. Novel approaches using biosensors and electrochemical sensors are being studied and presented within the context of this book.

Immunization against avian influenza remains an active area of research, despite a plethora of research articles and a wealth of information. The diversity of influenza virus strains and subtypes exacerbates the challenge for generating a universal vaccine against influenza. WHO makes recommendations for influenza vaccine composition for each flu season based on international surveillance systems and compares the ability of monovalent vaccine prototypes to elicit cross-reactive antibodies against prevalent circulating strains. Development of a universal vaccine to protect against the diverse and continuously evolving virus would be a shining beacon in the scientific virology community.

Additionally, production of influenza vaccine has been hampered by manufacturing difficulties and modest immunogenicity in humans. High-priority research goals include improving production speed and increasing quantity of vaccine. Areas of research include the use of cell culture systems, dose-sparing approaches, the use of adjuvants and live-attenuated viruses to induce more robust immune responses, as well as more contemporary delivery systems such as nanoparticles and recombinant vectors. Several such issues related to influenza vaccines are reviewed here.

Vulnerable populations such as pregnant females, the elderly, and those suffering from lung diseases warrant special attention regarding vaccine efficacy and safety. Thus vaccination outcomes in these populations are among the topics discussed in this book.

Dr. Manal Mohammad Baddour
Microbiology Dept.,
Faculty of Medicine
Alexandria University
Alexandria, Egypt

Section 1

Diagnostic Approaches

Chapter 1

Influenza Diagnosis with a Specific Emphasis on the M2e Antigen as a Diagnostic Tool

Yasemin Budama-Kilinc and Rabia Cakir-Koc

Additional information is available at the end of the chapter

http://dx.doi.org/10.5772/64786

Abstract

The therapy, observation, inclusiveness, and preclusion of related diseases all influence the diagnosis of influenza. Particularly, the pandemic duration and diagnosis time for influenza are extremely important. After the appearance of symptoms, antiviral medication must be initiated within 48 h. Cell culture, real-time polymerase chain reaction (PCR), flow cytometry, direct and indirect immunofluorescence methods, and the quick diagnosis test are all valuable approaches for the diagnosis of influenza. Different instruments, different time durations for the results, and different specialists characterize all these approaches. Antigen selection is of critical importance with regard to the specificity and sensitivity of these methods, especially the serological and rapid diagnosis tests. M2e, the highly conserved external domain of the influenza A M2 protein, is a potential differential diagnostic marker for influenza virus infection. This chapter reviews the studies that use M2e as a diagnosis agent, and it illuminates the role and importance of M2e in the diagnosis of influenza.

Keywords: M2e, diagnosis, peptide, antigen, virus culture, rapid immunochromotographic test, serological test, ELISA, PCR

1. Introduction

Influenza viruses can cause respiratory infections, and it is a major cause of morbidity and mortality worldwide [1]. Influenza is typically a mild disease that lasts for 1–2 weeks in most people [2], although in some cases it can be fatal [3]. The likelihood of developing complications is higher in certain risk groups, such as people with chronic health problems, children under 2 years old, and the elderly [4]. While 45–77% of those hospitalized due to influenza are under 65 years old, the patients who are older than 65 years are the most likely (60–90%) to die as a result of influenza [5–8].

The variable nature of the influenza has already caused several pandemics. The accurate and rapid diagnosis of influenza is therefore of great importance to the effective management of epidemic and pandemic periods [4]. As there are several respiratory pathogens that may cause clinical symptoms similar to those caused by influenza, a final diagnosis is difficult for doctors to establish [9]. As a result, sensitive and rapid diagnosis methods are needed to confirm the clinical diagnosis of influenza, as well as to improve the quality of monitoring systems. A variety of laboratory methods for the diagnosis of influenza are available (**Table 1**). Each of these methods has both advantages and disadvantages, and some or all of these factors may affect the selection of an appropriate diagnosis method [2].

Diagnosis method	Average acquisition time	Mechanism	Application opportunity	Sample required
Viral culture	3–7 days	Virus isolation	Limited	Bronchoalveolar lavage Nose and throat swab Nasopharyngeal aspirate
Molecular tests	1–2 days	RNA detection	Limited	Post-mortem tissue Bronchoalveolar lavage Nose and throat swab Nasopharyngeal aspirate
Rapid immunochromatographic tests	15–30 min	Antigen detection	Widespread	Bronchoalveolar lavage Nose and throat swab Nasopharyngeal aspirate
Serological tests	2 days	Antigen/antibody detection	Widespread	Serum

Table 1. Comparison of the diagnostic methods available for the influenza A virus.

In this chapter, the methods that have developed and used in the diagnosis of influenza will be evaluated in terms of their principles, sensitivity, specificity, time, advantages and disadvantages, and the antigens used for the diagnosis of influenza A.

2. Diagnosis methods for influenza A

There are four basic methods available for the diagnosis of influenza [10], each of which is detailed in **Table 1**.

http://dx.doi.org/10.5772/64786

2.1. Virus cultures

2.1.1. Classic virus cultures

Symptoms such as the deformation of cell morphology, cell necrosis, pouring from the cell location to the cell culture, and fusion in cells that are infected with the virus are, depending on the virus proliferation, referred to as the cytopathic effects (CPE) [11].

Virus cultures that use primary rhesus monkey kidney cells (PMK) or Madin-Darby canine kidney cells (MDCK) are commonly accepted to be one of the "gold standards" for laboratory diagnosis. Whether or not the cells are infected with the virus is determined by the cytopathic effects in the cell cultures and hemadsorption using immunofluorescence monoclonal antibodies against influenza [10].

2.1.2. Rapid shell vial virus cultures

Coverglasses are used in the rapid shell vial cell culture method to passage the cell lines onto them. The specimens are inoculated after the monolayer cell lines occur. The coverglasses are then stained with cause-specific FITC-marked monoclonal antibodies for about 24–48 h. Cytopathic effects are not expected with this method, unlike in standard tube cultures [12].

Influenza isolation with the rapid shell vial culture method provides an advantage with regard to its simplicity and speed when compared to traditional culture method [13]. Influenza shell vial cultures show results within 1–3 days after virus inoculation [12] (**Figure 1**).

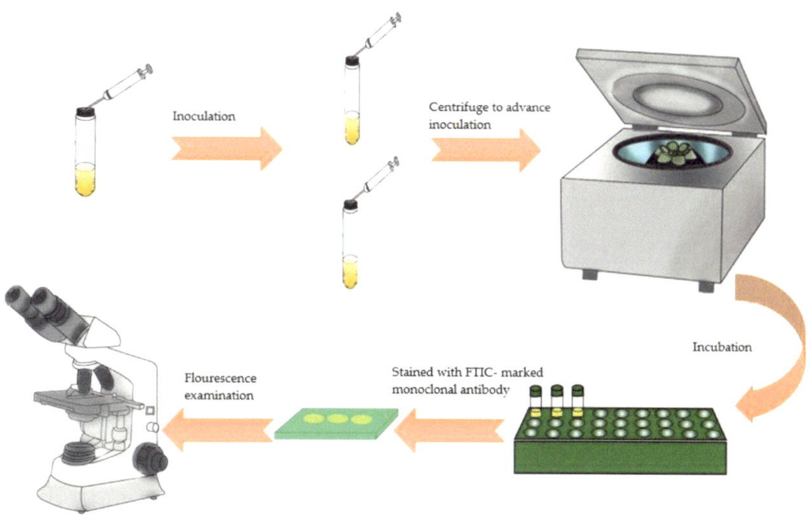

Figure 1. Schematic presentation of shell vial method.

The specificity of the rapid shell vial test is 100%. Although the time necessary to obtain the results is much shorter in this method than in traditional cell cultures, in many cases, the time is actually insufficient to begin optimal antiviral treatment [10].

2.2. Molecular methods

The genome of the influenza viruses consists of eight different parts of single-stranded negative sense RNA. This structure changes continuously and it contributes to the evaluation of the virus [14]. Major changes occur in the genes encoding the two major surface glycoproteins, namely the hemagglutinin (HA) and neuraminidase (NA) antigens. The HA antigens play a role in the connection of the virus to the cell, NA plays an essential role in release and spread of progeny virions, following the intracellular viral replication cycle [15]. There are 18 different hemagglutinin subtypes and 11 different neuraminidase subtypes, H1–H18 and N1–N11, respectively [16]. The high mutation rate causes the development of subtypes [17].

The extreme genetic variability of the influenza viruses leads to challenges in the design of molecular-based diagnosis tests. Most conserved sequences in the genome used to determine the RT-PCR primers can be used to identify individual strains of influenza virus [12]. A PCR that has been modified by the addition of the reverse transcription step is known as a reverse transcription-PCR (RT-PCR). In addition, the use of specific primers for significant types of HA and NA antigens can aid in the identification of subtypes of influenza viruses [17].

A RT-PCR can be performed in two different ways: (1) the one-step approach (reverse transcription and PCR), which is performed in a single tube; and (2) the two-step approach, which involves the transformation of RNA to cDNA and the amplification of the tested sequences. The two-step reaction process is more sensitive when compared with the one-step reaction. On the other hand, the one-step RT-PCR reaction is fast, and the minimal number of steps reduces the risk of contamination and so improves the reproducibility of the obtained results [12].

Many RT-PCR tests of the subtypes of influenza have shown greater sensitivity than other rapid diagnosis tests and conventional cell cultures. The RT-PCR activity does not change depending on the age of the patients. The rotation period of the RT-PCR for influenza is between 1 and 2 days. In addition, molecular tests require considerable skill and expertise, and they should hence be integrated into the laboratory processes [10].

2.3. Rapid immunochromatographic tests

Rapid diagnosis kits are immunochromatographic methods that include the use of monoclonal antibodies against preserved antigens or nucleoproteins that are localized with a membrane or impregnated onto a strip of influenza A or A and B [18].

Briefly put, according to these methods, the respiratory specimen is primarily treated with an extraction buffer and it is then applied to a filter paper or test strip depending on the test format. If influenza viral antigens are available, a visible color change is generated by the reaction of the antigens and influenza-specific monoclonal antibodies [19].

The sensitivity of the rapid diagnostic kits is approximately 70%, depending on the particular test kit used, the patient's age, and the sample collection time [20]. The specificity of the rapid diagnostic kits ranges from 76 to 100% [21]. In addition, many kits can distinguish between the influenza A and B strains, although they cannot subtype further [20].

Influenza A has a higher sensitivity in the rapid diagnosis test kits when compared with influenza B. Such rapid diagnosis kits are very convenient, and they have a high positive predictive value because of the spread of influenza in the community [21]. The most important advantage of these tests is the fact that they can provide results in approximately 10–30 min [10].

However, during periods of low influenza activity, the predictive value of the rapid diagnostic kits is also low, and false positive results are more likely. Therefore, the use of these tests during periods of high influenza activity is suggested [21]. In addition, more specific testing methods must be performed on patients who present with negative results according to the rapid influenza diagnostic kits during high influenza periods. The major disadvantage of these tests is their limited shelf life of approximately 1–2 years. The inadequate collection of samples and the misinterpretation of test strips by inexperienced personnel may also lead to errors [10].

2.4. Serological tests

Serological methods are all based on determining the antibody response in the sera or specific antigens or gene sequences of influenza virus. Specific, sensitive, and validated serological assays can be used for diagnosis of influenza, the identification of the source of infection, the epidemiology studies, and the identification of asymptomatic cases. Serological methods have also been utilized at prescreening of influenza disease [22].

The immunology of tested population and sensibility and specificity of the tests have major role on interpret results of serological tests [23]. Each type of serological methods have own advantages, disadvantages, and unique characteristics [24]. The serological diagnosis of influenza infection is based on agar gel immunodiffusion, radioimmunoassay, immunofluorescence antibody tests, hemagglutination inhibition, enzyme-linked immunoassay (EIA), complement fixation, and an increase of specific antibody titer between acute and healing serum samples as measured by neutralization tests [10, 17, 25].

2.4.1. Direct immunofluorescence antibody test (DFA)

In this method, antibodies are labeled with fluorescent compounds called fluorophores. Fluorophores are generally organic molecules with cyclic structure. Fluorescein and rhodamine are examples of the most used molecules.

In this method, the antigen in the suspected material is fixed on slides and specifically labeled antibodies placed onto the antigen. Fluorescence labeled (FITC) "monoclonal antibodies" are considered positive due to the luminescence in the presence of agent in patients' samples [12, 25–27]. DFA test is developed for antigen detection in tissue or body fluids and used successfully for diagnosis of influenza. Among children who have high fever and spread lots of influenza viruses, DFA sensitivity is commonly higher [26] (**Figure 2**).

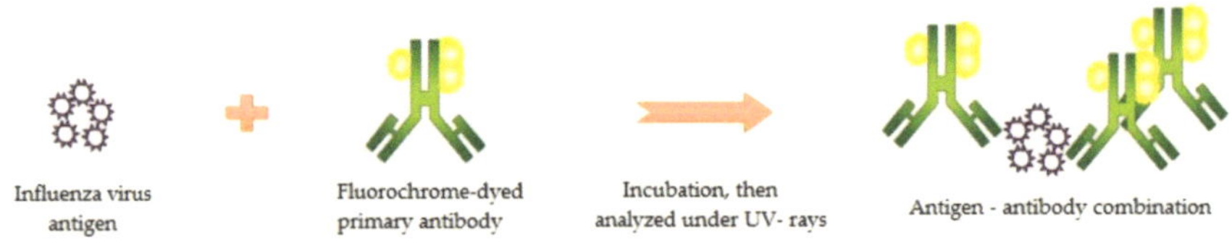

Figure 2. Schematic presentation of direct immunofluorescence antibody test.

2.4.2. Indirect immunofluorescence antibody test (IFAT)

In an indirect immunofluorescence assay, antibodies against influenza labeled with fluorescence dyes are used [10, 27, 28]. Influenza A virus particles are fixed on a slide and then the suspected serum is added. FITC conjugated anti-human IgG antibodies are added and examination is made under a microscope [29]. If there is a homologous antibody against the virus on the slide in the influenza suspected serum, a yellow-green glow is seen under a microscope (i.e., a positive reaction) [10, 12].

In principle, the serum antibodies react with immunofluorescence allow for the rapid diagnosis. The sensitivity of the IFA test is 70–90%, while the specificity is above 90% for diagnosis of influenza [20]. There are individual differences in the reporting methods for the different immunofluorescence tests, since this test faces the issue of subjectivity in the reading of slides. To overcome this problem, the IFAT should be reported by experienced clinical laboratorians [30, 31] (**Figure 3**).

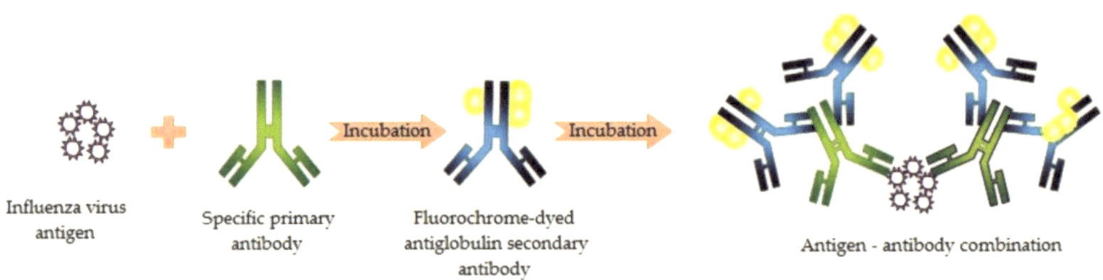

Figure 3. Schematic presentation of indirect immunofluorescence antibody test.

2.4.3. Radioimmunoassay (RIA)

Radioimmunoassay test is used to search for both an antibody against influenza and virus or viral antigen, immunoglobulins are conjugated with radioactive material (radioisotopes ^{14}C, ^{125}I, etc.). In positive reactions, the immune complex that occurs when the influenza antigen and specific antibody couple gains radioactivity. This radioactivity is determined by special counters (such as a gamma counter detector). When the results are evaluated according to a curve known as the standard curve, an overall result can be seen. The degree of determined

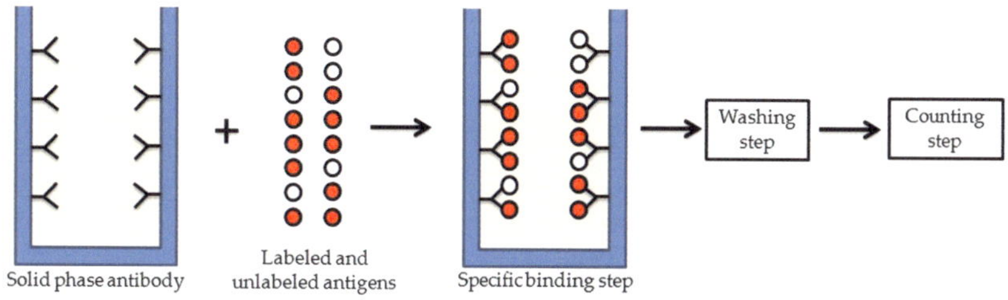

Figure 4. Principle of RIA. Labeled antigen competes with patient antigen for a limited number of binding sites on solid-phase antibody.

radioactivity could be measured in this way. In negative reactions, radioactivity cannot be detected [27, 32].

RIA is a very sensitive and precise technique for detection low amounts of analytes. Otherwise, the health hazard of radioactive substances is most important limitation of all RIA techniques due to disposal problems, short half-life, and the need for expensive equipment [31] (**Figure 4**).

2.4.4. Agar gel immunodiffusion (AGID)

The AGID detects antibodies against all influenza A viruses, regardless of subtype. The principle of the AGID test is the simultaneous migration of antigen and antibodies toward each other through an agar gel matrix. Influenza antigens and antibodies form a precipitate in to gel matrix and precipitation line is visualized. Various parameters such as electrolyte concentration, pH, and temperature can affect precipitate formation [33]. Also, concentrations of the antigen or antibodies cause shift the location of the line [34]. The immunodiffusion method can be performed in three different ways, namely simple diffusion (the Oudin method), unidirectional diffusion (the Mancini method), and bidirectional diffusion (Ouchterlony) [35]. The advantages of this method are simplicity, low cost, and inessential specialized laboratory equipment [36].

2.4.5. Neutralization test

The neutralization assay determines that patients' antibody can neutralize the infectivity of a given influenza virus strain. Sera that contain specific neutralizing antibodies prevent the cytopathic effects of influenza virus [27]. Influenza viruses cause CPE via proliferation in cells form plaques (i.e., the CPE focus) on nutrient agarose-coated cells [19]. If the virus is cultured on monolayer cells after being stirred with antiviral homologous antibodies formed against itself and then left at room temperature for 30–40 min, plaques either do not form (i.e., plaque neutralization) or else the number of plaques decreases in those cells coated with nutrient agar (i.e., plaque reduction). A reduction in the number of plaques of 50% or more is considered a positive reaction. If the virus encounters a homologous antibody carrying serum, then plaque formation is seen because the neutralization does not occur [12].

The influenza subtypes can be defined by using a type-specific antiviral immune serum. The neutralization reaction is also utilized as a protection test in animals [27].

The neutralization test has several advantages which it can identify functional, strain-specific antibodies in sera [37]. However, it cannot be used routinely since it is time-consuming and laborious.

2.4.6. Complement fixation (CF) test

The complement fixation test (CFT) is one of the classical influenza diagnostic assays, which mainly detects IgG antibodies [38].

In this test, the primarily influenza suspected serum (titrated), then the known viral antigen (titrated), and later the complement (fresh guinea pig serum titer) are added. They are thoroughly mixed and then allowed to stand. At this stage, if a homologous antibody against influenza is present in the serum, the antibody couples with the antigen and the complement binds with this complex. If there is no antibody present, coupling with the antigen does not occur and hence the complement cannot connect and so remains free. A mixture known as the hemolytic system (hemolytic serum + sheep red blood cells) is added to the tubes to determine whether or not the complement is attached. If there is no hemolysis in the erythrocytes, the complement is held in the first stage or, in other words, in the antibody-antigen complex. This indicates the presence of an antibody in the influenza suspected patient's serum (i.e., a positive reaction) [12, 39].

CFT is useful test for diagnosis of acute virus infection, however, it is quite complex, less sensitive, very labor intensive, and is not suitable for automation.

2.4.7. Hemagglutination (HA) vs. hemagglutination inhibition (HI)

The hemagglutination inhibition test is an important diagnostic tool in certain infections especially influenza. The hemagglutinin protein on the surface of the virus may cause agglutination in the presence of erythrocytes [40]. Blocking of this aggregation by specific antibodies in the patient's serum is named as hemagglutination inhibition test [37].

The HA agglutination test is the conventional method for the determination of influenza viruses, while the HI test is commonly used for typing [40]. If the sera from individuals suspected of carrying the disease have virus-specific antibodies against the virus, then these antibodies prevent HA by neutralizing the HA property of the virus when the antibodies and the virus come into contact with each other. In test tubes, erythrocyte aggregate occurs on the bottom in the form of a round point [19].

In the HI test, the numbers of antibodies within the serum are proportional to the amount of HI titers. The HI titers in the serum may remain at the initial dilution if there is less antibody present, although the titers in the serum will reach different dilutions if there is too much antibody present [39, 41].

The hemagglutination inhibition assay is a reliable, relatively simple, and inexpensive technique to antigenically characterize isolates of influenza viruses [37]. Whereas the HI test is very useful in epidemiological surveys, it is not suitable for routine diagnosis of influenza [42]. Nowadays, this assay is widely used and is replaced by more modern immunoassays [38].

2.4.8. Enzyme-linked immunosorbent assay (ELISA)

In enzyme immunoassays, enzyme-conjugated antibodies are generally used for detection of viral antigens. These groups of tests, antigen or antibody are bound to solid phase as microtiter plates, nitrocellulose membranes, and magnetic latex beads [31]. Patient serum is added to antigen bounded solid phase and an enzyme-labeled antiglobulin is added. If anti-influenza antibody is present in patient's serum, enzyme-labeled secondary antibody reacts and chromogenic substrate causes color change [27].

The specific antigens as HA, NA, NP, and M protein of influenza are widely used ELISA. The sensitivity of EIA varies between 64 and 78% [43]. Because of the high specificity, sensitivity, simplicity, and low cost, ELISA is one of the most common used immunoassays in the clinical laboratory [31].

3. Antigens that are used in diagnosis

The methods used in the diagnosis of influenza (except for viral cultures) are based on the determination of the antigen of the virus, the determination of antibodies against the antigen in the patient, or the determination of the gene region of the selected antigen as in molecular methods [40]. In all these methods, the target antigenic structures are used as important selection criteria that affect the specificity and sensitivity of the method. Nucleoproteins and neuraminidase are used in the viral commercial diagnostic kits (rapid tests) popular in commercial studies and academic research. Due to the virus undergoing changes, the use of these antigens in the diagnosis tests affects the obtained results. For this reason, it is also important to use the conserved regions of influenza A in diagnosis [44].

Therefore, in this part of the chapter, the M2 protein, the most conserved structure of influenza A, will be evaluated in terms of its diagnostic importance by considering its biological functions.

3.1. Definition of M2e protein

In influenza A viruses, one of the most important structural proteins is matrix protein 2 (M2) [45]. The M2 protein, the internal membrane protein, is made up of an ectodomain part, which is a single membrane spanning domain located at the N-terminus, and a cytoplasmic tail, which is found in the C-terminal [46].

While the N-terminus domain is 24 amino acids long, part of it is located at the outer side of the membrane surface (M2e), while the 54 amino acids long C-terminus is situated in the cytoplasmic side and the remaining 19 amino acids sequence the lipid bilayer [46] (**Figure 5**).

From the first human influenza A strain that was isolated in 1933 to the present day, no amino acid mutation has been found in the extracellular domain of the M2 protein [47]. In all subtypes of the influenza A viruses, the extracellular domain of the M2 protein, M2e, is significantly conserved with an unchanged SLLTEVET (residues 2e9) sequence at the N-terminal [48]. The M2e protein consists of a homotetramer structure with disulfide linkages that are held together by noncovalent interactions [49]. The M2e protein is conserved in all types of influenza A viruses. Despite appearing in small amounts on the surface of mature virions, this protein is majorly expressed on the surface of infected cells [46].

The peptide epitope of the influenza A virus M2e protein is: Met-Ser-Leu-Leu-Thr-Glu-Val-Glu-Thr-Pro-Ile-Arg-Asn-Glu-Trp-Gly-Cys-Arg-Cys-Asn-Asp-Ser-Ser.

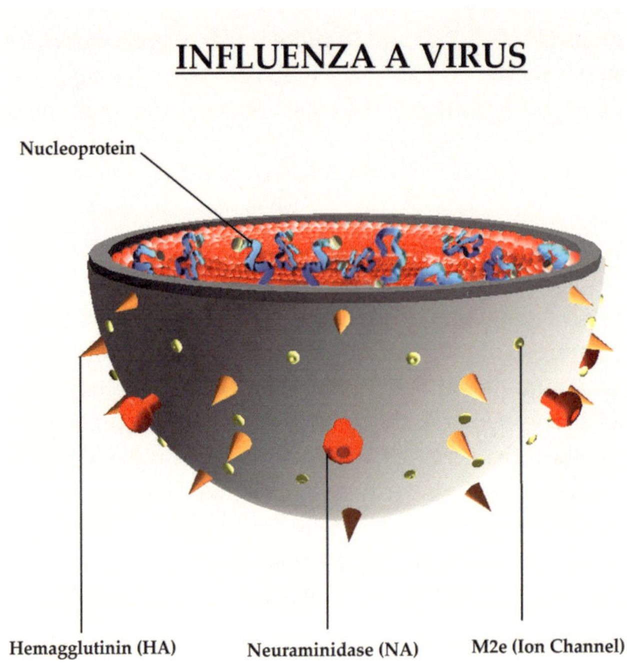

Figure 5. Schematic presentation of influenza A virus structure.

3.2. Biological function of M2e

The main functions of the M2e protein are: (i) functioning as a proton channel; (ii) playing a role in viral replication; and (ii) defending the maturation of HA and structural integrity [48].

The M2e protein is not required for viral replication, but during viral disintegration, it does act as an ion channel that allows the entry of protons into the virions [50]. M2 also plays an effective role in virus morphogenesis and assembly.

M2e stabilizes the newly synthesized HA molecules by adjusting the pH toward the secretion pathway [51]. M2 transport protons reduce the interior pH of the virions via a receptor-mediated endocytosis procedure during the entry of the virus [52].

3.3. Immunological responses against M2e

Mucosal and systemic immunity play a role in the body's resistance to infection. Influenza-specific lymphocytes have been detected in the blood and lower respiratory secretions of influenza patients [53]. A short-term primary cytotoxic T-cell response can be detected after 1–2 weeks (infection with influenza viruses leads to virus-specific B cell as well as T-cell responses) [54]. Antibodies occur against type-specific internal proteins, NA, and M1, as well as against viral surface glycoproteins such as HA and NA. The neutralizing antibodies against HA are the first immune constituents to protect the host from infections caused by the influenza viruses [55, 56].

M2 is a significantly expressed structural protein on the surface of infected cells. M2e is a small portion with a low immunogenicity in its native form [52]. The relatively small size of M2e and its low abundance in virions when compared to other glycoproteins like HA and NA are possible explanations for the low reactivity of M2e [57]. Anti-M2e antibodies can develop in some infected patients [52]. The host's adaptive immune system attracts the virus. At the same time, the infection of humans with influenza A viruses stimulates a weak anti-M2 antibody response for a short duration of time [58]. The anti-M2e antibodies' seroprevalence is increased with age, which is an auxiliary factor in this pre-existing immunity against M2 [59].

M2e-specific antibodies act through the antibody dependent cell cytotoxicity, and the innate or complementary immune system promotes the killing of infected cells. Specific M2e antibodies prevent the release of viral particles toward the extracellular fluid or else stimulate the uptake by phagocytic cells through the Fc receptors via connecting to the viral cell [44, 52].

3.4. Studies that have used M2e in the diagnosis of influenza

Ingrole et al. chose to use M2e in their study based on its preserved region. The use of an elastin-like particle led to the increase in size of the produced antibody. M2e can easily be recognized by the M2e-specific antibodies due to the conjugation of M2e and ELP (elastin-like particles) [60].

Khurana et al. conducted an experiment based on HA2 (488–516), PB1-F2 (2–75), and M2 (2–24) peptides, which have the most conserved regions of the H5N1 strain. In their study, experiments were carried out with ELISA and rapid diagnostic kits, and the effects of these peptides were investigated. In the study that used rapid diagnostic kits, the attachment to the HA2 and M2 peptide bands was observed to be positive in the serum of infected patients. In the ELISA study, there was no reactivity against H5N1 in patients who were vaccinated with a vaccine that did not include the M2e peptide [61].

Denis et al. investigated the use of the papaya mosaic virus as a carrier of the conserved and small amount M2 peptide instead of HA and NA peptides in a vaccine study. Papaya mosaic virus conjugated virus-like particles have been observed to increase the production of the antibody against the M2 peptide. Specific bindings were observed against M2e in both ELISA and MCDK cell culture experiments [62].

Wolf examined the effect of M2e-based multiple antigenic peptides on the production of antibodies via ELISA and ELISPOT techniques. The specificity to the M2e peptide was measured in antibody secreting cells by ELISPOT assay and, as a result, a higher formation of immunoglobulin levels was observed [63].

Hadifar et al. used an ELISA method based on the distracted intravenous access (DIVA) test against H5N1 in their study. The M2e antigenicity of the monomers that form when infected in a natural way to be limited is developed with the DIVA test method. The use of the tetramer structure of M2e instead of the M2e monomer increased the efficiency of the ELISA and other tests mentioned in this study [64].

Tarigan et al. used the single M2e peptide (sp-M2e) ELISA and multiple antigenic forms of the M2e ELISA methods, and the sensitivity of these tests in the diagnosis of M2e was compared. The degrees of M2e were measured by ELISA in order to use the M2e as a target in the DIVA test during pandemics. Although both ELISA techniques have specificity in the diagnosis of the M2e peptide, the MAP-M2e ELISA technique has higher specificity and sensitivity in the diagnosis of M2e [65].

Black et al. determined the influenza A (H2N2) M2 expression of recombinant baculovirus via an indirect immunofluorescent antibody assay (IFA) in a study conducted in 1993. The formation of an antibody against M2e was determined using the EIA test [54].

4. Future aspects

In a study conducted by the US Food and Drug Administration (FDA), the analytical performance of the 11 most widely used influenza diagnostic tests on the market was evaluated in a comprehensive manner. In experiments conducted using 23 different influenza subtypes that have been in circulation recently, although most brands could detect the viral antigen in samples that included a high concentration of influenza virus, it was found that detection based on subtypes of the virus is limited in lower concentrations. It was further suggested that physicians should be careful of negative results when using rapid diagnosis tests for the diagnosis of influenza [66].

Peptide-based enzyme immunoassays are widely used in the sero-diagnosis of bacterial and viral infections. These tests can be easily applied due to their enhanced advantages, namely simplicity, specificity, sensitivity, and relative inexpensiveness.

Despite the genetic differentiation of the influenza A virus, it has been shown that the peptide region formed by the 24 amino acids of the M2e protein located on the surface of the virus is the most conserved region in all strains, and it has therefore been used as a potential diagnosis marker in various studies [56, 57, 67, 68]. Although M2e is normally found in small quantities on virus particles, it is secreted abundantly on the cell surface infected by the virus and, in particular, it will provide a significant advantage in the detection of the disease during pandemic periods [61]. Therefore, diagnosis tests that are developed based on M2e will be able to detect different subtypes of the influenza viruses.

http://dx.doi.org/10.5772/64786

Acknowledgements

The authors would like to thank The Scientific and Technological Research Council of Turkey (TUBİTAK) for their support the named "Development of Rapid Diagnostic Kit with Immunochromatographic Method of Depending on IgY Antibody Specific in (M2e) Peptide for Diagnosis of Influenza A Infection" (Project No. 115S132).

Author details

Yasemin Budama-Kilinc* and Rabia Cakir-Koc

*Address all correspondence to: yaseminbudama@gmail.com

Department of Bioengineering, Chemical and Metallurgical Engineering Faculty, Yildiz Technical University, Esenler, Istanbul, Turkey

References

[1] Kunisaki, K.M. and E.N. Janoff, Influenza in immunosuppressed populations: a review of infection frequency, morbidity, mortality, and vaccine responses. The Lancet Infectious Diseases, 2009. 9(8): p. 493–504.

[2] Ellis, J.S. and M.C. Zambon, Molecular diagnosis of influenza. Reviews in Medical Virology, 2002. 12(6): p. 375–389.

[3] Morens, D.M., J.K. Taubenberger, and A.S. Fauci, Predominant role of bacterial pneumonia as a cause of death in pandemic influenza: implications for pandemic influenza preparedness. Journal of Infectious Diseases, 2008. 198(7): p. 962–970.

[4] Steininger, C., et al., Effectiveness of reverse transcription-PCR, virus isolation, and enzyme-linked immunosorbent assay for diagnosis of influenza A virus infection in different age groups. Journal of Clinical Microbiology, 2002. 40(6): p. 2051–2056.

[5] Irwin, D.E., et al., Impact of patient characteristics on the risk of influenza/ILI-related complications. BMC Health Services Research, 2001. 1(1): p. 1.

[6] Barker, W.H., Excess pneumonia and influenza associated hospitalization during influenza epidemics in the United States, 1970–78. American Journal of Public Health, 1986. 76(7): p. 761–765.

[7] Bridges, C.B., et al., Prevention and control of influenza. Recommendations of the Advisory Committee on Immunization Practices (ACIP). MMWR. Recommendations

and Reports: Morbidity and Mortality Weekly Report. Recommendations and Reports/ Centers for Disease Control, 2002. 51(RR-3): p. 1–31.

[8] Perrotta, D.M., M. Decker, and W.P. Glezen, Acute respiratory disease hospitalizations as a measure of impact of epidemic influenza. American Journal of Epidemiology, 1985. 122(3): p. 468–476.

[9] Montalto, N.J., An office-based approach to influenza: clinical diagnosis and laboratory testing. American Family Physician, 2003. 67(1): p. 111–118.

[10] Gavin, P.J. and R.B. Thomson, Review of rapid diagnostic tests for influenza. Clinical and Applied Immunology Reviews, 2004. 4(3): p. 151–172.

[11] Albrecht, T., et al., Effects on cells. 1996.

[12] Kim, D.-K. and B. Poudel, Tools to detect influenza virus. Yonsei Medical Journal, 2013. 54(3): p. 560–566.

[13] Espy, M., et al., Rapid detection of influenza virus by shell vial assay with monoclonal antibodies. Journal of Clinical Microbiology, 1986. 24(4): p. 677–679.

[14] Webster, R.G., et al., Evolution and ecology of influenza A viruses. Microbiological Reviews, 1992. 56(1): p. 152–179.

[15] Matrosovich, M.N., et al., Neuraminidase is important for the initiation of influenza virus infection in human airway epithelium. Journal of Virology, 2004. 78(22): p. 12665–12667.

[16] Quan, F.-S., et al., Progress in developing virus-like particle influenza vaccines. Expert Review of Vaccines, 2016: p. 1–13.

[17] Wozniak-Kosek, A., B. Kempińska-Mirosławska, and G. Hoser, Detection of the influenza virus yesterday and now. Acta Biochimica Polonica, 2014. 61(3): p. 465–470.

[18] Hurt, A.C., et al., Performance of six influenza rapid tests in detecting human influenza in clinical specimens. Journal of clinical virology, 2007. 39(2): p. 132–135.

[19] Chen, H., et al., Evaluation of a rapid detection influenza virus A antigens kit using paired serum antibody test. Yonsei Medical Journal, 2013. 54(2): p. 476–479.

[20] Foo, H. and D.E. Dwyer, Rapid tests for the diagnosis of influenza. Australian Prescriber, 2009. 32(3).

[21] Boivin, G., I. Hardy, and A. Kress, Evaluation of a rapid optical immunoassay for influenza viruses (FLU OIA test) in comparison with cell culture and reverse transcription-PCR. Journal of Clinical Microbiology, 2001. 39(2): p. 730–732.

[22] Vemula, S.V., et al., Current approaches for diagnosis of influenza virus infections in humans. Viruses, 2016. 8(4): p. 96.

[23] Miller, E., et al., Incidence of 2009 pandemic influenza A H1N1 infection in England: a cross-sectional serological study. The Lancet, 2010. 375(9720): p. 1100–1108.

[24] Desvaux, S., et al., Evaluation of serological tests for H5N1 avian influenza on field samples from domestic poultry populations in Vietnam: consequences for surveillance. Veterinary Microbiology, 2012. 156(3): p. 277–284.

[25] Aksakal, B.B.Z.İ.A., Avian İnfluenza Tip A Virüsleri: Etiyoloji, Teshis ve Korunma.

[26] Nitsch-Osuch, A., A. Wozniak-Kosek, and L.B. Brydak, Accuracy of rapid influenza diagnostic test and immunofluorescence assay compared to real time RT-PCR in children with influenza A (H1N1) pdm09 infection Wiarygodność szybkiego testu diagnostycznego i metody immunofluorescencji bezpośredniej w odniesieniu do real-time RT-PCR u dzieci z grypą wywołaną wirusem typu A (H1N1) pdm09. Journal Cover, 2016. 70.

[27] di BS, K., C. Hoffmann, and W. Preiser, Influenza Report 2006.

[28] Wang, B., et al., Protective efficacy of a broadly cross-reactive swine influenza DNA vaccine encoding M2e, cytotoxic T lymphocyte epitope and consensus H3 hemagglutinin. Virology Journal, 2012. 9(1): p. 1.

[29] Allwinn, R., et al., Determination of serum antibodies against swine-origin influenza A virus H1N1/09 by immunofluorescence, haemagglutination inhibition, and by neutralization tests: how is the prevalence rate of protecting antibodies in humans? Medical Microbiology and Immunology, 2010. 199(2): p. 117–121.

[30] Read, M.C., Influenza Report 2006.

[31] Stevens, C.D., Clinical immunology & serology: a laboratory perspective. 2009: FA Davis.

[32] Sarkkinen, H., P. Halonen, and A. Salmi, Detection of influenza A virus by radioimmunoassay and enzyme-immunoassay from nasopharyngeal specimens. Journal of Medical Virology, 1981. 7(3): p. 213–220.

[33] Beard, C., Demonstration of type-specific influenza antibody in mammalian and avian sera by immunodiffusion. Bulletin of the World Health Organization, 1970. 42(5): p. 779.

[34] Harlow, E. and D. Lane, A laboratory manual. New York: Cold Spring Harbor Laboratory, 1988: p. 579.

[35] Grist, N.R., et al., Diagnostic methods in clinical virology. 1979: Blackwell Scientific Publications, Osney Mead, Oxford OX2 OEL.

[36] Jenson, T.A., Agar Gel immunodiffusion assay to detect antibodies to type A influenza virus. Animal Influenza Virus, 2014: p. 141–150.

[37] Klimov, A., et al., Influenza virus titration, antigenic characterization, and serological methods for antibody detection. Influenza Virus: Methods and Protocols, 2012: p. 25–51.

[38] Vainionpää R., W.M., Leinikki P., Diagnostic techniques: serological and molecular approaches, in Reference module in biomedical sciences. 2015, Elsevier.

[39] Julkunen, I., R. Pyhälä, and T. Hovi, Enzyme immunoassay, complement fixation and hemagglutination inhibition tests in the diagnosis of influenza A and B virus infections. Purified hemagglutinin in subtype-specific diagnosis. Journal of Virological Methods, 1985. 10(1): p. 75–84.

[40] Amano, Y. and Q. Cheng, Detection of influenza virus: traditional approaches and development of biosensors. Analytical and Bioanalytical Chemistry, 2005. 381(1): p. 156–164.

[41] Serter, P.D.N., Genel Mikrobiyoloji Ve Immünoloji: Anadolu Universitesi.

[42] Garin, B., E. Plateau, and S. Gillet-Forin, Serological diagnosis of influenza A infections in the horse by enzyme immunoassay. Comparison with the complement fixation test. Veterinary Immunology and Immunopathology, 1986. 13(4): p. 357–363.

[43] Allwinn, R., et al., Laboratory diagnosis of influenza–virology or serology? Medical Microbiology and Immunology, 2002. 191(3–4): p. 157–160.

[44] Staneková, Z. and E. Varečková, Conserved epitopes of influenza A virus inducing protective immunity and their prospects for universal vaccine development. Virology Journal, 2010. 7(1): p. 1.

[45] Cho, K.J., et al., Structure of the extracellular domain of matrix protein 2 of influenza A virus in complex with a protective monoclonal antibody. Journal of Virology, 2015. 89(7): p. 3700–3711.

[46] Liu, W., H. Li, and Y.-H. Chen, N-terminus of M2 protein could induce antibodies with inhibitory activity against influenza virus replication. FEMS Immunology & Medical Microbiology, 2003. 35(2): p. 141–146.

[47] Stepanova, L.A., et al., Protection against multiple influenza A virus strains induced by candidate recombinant vaccine based on heterologous M2e peptides linked to flagellin. PLoS One, 2015. 10(3): p. e0119520.

[48] Du, L., Y. Zhou, and S. Jiang, Research and development of universal influenza vaccines. Microbes and Infection, 2010. 12(4): p. 280–286.

[49] Holsinger, L.J. and R. Alams, Influenza virus M2 integral membrane protein is a homotetramer stabilized by formation of disulfide bonds. Virology, 1991. 183(1): p. 32–43.

[50] Lamb, R. and R. Krug, Orthomyxoviridae: the viruses and their replication. Fields Virology, 2001. 1: p. 1487–1531.

[51] Webby, R. and R. Webster, Emergence of influenza A viruses. Philosophical Transactions of the Royal Society of London. Series B: Biological Sciences, 2001. 356(1416): p. 1817–28.

[52] Ebrahimi, S.M. and M. Tebianian, Influenza A viruses: why focusing on M2e-based universal vaccines. Virus Genes, 2011. 42(1): p. 1–8.

[53] Huleatt, J.W., et al., Potent immunogenicity and efficacy of a universal influenza vaccine candidate comprising a recombinant fusion protein linking influenza M2e to the TLR5 ligand flagellin. Vaccine, 2008. 26(2): p. 201–214.

[54] Black, R.A., et al., Antibody response to the M2 protein of influenza A virus expressed in insect cells. Journal of General Virology, 1993. 74(1): p. 143–146.

[55] Cox, N.J., et al., Orthomyxoviruses: influenza. Topley and Wilson's microbiology and microbial infections, 1998.

[56] Tompkins, S.M., et al., Matrix protein 2 vaccination and protection against influenza viruses, including subtype H5N1. Matrix, 2007.

[57] Neirynck, S., et al., A universal influenza A vaccine based on the extracellular domain of the M2 protein. Nature Medicine, 1999. 5(10): p. 1157–1163.

[58] De Filette, M., et al., Improved design and intranasal delivery of an M2e-based human influenza A vaccine. Vaccine, 2006. 24(44): p. 6597–6601.

[59] Fiers, W., et al., M2e-based universal influenza A vaccine. Vaccine, 2009. 27(45): p. 6280–6283.

[60] Tao, W. and H.S. Gill, M2e-immobilized gold nanoparticles as influenza A vaccine: Role of soluble M2e and longevity of protection. Vaccine, 2015. 33(20): p. 2307–2315.

[61] Khurana, S., et al., H5N1-SeroDetect EIA and rapid test: a novel differential diagnostic assay for serodiagnosis of H5N1 infections and surveillance. Journal of Virology, 2011. 85(23): p. 12455–12463.

[62] Denis, J., et al., Development of a universal influenza A vaccine based on the M2e peptide fused to the papaya mosaic virus (PapMV) vaccine platform. Vaccine, 2008. 26(27): p. 3395–3403.

[63] Wolf, A.I., et al., Vaccination with M2e-based multiple antigenic peptides: characterization of the B cell response and protection efficacy in inbred and outbred mice. PLoS One, 2011. 6(12): p. e28445.

[64] Hadifar, F., et al., Multimeric recombinant M2e protein-based ELISA: a significant improvement in differentiating avian influenza infected chickens from vaccinated ones. PLoS One, 2014. 9(10): p. e108420.

[65] Tarigan, S., et al., Characterization of the M2e antibody response following highly pathogenic H5N1 avian influenza virus infection and reliability of M2e ELISA for

identifying infected among vaccinated chickens. Avian Pathology, 2015. 44(4): p. 259–268.

[66] Shively, R. Evaluation of 11 commercially available rapid influenza diagnostic tests — United States, 2011–2012. Morbidity and Mortality Weekly Report (MMWR) 2012. Available from: http://www.cdc.gov/mmwr/preview/mmwrhtml/mm6143a3.htm.

[67] Liu, W., et al., Sequence comparison between the extracellular domain of M2 protein human and avian influenza A virus provides new information for bivalent influenza vaccine design. Microbes and Infection, 2005. 7(2): p. 171–177.

[68] Fiers, W., et al., A "universal" human influenza A vaccine. Virus Research, 2004. 103(1): p. 173–176.

Chapter 2

Application of the New Generation of Sequencing Technologies for Evaluation of Genetic Consistency of Influenza A Vaccine Viruses

Ewan Peter Plant, Tatiana Zagorodnyaya,
Elvira Rodionova, Alin Voskanian-Kordi,
Vahan Simonyan, Zhiping Ye and Majid Laassri

Additional information is available at the end of the chapter

http://dx.doi.org/10.5772/64371

Abstract

For almost half a century, Sanger sequencing has been the conventional method for sequencing DNA. However, its utility for sequencing heterogeneous viral populations is limited because it can only detect mutations that are present in a significant portion of the DNA molecules. Several molecular methods that quantify mutations present at low levels in viral populations were proposed for evaluation of genetic consistency of viral vaccines; however, these methods are only suitable for single site polymorphisms, and cannot be used to screen for unknown mutations.

Next-generation (deep) sequencing methods have enabled the determination of sequences of the entire viral population, including minority components. They enable not only sequencing, but also accurate quantification of mutations. This technique has great value for monitoring the genetic consistency of viral vaccines. Recently, a number of new deep sequencing platforms were introduced (MiSeq, Iron Torrent, etc.) that made such an analysis quite affordable for individual research labs. Here, we review the use of current deep sequencing approaches for influenza virus studies, focusing on the evaluation of the genetic consistency of influenza A vaccine viruses. We also describe a new bioinformatic tool to analyze deep sequencing data and identify artifacts from the true mutants.

Keywords: deep sequencing, DNA and RNA libraries, influenza viruses, mutational profiles, sequence heterogeneity

1. Introductory comments on influenza viruses and vaccines

1.1. Influenza viruses

Influenza A viruses are the causative agents of seasonal epidemics and periodic pandemics. There are many serotypes that infect birds, especially waterfowl, and a few serotypes that infect mammals, including humans. Although some influenza A strains from birds and pigs have jumped the species barrier to infect humans, the majority of human infections are caused by the spread of endemic strains. The endemic strains are continually evolving being one of the reasons that influenza A infections remain a persistent problem. Strains of influenza virus that are used in vaccine production are prone to mutations during the manufacturing process, which can cause breaches in the consistency of vaccine quality. Such mutations can lead to changes in the antigenic structure of the virus and thus affect vaccine effectiveness.

Influenza A viruses belong to the Orthomyxoviridae family of viruses [1]. There are several common features shared among the viruses in this family: they are all negative sense, single-stranded RNA viruses that replicate in the nucleus of the host cell. The influenza A virus genome is comprised of eight RNA segments that encode more than 11 proteins. Two of the segments each encode a major antigenic protein. The fourth largest segment encodes a hemagglutinin (HA) protein and the sixth largest segment encodes a neuraminidase (NA) protein. The different subtypes and strains of influenza A viruses are distinguished by the HA and NA proteins that coat the surface of the virus. There are at least 18 different HA types and 11 NA types [2]. The segmented nature of the viral genome enables two viruses co-infecting the same cell to exchange their segments to produce reassortant progeny. Replication of influenza A viruses also results in mutated viral genomes because of the high error frequency of the RNA polymerase and actions by host defensive elements [3, 4]. Mutations contribute to the emergence of new endemic strains and reassortment may lead to the emergence of epidemic or pandemic strains.

The presence of mutations in influenza A populations has been examined in a variety of contexts. Several groups have isolated clones and used Sanger sequencing to identify mutations. Isolation of a sufficient number of clones has resulted in estimates of the mutation frequencies ranging from 6×10^{-4} to 2×10^{-6} [3, 5, 6]. Although the information about heterogeneity is of great interest, caution must be exercised to ensure that it is accurately reflected in sequence databases. The presence of errors in influenza databases has been noted [7, 8]. To limit discrepancies, some groups have used next-generation sequencing (NGS) to identify sequence heterogeneities [9–12]. Additional technologies such as multisegment reverse-transcription PCR have also been employed [13]. These studies revealed several interesting things. For example, it has been found that differences in viral sequences may occur after a single passage [14], that the same antigenic variants can be detected in different individuals [15], and that oseltamivir resistant and sensitive viruses can be found together as part of heterogeneous viral populations [16].

Most human infections are caused by influenza B viruses and the influenza A serotypes H1N1 and H3N2. In addition to the endemic human influenza transmission, there are cases reported

http://dx.doi.org/10.5772/64371

each year of influenza A infections originating from an animal. Influenza A (H3N2) variant viruses from swine are sometimes transmitted to humans, especially those in close contact with pigs in agricultural settings [17]. Poultry workers are also frequently seropositive for a variety of different avian influenza strains [18–20] suggesting infrequent but detectable transmission. In most cases, there is no person-to-person transmission of the animal viruses. Nevertheless candidate vaccine viruses (CVVs) are prepared each year against some of these viruses to provide a prophylactic option in the event of an outbreak (http://www.who.int/influenza/en/). The CVVs for vaccines against endemic strains and potentially pandemic strains are provided to vaccine manufacturers for use as seed viruses in the manufacturing process.

1.2. Influenza vaccine production

There are several different methods that are used to produce influenza vaccines. Errors may be introduced into the antigenic protein during the replication of the seed virus, no matter which production method is used. The different licensed vaccines are produced from influenza virus grown in eggs or cell culture, or from recombinant viruses expressing the influenza HA from an alternative viral backbone grown in cell culture. Contemporary strains isolated from patients during the current epidemic season normally do not always grow well in cell substrates used for vaccine production. To increase virus yields they are recombined with reference high-growth strains, such that the CVVs have HA and NA-coding RNA segments from the contemporary strain, and RNA segments coding for replicative proteins from the high-growth reference virus. HA is the primary protective antigen and is responsible for binding the cellular receptor. Receptor properties in human and chicken cells differ, forcing the virus HA to adapt to the new receptor, leading to changes in the antigenic specificity potentially affecting vaccine potency.

The most common manufacturing process used in FDA-licensed vaccines is to grow influenza virus in eggs and then inactivate the virus. The inactivated virus is purified and then diluted to the desired potency for filling vials or syringes. Live attenuated influenza vaccines (LAIV) are also grown in eggs but are administered as a nasal spray. Codon deoptimization has also been proposed as a method for creating attenuated viruses [21, 22]. Unlike the current licensed products these may be grown in cell culture.

Some inactivated influenza vaccines are grown in cells. Production of cell-grown vaccines currently uses the same egg isolated seed virus that is used for egg inactivated vaccine production. The cell-grown viruses are harvested, inactivated, and filled into vials or syringes for distribution in a similar manner to the egg grown viruses. The production of recombinant viruses to prepare HA does not require a live seed virus. The HA sequence is cloned into the virus used for production. Although the frequency of errors during replication may differ from that of an influenza virus, the concern still remains. Even if vaccine strains are produced using cloned DNA sequences or synthetic sequences, there is still the possibility of errors arising during amplification of the seed virus. Errors may emerge because of inaccuracies inherent in the replication system or as a response to the host cell defenses.

1.3. Influenza vaccine seed viruses

The seed viruses used to produce influenza vaccines are derived from different sources. Because the influenza virus spreads throughout the world and strains are continually evolving, a network of academic, governmental, and commercial organizations work together to produce new seed viruses. New virus isolates are collected by National Influenza Centers and sent to the World Health Organization Collaborating Centers (WHO CCs). The viruses are typed according to strain and subtype using antigenic and genetic analyses. Viruses are usually isolated in Madin-Darby Canine Kidney Epithelial Cells (MDCK cells) and then amplified in eggs. It is important that the seed virus is as close in sequence and antigenicity to the original isolate as possible. To this end, the egg-amplified virus is used to immunize ferrets for the production of antiserum. The antiserum is then used for antigenic typing of viruses. Such analyses are used to determine how well the strains used in the influenza vaccine are matched to the currently circulating strains.

To produce sufficient quantities of vaccine, the CVVs must have good growth characteristics. Ideally, the viruses should replicate efficiently, have a high antigen (primarily hemagglutinin) to total protein ratio and not have increased pathogenicity. Many viruses do not produce high yields in eggs without adaptation. Some viruses have been propagated for many years and have well-known growth characteristics. They include the influenza A strains Puerto Rico/8/1934, cold-adapted A/Ann Arbor/6/1960, A/Leningrad/134/17/1957 and variants of these viruses. Where appropriate these strains have been used as a backbone for influenza A CVVs. Combining the high yield characteristics with the antigenic characteristics of contemporary strains facilitates vaccine production. Reassortant viruses with the desired antigenicity and growth characteristics are produced by two different methods; classical reassortment and genetic reassortment. Dr. Kilbourne of the New York Medical College (NYMC) developed the classical method to create reassortant viruses that expressed the HA and NA from a seasonal strain in the background of a high-growth virus [23]. This method involves co-culture of a contemporary virus and a high yield strain with antibodies to select against the HA and NA of the high yielded strain. Although the resulting viruses have the desired HA and NA genomic segments, the remaining segments may come from either the high-growth strain or the contemporary strain. Another approach based on genetic engineering allows the production of viruses from plasmids expressing the eight influenza virus segments. Genetic engineering also allows the expression of HA and NA proteins in a vector-based system such as a baculovirus. The desired genetic sequence of HA engineered in this system may be incompatible with baculovirus components, which can result in changes as more efficient mutants displace the parental virus (the so-called gene constellation effect) [24].

All CVVs go through several rounds of replication at manufacturers' facilities as they produce their own virus stocks, working seed, and the final product. Some changes to the virus may occur during manufacture so tests to verify the identity, purity, potency and stability of vaccine lots are required. The potency of inactivated influenza vaccines and influenza vaccine produced from recombinant viruses is determined using standardized reagents supplied by national regulatory authorities. The potency of a live-attenuated virus is calculated from the

http://dx.doi.org/10.5772/64371

amount of viable attenuated virus. Genetic characterization of the vaccine viruses is currently achieved by partial genome sequencing or restriction analysis.

It has been suggested that most of the differences between natural isolates and vaccine seed viruses occur during the selection and clonal isolation of the candidate virus prior to manufacture [25]. The fidelity of replication will vary among viruses and es and will depend on other factors such as the host cell line and multiplicity of infection used. There are some limits on the number of times that seed viruses may be passaged so that mutations are less likely to occur. The European Pharmacopoeia monograph 0158 for inactivated influenza vaccines states that the seed virus should not be passaged more than 15 times. However, because regulations tend to lag behind scientific development, there is no universally accepted guideline for influenza vaccine manufacture that covers egg-derived, cell-derived, and synthetic reassortant viruses.

2. Importance of the evaluation of genetic consistency of influenza A vaccine viruses

Virus populations are comprised of genetically variable viruses and this can affect their replication, evolution, attenuation, and pathogenesis [26, 27]. Having an understanding of the mutations present, even at low levels, in a virus population is important for our understanding of how the viruses grow and cause infections. It has recently been shown that an influenza population containing two variants involved in cell exit grows better than populations containing either variant alone [28]. Although good growth properties are a desirable feature in vaccine seed viruses, it is critical that other parts of the genome, such as those causing attenuation or encoding the major antigenic regions, remain stable. Consistency of manufacture is important and having suitable means to assess genetic consistency is valuable. New assays capable of assessing entire viral genomes, and detecting mutations present at a low level, are needed.

The emergence of mutations in the course of vaccine manufacture was shown to contribute to partial reversion to virulence in the oral polio vaccine (OPV). Mutant analysis by PCR and restriction enzyme cleavage (MAPREC) is used to control batches of oral polio vaccine for the presence of neurovirulent mutations [29, 30] and has been expanded to be used for other viruses [31, 32]. Mutations emerging during virus growth may also change antigenic properties and therefore affect protective potency of live and inactivated vaccines. New approaches that can be used not only for monitoring genetic stability of live vaccines, but also for controlling consistency of inactivated vaccines are needed. Influenza vaccines are manufactured in embryonated chicken eggs or cell culture. There is evidence that vaccine seed viruses adapt to grow efficiently in the different substrates and this can lead to changes in the receptor-recognition site of viral hemagglutinin, which is the major protective antigen [33–36]. For this reason, it is important to monitor the changes that may take place in major protective epitopes of the virus. It is also important to know that mutations responsible for attenuated phenotypes are maintained. Knowing which mutations are emerging during virus growth in production substrates could also be used to optimize genetic structure of vaccine strains. Consistently accumulating mutations have higher fitness, and if they have no deleterious properties, their incorporation into the genome of vaccine virus could increase its yield and improve vaccine potency. Given these concerns it is imperative to screen genomes of viral vaccines for emerging mutations.

3. Methods used for evaluation of genetic consistency of vaccine viruses

As mentioned above viral populations are highly heterogeneous, and even small quantities of mutants in virus stocks may affect their biological properties. Although PCR and restriction analysis of reassortant influenza viruses can demonstrate which parental strain each genomic segment was derived from, it cannot detect new mutations. Even traditional sequencing methods are not sensitive enough to detect small amounts of mutants, and highly sensitive PCR-based methods can only analyze one or few known mutations at a time.

Conventional sequencing approaches are suitable for discovery of mutations that are present in substantial amounts, usually around 20–25% [37]. Determining the actual frequency using conventional sequencing requires the labor- and time-intensive analysis of a large number of virus clones (plaques).

There are indirect approaches based on analysis of electrophoretic mobility in gels [38], which are insufficiently sensitive and do not allow mutations to be located accurately. Mass spectrometry (MALDI-TOF) [39] and hybridization with microarrays of short oligonucleotides [40–42] are sensitive, but are laborious and may require follow-up by direct sequencing. A highly sensitive mutant analysis by PCR and MAPREC [29–31] can detect and quantify mutants at levels as low as 0.1% of the viral population. Recently we developed a quantitative allele-specific PCR (asqPCR) [43] for detection of a low level of mutants in viral vaccines. RT-PCR has been proposed as a method for checking the homogeneity of influenza vaccine seed candidates [44]. However, these methods are only suitable for analysis of one known mutation at a time.

Several versions of high-throughput sequencing technology, known also as deep or massively parallel sequencing (MPS) have been used to assess influenza vaccine viruses. These technologies enable rapid generation of large amounts of sequence information [45]. Three different platforms for deep sequencing are used widely at present time: the Roche/454 FLX [46] (http://www.454.com/) (http://454.com/products/technology.asp), the Illumina/Solexa Genome Analyzer [47]) (http://www.illumina.com/technology/next-generation sequencing/sequencing-technology.html), and the Applied Biosystems SOLiD TM System (http://www.thermofisher.com/us/en/home/brands/applied-biosystems.html). Two new sequencing platforms that are improved to sequence long reads have been developed recently: the Pacific Biosciences SMRT Sequencing (http://www.pacb.com/smrt-science/smrt-sequencing/) [48] and Oxford Nanopore Technologies MinION (https://www.nanoporetech.com/technology/the-minion-device-a-miniaturised-sensing-system/the-minion-device-a-miniaturised-sensing-system).

These systems are also called "single molecule" sequencers and do not require any amplification of DNA fragments prior to sequencing.

The deep sequencing technologies were shown to be suitable for analysis of heterogeneities in viral populations [49]. It can produce huge sequencing information in one run. They are used for *de novo* sequencing of large genomes, metagenomics studies (virome, microbiome, etc.), screening for genomic markers, and many other applications [50–58]. Previously, it was demonstrated that deep sequencing can be used to monitor the genetic stability of oral polio vaccines, and could replace the WHO-recommended MAPREC assay for lot release of OPV [59]. Recently we showed that deep sequencing is suitable for evaluation of genetic consistency of influenza vaccine viruses [36, 60].

4. Description of the most used deep sequencing platforms

Deep or massively parallel sequencing refers to several high-throughput methods for DNA sequencing that are often referred to as NGS. They have dramatically improved the ability of biotechnology, scientific, and healthcare researchers to analyze viruses by allowing users to have massive sequencing information for the entire genomes. The high-throughput sequencing field has witnessed the rise of many technologies capable of massive genomic analysis. In the virology field, deep sequencing has made it simple to sequence full viral genomes. Likewise, identification and classification of novel and known viruses, unbiased characterization of viral populations without the need for virus culturing (viromes), molecular epidemiology, viral diversity and evolution, transmission and pathogenesis, and medical virology have greatly benefited from the use of deep sequencing. The cost of deep sequencing has decreased to an affordable price due to the competition between vendors and the ability to analyze multiple samples run in one lane of the sequencing flow cell. This has allowed virologists to study a huge number of viral samples, including mixture of viral populations, and study low-level mutants in a wide range of viruses [36, 59–61].

There are several platforms for deep sequencing. The most widely used sequencing platforms are the Roche/454 FLX [46] (http://www.454.com/), the Illumina/Solexa Genome Analyzer [47] (http://www.illumina.com/technology/next-generation-sequencing/solexa-technology.html), and the Applied Biosystems SOLiD System (http://www.appliedbiosystems.com/absite/us/en/home/applications-technologies/solid-next-generation-sequencing/next-generation-systems/solid-4-system.html?CID=FL-091411_solid4).

The differences between these platforms include DNA library preparation procedures and chemistry, the sequencing reactions on the amplified strands, the length of reads, the amount of data generated per run, the hardware, the software engineering and the technology used to amplify single strands of a fragment from the library.

In general the DNA libraries of fragment targets are generated, and adaptors containing universal priming sites are ligated to the fragmented target ends, allowing complex genomes to be amplified with PCR primers. After ligation, the DNA is separated into single strands and attached or immobilized to a solid surface or support. The immobilization of spatially separated template sites allows thousands to billions of sequencing reactions to be performed simultaneously.

Immobilization and separation of the millions of molecules to different surfaces can be achieved by a variety of methods including the Polonator and PicoTiter Plate [47, 62–64]. Attachment of forward and reverse primers to a slide and use of solid-phase amplification also result in the enrichment and amplification of separate template strands [47] (Illumina/Solexa).

Two newer sequencing platforms with longer reads differ from those described above. They are sometimes referred to as "single molecule" sequencers because they sequence molecule by molecule and do not require any amplification of DNA fragments prior to sequencing. The Pacific Biosciences system involves the attachment of a DNA polymerase to the DNA molecule. During the sequencing phase the polymerase adds bases labeled with a fluorophore. The fluorescence unique to each base is recorded and, as each new base is added, the fluorescent label is removed [48]. It generates long sequencing reads (10–15 kb long) from single molecules of DNA, very quickly.

The Oxford Nanopore system runs the sample through very small (1 nm wide) pores. As the DNA passes through these nanopores, the Oxford machine records the electrical charge that is associated with each individual base pair of DNA, like a signature. It produces longer reads (>100 kb long).

A detailed description of the most used two deep sequencing platforms for analysis of influenza viruses and their vaccines is given below.

4.1. Roche/454 FLX pyrosequencer

The Roche/454 FLX sequencing [46] is based on the use of the pyrosequencing technology (http://my454.com/products/technology.asp), in which the incorporation of each nucleotide by DNA polymerase results in the release of pyrophosphate that initiates a cascade of enzymatic reactions that converts the pyrophosphate to a light signal. This light is recorded by CCD camera. This approach, as with most NGS procedures, starts with DNA library preparation; the library DNAs with 454-specific adaptors are denatured into single strands and mixed with agarose beads whose surfaces carry oligonucleotides complementary to the 454-specific adapter sequences on the fragment library, so each bead is associated with a single fragment. The DNA fragments captured by beads are amplified by emulsion PCR (ePCR) [65] to produce approximately one million copies of each DNA fragment on the surface of each bead. These amplified single molecules are then sequenced on a picotiter plate (a fused silica capillary structure) that holds a single bead in each of several hundred thousand single wells, which provides a fixed location at which each sequencing reaction can be monitored.

Individual dNTPs are added to the template in the presence of a DNA polymerase. The sequencing reaction releases pyrophosphate (PPi) after the incorporation of a complementary nucleotide. The released PPi is used by an ATP sulfurylase to release ATP from adenosine 5'-phosphosulfate. The ATP is then used to generate light by converting luciferin into oxyluciferin [66]. Unincorporated dNTPs are degraded by an apyrase, and dATPαS (which is not a substrate for luciferase) is used instead of dATP. This pyrosequencing reaction is repeated during the sequence of the entire target DNA. This sequencing technology can now produce sequencing reads with up to 1000 bp in length (http://454.com/products/gs-flx-system/).

These raw reads are processed by the 454 analysis software and then filtered to remove poor-quality sequences, mixed sequences, and sequences without the initiating TCGA sequence. Recently, the 454-FLX system was upgraded to reach 99.9% of accuracy after filter and an output of 14 Gb of data per run within 24 h.

4.2. Illumina genome sequencer

The Illumina sequencing [47] method begins with Illumina library preparation flanked with Illumina-specific adapters. Sequencing templates are immobilized on a proprietary flow cell surface that contains immobilized oligos with sequence complementary to those of the adapters, and designed to present the DNA in a manner that facilitates access to enzymes while ensuring high stability of surface-bound template and low non-specific binding of fluorescently labeled nucleotides. Solid-phase amplification of each single strand DNA from library is performed by bridge amplification, which results in the generation of several million dense clusters of single-stranded DNA in each channel of the flow cell.

The Illumina system sequences DNA in the presence of four reversible terminator-bound dNTPs [47]. At each sequencing step, a fluorescently labeled dNTP is added to the molecule. The fluorescent signal is recorded and then the fluorophore is removed to allow sequencing to continue. The base calls correlate with the signal intensity. Illumina sequencing technology can now produce sequencing reads with up to 600 bp in length (http://www.illumina.com/systems/sequencing.html). The sequencing results are generated in files in which each raw read base has an assigned quality score so that the software can apply a weighting factor in calling differences and generating confidence scores. Illumina data collection software enables users to align sequences to a reference in resequencing applications. This software suite includes the full range of data collection, processing, and analysis modules to streamline collection and analysis of data.

4.3. Deep sequencing data analysis

The massively parallel scale of sequencing implies a similarly massive scale of computational analysis. The conventional pipeline for analysis of next-generation sequencing data includes the following stages: quality control and source data filtering; alignment (mapping); reference profiling (variant-calling, pileup); followed by single-nucleotide polymorphism (SNP) calling (genotyping); and some form of clusterization or classification analysis of samples to discover up or down expression of genes, detect overabundance of SNP positions and correlate those with function and phenotype. Because of the sheer size of the data and amount of calculations needed, such analyses place significant demands on the information technology (IT) infrastructure. Lack of computational power, insufficiency of actively accessible storage facilities in laboratory information management systems (LIMS) and deficiency in network capacity to move data add significantly to the overhead required for high-throughput data production.

The hardware aspect of next-generation sequencing is complicated by the imperfections of current sequence analysis tools, which are suited to shorter sequence read data. There are multiple implementations for all of the stages of the analysis, and some of those are considered to be industry standard tools, running formidable amount of bio-medical analytics. Large-scale analysis of thousands of samples using variety of available tools highlighted important issues with data quality, pre-analytic quality controls, software reproducibility and post-analytic quality controls. Existing data analysis pipelines and algorithms must be modified to accommodate extra-large amounts of short read sequences and combination of shorter and longer read technologies.

To analyze the deep sequencing data for genetic consistency evaluation of influenza vaccine viruses, we have used the corresponding viral reference sequences from NCBI GenBank as a template for alignment of individual sequencing reads. First, sequencing reads with low quality (Phred) score are removed from the data set, and the remaining sequences aligned with reference influenza virus sequence using custom software: The High-performance Integrated Virtual Environment (HIVE, https://hive.biochemistry.gwu.edu/dna.cgi?cmd=main) computer cluster [67, 68].

To create a quantifiable measure comparing the quality of the sequencing and mapping at different positions on a genome, we developed a metrics for assessing positional variant-call quality. To do that, first a histogram is built at every position of a genome where the number

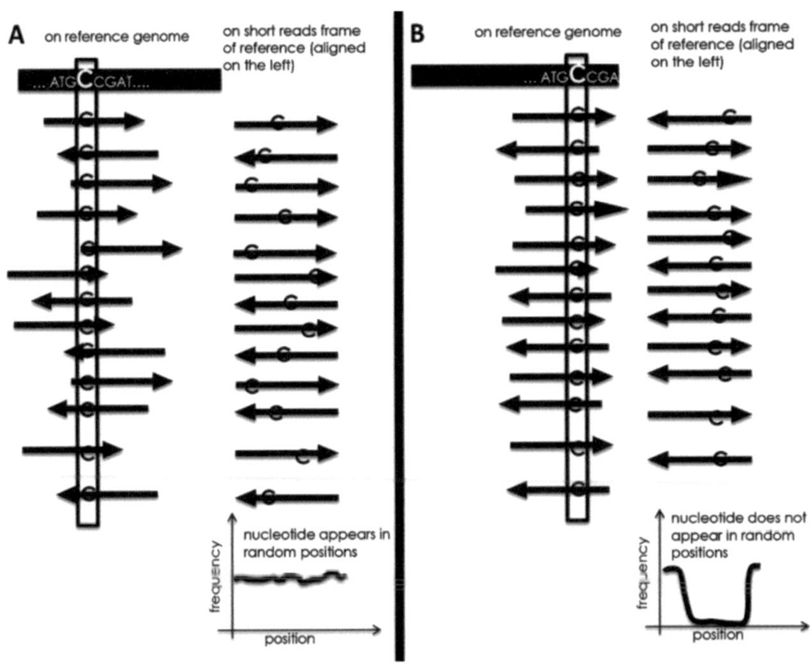

Figure 1. Explanation of entropy computation. For all bases aligned to a particular reference position, the coordinates on a read-frame are accumulated into a positional frequency histogram. For a non-biased position, such distribution is more or less uniform (A). For terminally biased base calls such frequency distribution is skewed towards ends (B) and the Shannon's entropy values drop closer to zero.

of times a base has occurred at a given read-position is accumulated. Additionally, positions of insertion and deletions are also collected in similar histogram. The underlying assumption of the next-generation sequencing method is that the DNA amplification and digestion procedure is random and the short sequences produced by DNA digestion are not strongly biased and not sequence dependent. The default assumption is that a particular variant call should be confirmed by different positions on many reads thus rendering the histogram distribution to be uniform along the entire length of sequence read.

Post-alignment quality control includes identification of mutations distributed non-randomly along individual sequencing reads, which may indicate artifacts in PCR amplification or DNA sequencing procedures (**Figure 1A** and **B**). Biased distribution of mutations along sequencing reads was revealed by calculating Shannon entropy values [69]. Low entropy value suggests that a mutation could be an artifact produced in sequencing procedures. This means that there is an abnormal bias in distribution of this mutation. This entropy-based post-alignment quality control value is calculated on the basis of the equation below. It is based on the normalized first order momentum of logarithmic probability distribution for a particular base (*b*) at a particular position (*r*) of reference genome:

$$Entropy(b,r) = -\frac{\sum_L p_i(b) \times log(p_i(b))}{\log(L^{-1})}$$

where L is the length of the longest read, p_i(b) is the frequency distribution of a base b in the reference frame of the reads mapped at the location r. The index i runs over all of the available positions from 1 to L. The denominator makes sure the Shannon's entropy is normalized to a unit value of 1 as the maximum value for entirely uniform distribution. In contrast singular value distribution would have a value for entropy equal to zero. This value is computed for all of the reference positions for every base.

Finally, aligned sequencing reads were used to compute SNP profiles for the entire viral genome.

5. The use of deep sequencing for evaluation of genetic consistency of influenza A vaccine viruses

Influenza A viruses are enveloped, single-stranded RNA viruses belonging to the Orthomyxoviridae family [70], which also contains four other viral species: influenza B virus, influenza C virus, thogotovirus, and isavirus. The segmented genome of influenza A virus is about 13.6 kb in size and encodes for at least 11 proteins. Its genome is highly variable due to the low fidelity of RNA polymerase and reassortment between co-infecting strains [71]. New virus mutants emerge continuously allowing viruses to survive in presence of the host immunity and cause repeated annual epidemics and occasionally pandemics. Because of this frequent change of the antigens, influenza vaccines must be frequently reformulated to include antigens of the currently circulating strains. Both live and inactivated influenza vaccines are produced mostly by reassortment with high-growth strains for vaccine production [72, 73]. As stated above, adaptation to growth in different cells can lead to changes in viral receptor-binding region, and also in protective epitopes. Therefore, it is desirable to monitor genetic stability of viruses used in vaccine manufacture to ensure that their antigenic structure remains unchanged.

Deep sequencing technology has opened up the possibility for the characterization of viral genomes directly from samples [74, 75]. The viral metagenome or "virome" refers to the collection of viruses found in a particular sample from humans, animals, plants or from a specific environmental sample. Virome studies can lead to the discovery of new viruses and/or to their association with known or novel diseases. Numerous viruses have been identified as part of the virome study, including influenza A viruses [2].

The deep sequencing technologies are a great tool to investigate genetically complex populations of influenza viruses and to detect minority mutant variants with clinical or epidemiological relevance. Deep sequencing-based methods have recently been applied for the assessment of influenza A viruses diversity and their dynamics of evolution [60, 76, 77]. Others have focused on the evolution of avian influenza strains with potential to become pandemic in humans [78–82], as well as the detection of virulence signatures [83] and reassortment patterns [84]. Other studies have investigated the transmission and adaptation of avian influenza viruses to humans, as part of preparedness for a potential influenza pandemic [12, 53, 85–98].

As it is crucial to study transmission and adaptation of avian influenza viruses, and swine strains for epidemics and pandemics in humans, many studies based on the use of deep sequencing techniques have described avian and swine influenza virus evolution [99–103]. Other studies have investigated the predominance and spread of different human influenza viruses in specific geographic areas [16, 104–106].

Study of drug escape variants is an important aspect of epidemiological and clinical virology. Sanger sequencing can only detect mutations present in around 20% of the viral population [37, 107–109], which excludes it for quantitation of low-level viral mutant variants. Using deep sequencing to detect low portion of mutant drug resistant variants at levels as low as 0.1% of the virus population has been demonstrated [110–116]. Other studies have focused on the use of deep sequencing for surveillance of drug resistance-associated mutations for both NA inhibitors and adamantanes [117–127]. Deep sequencing has also been used for the detection and subtyping of human influenza A viruses and reassortants [61, 84].

Recently, deep sequencing based methods have been proposed for the assessment of influenza A viruses antigenic stability [128] using complete influenza A genomes and exploiting the ability to detect and quantify mutations in heterogeneous viral populations. Deep sequencing was used to study the evolution of influenza A viruses in the vaccinated pigs. The genetic diversity and evolution of the virus at an intra-host level was analyzed directly from nasal swabs collected during infection [129]. The obtained results demonstrated remarkable diversity of influenza A viruses, and rapid change of these viruses during infection of vaccinated pigs. These types of complex studies can be done only by high throughput sequence analysis.

To evaluate the genetic stability in influenza vaccine viruses, we have used a deep sequencing approach that was recently qualified for quantitation of all mutants in the entire genome including those that are present at low level in viral populations [59]. Recently, we explored the utility of deep sequencing methods for monitoring the consistency of influenza A vaccines [36, 60]. Also in the same study, we proposed new protocols for simultaneous amplification of all segments of influenza A genomes and new bioinformatic tools to analyze the data and to identify artifacts generated during PCR amplification and deep sequencing procedures. Amplification of the entire genome of influenza viruses presents a challenge because of the difference in size and sequence composition of the eight genomic segments.

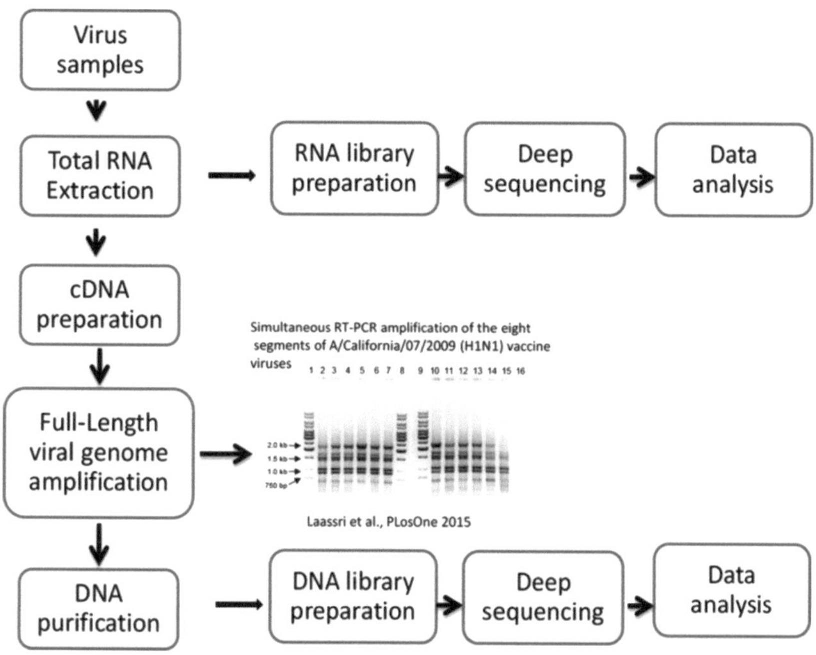

Figure 2. General steps followed for RNA/DNA libraries sequencing of influenza A/California/07/2009 (H1N1) vaccine viruses.

We described PCR conditions that allow to amplify all genomic segments of influenza A virus in one reaction [60] that was optimized subsequently during an analysis of the A/California/07/2009 (H1N1) vaccine viruses (derived from X-179A, X-181, 121XP viruses) [36]. We have used both the total RNA (without specific amplification of viral cDNA) and DNA amplicon, for RNA and DNA libraries preparation, respectively, and both protocols were compared for consistency in mutant variants quantitation.

The protocols for deep sequencing of viral DNA libraries and whole-RNA libraries used to determine quantitative profiles of mutations along the entire genome of viruses of influenza

A/California/07/2009 (H1N1) vaccine viruses were described [36]. The steps followed to perform the deep sequencing are presented in **Figure 2** and can be summarized as follows: The PCR product was purified by QIAquick PCR Purification Kit (Qiagen) and fragmented by an ultrasonicator (Covaris) to generate the optimal fragment sizes needed for Illumina sequencing, then the fragmented DNAs were used for library preparation with NEBNext® DNA Sample Prep Reagent Set 1 (New England BioLabs).

For preparation of Illumina sequencing libraries from total RNA, the NEBNext mRNA Sample Prep Master Mix Set 1 (New England BioLabs) was used. Briefly, total RNA (extracted as mentioned above) was fragmented as described above to generate the optimal fragment sizes. Double-stranded cDNA was prepared and ligated to the Illumina paired end adaptors. Finally, the libraries were amplified using 15 cycles of PCR with multiplex indexed primers and purified with magnetic beads using Agencourt Ampure Beads (Beckman Coulter). Deep sequencing was performed at Macrogen (Seoul, Korea) using HiSeq2000 (Illumina) or at our laboratory using MiSeq (Illumina).

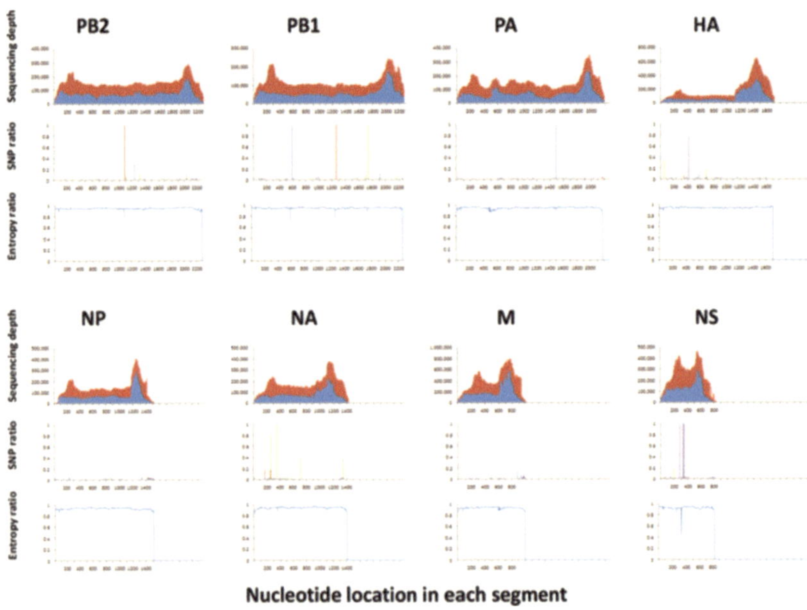

Figure 3. Sequencing analysis of the entire genome of the influenza A/California/07/2009 (H1N1) vaccine virus reassortant tenth passage in eggs sequenced by HiSeq (Macrogen) using 101 bp paired-end Illumina/Solexa sequencing technology. Computations were made by in-house custom software HIVE-align. For each segment, the charts of the depth of sequencing coverage distribution (the number of times every nucleotide was sequenced on ordinate plotted against the position on genome—abscissa), SNP profile (the ratio of mutants on ordinate plotted against the position on genome—abscissa), and entropy were built.

The sequencing data analysis was done using custom software, a highly integrated virtual environment (HIVE) computer cluster (https://hive.biochemistry.gwu.edu/dna.cgi?cmd=main) as described above. The RNA sequences of X-179A, X-181, 121XP, A/California/07/2009 (H1N1), and A/PR/08/34 viruses deposited in NCBI GenBank were used as references for alignment of the viral sequence reads. We analyzed the depth of sequencing, the single-nucleotide polymorphism profile, and entropy (that allow us to distinct between bias and true mutation) for each segment of influenza virus (see **Figure 3**, for example), the data analysis resulted also on generation of consensus sequences for each segment.

The deep sequencing results revealed several heterogeneities in most genomic segments, and several mutations led to amino acid changes. Deep sequencing of whole-RNA libraries was found to be more reproducible than sequencing of DNA libraries. This may be due to errors introduced during PCR amplification by DNA polymerase and non-specific alignment of primers [36].

The deep sequencing of the X-179A passaged viruses [36] identified several mutations in HA and NA genes. In HA two non-synonymous mutations; Pro_{314}Gln (in 17% of the virus population) and Asn_{146}Asp (in 78% of the virus population) were identified. The Asn_{146}Asp mutation is found in the antigenic site Sa; it was detected at 11% in the A/California/07/2009 (H1N1) strain and as the dominant residue in the X-181 virus [36]. One X-179A stock contained the Lys_{328}Thr mutation at a low level (9%). Viruses derived from X-179A were heterogeneous and contained some complete nucleotide substitutions in comparison to their published sequences in PB2, PB1, NP, and in NS segments [36]. The X-181 virus was developed from the X-179A seed lot by another round of reassortment, and also is subjected to several passages in eggs. Deep sequencing results [36] showed that the G_{756}T (Glu_{252}Asp, present at 47%) mutation emerged in HA of the passaged X181 virus, and it is located in the conserved region of the antigenic site Ca [36].

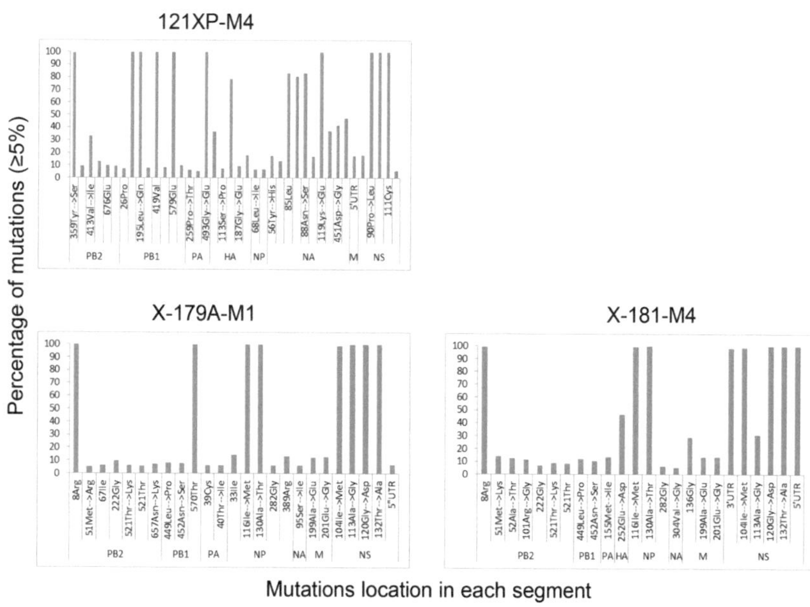

Figure 4. Percent of mutations (≥5%) emerged in X-179A-M1, X-181-M4, and 121XP-M4 viruses (derived from X-179A, X-181, and 121XP viruses, respectively) passaged 10 times in embryonated chicken eggs.

Unlike the X-179A and X-181 viruses, 121XP was developed by reverse genetics [130]. The deep sequencing of 121XP virus passaged 10 times in eggs (121XP-M4 virus) showed that this virus is more heterogenic than X-179A and X-181 viruses passaged 10 times in eggs (X-179A-M1 and X-181-M4 viruses respectively; **Figure 4**) [36]. In the passaged 121XP virus, the mutation $Lys_{226}Glu$ was emerged at low level (18%) in Ca antigenic site of HA, which is very close to the region that participates in the modulation of HA receptor specificity and that enables H3 influenza viruses to switch specificity from avian to human [131–133]; another mutation $Lys_{136}Asn$ was emerged at a high level (78%) close to the HA antigenic site Sa within the sialic acid-binding pocket [134]. Recently a similar deep sequencing approach was used to study the genetic and potential antigenic diversity of influenza viruses infecting humans, some of whom became infected despite recent vaccination [15].

We found that the deep sequencing approach based on RNA library preparation was effective and reproducible for detection of low quantities of mutants in the entire genome of influenza A vaccine viruses [36]. The deep sequencing approach revealed that the viruses derived from three pandemic A/Ca/07/2009 (H1N1) vaccine viruses have varying levels of sequence heterogeneities some of them in antigenic sites, which may affect their efficacy.

6. Conclusions

In the last few years, the use of deep sequencing has expanded largely to tackle problems in many fields of virology. The greatest benefit of deep sequencing is its ability to detect minor mutant variants, as low as 0.1% of virus population [36, 59, 60, 110, 111, 113, 114]. The deep sequencing approach based on RNA library preparation is effective and reproducible for detection of low quantities of mutants in the entire genome of influenza A vaccine viruses [36], and eliminates the need for full-length amplification. The deep sequencing platforms are improving continuously to combine low error rates with long reads and relatively low cost. It played a key role in the discovery of many new viruses, the characterization of virus populations in humans and the potential of their association with the pathogenesis of several diseases. As described here, there is no doubt that the deep sequencing is facilitating and accelerating the evaluation of the genetic consistency of vaccine viruses. It is an important tool for monitoring vaccine consistency during manufacture and after vaccination. Deep sequencing-based assays are already being implemented for the genetic consistency evaluation of oral polio vaccine and influenza A vaccine viruses [36, 59, 60]. The ability to quantify potentially undesirable mutations in vaccine batches makes this method suitable for quality control to ensure manufacture of safe and effective vaccines.

Acknowledgements

We thank Dr. Konstantin Chumakov and Dr. Christian Sauder for their critical review of this chapter. The contents of this chapter represent solely the opinion of authors and do not represent the official view of FDA.

http://dx.doi.org/10.5772/64371

Author details

Ewan Peter Plant, Tatiana Zagorodnyaya, Elvira Rodionova, Alin Voskanian-Kordi, Vahan Simonyan, Zhiping Ye and Majid Laassri*

*Address all correspondence to: majid.laassri@fda.hhs.gov

Center for Biologics Evaluation and Research, US Food and Drug Administration, Silver Spring, MD, USA

References

[1] Lamb, R.A. and R.M. Krug, Orthomyxoviridae: the viruses and their replication, in Fields virology, D.M.K. Bernard, N. Fields, P.M. Howley, Editor. 1996, Philadelphia: Lippincott-Raven Publishers, pp. 1353–96.

[2] Tong, S., et al., New world bats harbor diverse influenza A viruses. PLoS Pathog, 2013. 9(10): p. e1003657.

[3] Cheung, P.P., et al., Comparative mutational analyses of influenza A viruses. RNA, 2015. 21(1): pp. 36–47.

[4] Gutierrez, R.A., et al., Biased mutational pattern and quasispecies hypothesis in H5N1 virus. Infect Genet Evol, 2013. 15: pp. 69–76.

[5] Nobusawa, E. and K. Sato, Comparison of the mutation rates of human influenza A and B viruses. J Virol, 2006. 80(7): pp. 3675–8.

[6] Parvin, J.D., et al., Measurement of the mutation rates of animal viruses: influenza A virus and poliovirus type 1. J Virol, 1986. 59(2): pp. 377–83.

[7] Krasnitz, M., A.J. Levine, and R. Rabadan, Anomalies in the influenza virus genome database: new biology or laboratory errors? J Virol, 2008. 82(17): pp. 8947–50.

[8] Suarez, D.L., N. Chester, and J. Hatfield, Sequencing artifacts in the type A influenza databases and attempts to correct them. Influenza Other Respir Viruses, 2014. 8(4): pp. 499–505.

[9] Roedig, J.V., et al., Impact of host cell line adaptation on quasispecies composition and glycosylation of influenza A virus hemagglutinin. PLoS One, 2011. 6(12): p. e27989.

[10] Van den Hoecke, S., et al., Analysis of the genetic diversity of influenza A viruses using next-generation DNA sequencing. BMC Genomics, 2015. 16: p. 79.

[11] Wang, J., et al., MinION nanopore sequencing of an influenza genome. Front Microbiol, 2015. 6: p. 766.

[12] Watson, S.J., et al., Viral population analysis and minority-variant detection using short read next-generation sequencing. Philos Trans R Soc Lond B Biol Sci, 2013. 368(1614): p. 20120205.

[13] Zou, X.H., et al., Evaluation of a single-reaction method for whole genome sequencing of influenza A virus using next generation sequencing. Biomed Environ Sci, 2016. 29(1): pp. 41–6.

[14] Lee, H.K., et al., Comparison of mutation patterns in full-genome A/H3N2 influenza sequences obtained directly from clinical samples and the same samples after a single MDCK passage. PLoS One, 2013. 8(11): p. e79252.

[15] Dinis, J.M., et al., Deep sequencing reveals potential antigenic variants at low frequency in influenza A-infected humans. J Virol, 2016. 90(7): 3355–3365.

[16] Fordyce, S.L., et al., Genetic diversity among pandemic 2009 influenza viruses isolated from a transmission chain. Virol J, 2013. 10: p. 116.

[17] Nelson, M.I., et al., Evolutionary dynamics of influenza A viruses in US Exhibition Swine. J Infect Dis, 2016. 213(2): p. 173–82.

[18] Di Trani, L., et al., Serosurvey against H5 and H7 avian influenza viruses in Italian poultry workers. Avian Dis, 2012. 56(4 Suppl): pp. 1068–71.

[19] Heidari, A., et al., Serological evidence of H9N2 avian influenza virus exposure among poultry workers from Fars province of Iran. Virol J, 2016. 13(1): p. 16.

[20] Huang, S.Y., et al., Serological comparison of antibodies to avian influenza viruses, subtypes H5N2, H6N1, H7N3 and H7N9 between poultry workers and non-poultry workers in Taiwan in 2012. Epidemiol Infect, 2015. 143(14): pp. 2965–74.

[21] Broadbent, A.J., et al., Evaluation of the attenuation, immunogenicity, and efficacy of a live virus vaccine generated by codon-pair bias de-optimization of the 2009 pandemic H1N1 influenza virus, in ferrets. Vaccine, 2016. 34(4): pp. 563–70.

[22] Fan, R.L., et al., Generation of live attenuated influenza virus by using codon usage bias. J Virol, 2015. 89(21): pp. 10762–73.

[23] Kilbourne, E.D., Future influenza vaccines and the use of genetic recombinants. Bull World Health Organ, 1969. 41(3): pp. 643–5.

[24] Plant E.P. and Z. Ye., Gene constellation of influenza vaccine seed viruses in Current issues in molecular virology – viral genetics and biotechnological applications, V. Romanowski, Editor. 2013, InTech, pp 213–237.

[25] Buonagurio, D.A., et al., Genetic stability of live, cold-adapted influenza virus components of the FluMist/CAIV-T vaccine throughout the manufacturing process. Vaccine, 2006. 24(12): pp. 2151–60.

[26] Domingo, E., et al., The quasispecies (extremely heterogeneous) nature of viral RNA genome populations: biological relevance---a review. Gene, 1985. 40(1): pp. 1–8.

[27] Hansen, H., et al., Recombinant viruses obtained from co-infection in vitro with a live vaccinia-vectored influenza vaccine and a naturally occurring cowpox virus display different plaque phenotypes and loss of the transgene. Vaccine, 2004. 23(4): pp. 499–506.

[28] Xue, K.S., et al., Cooperation between distinct viral variants promotes growth of H3N2 influenza in cell culture. eLife 2016;5: p. e13974.

[29] Chumakov, K.M., Molecular consistency monitoring of oral poliovirus vaccine and other live viral vaccines. Dev Biol Stand, 1999. 100: pp. 67–74.

[30] Chumakov, K.M., et al., Correlation between amount of virus with altered nucleotide sequence and the monkey test for acceptability of oral poliovirus vaccine. Proc Natl Acad Sci U S A, 1991. 88(1): pp. 199–203.

[31] Bidzhieva, B., M. Laassri, and K. Chumakov, MAPREC assay for quantitation of mutants in a recombinant flavivirus vaccine strain using near-infrared fluorescent dyes. J Virol Methods, 2011. 175(1): pp. 14–9.

[32] Laassri, M., et al., Microarray hybridization for assessment of the genetic stability of chimeric West Nile/dengue 4 virus. J Med Virol, 2011. 83(5): pp. 910–20.

[33] Gambaryan, A.S., et al., Effects of host-dependent glycosylation of hemagglutinin on receptor-binding properties on H1N1 human influenza A virus grown in MDCK cells and in embryonated eggs. Virology, 1998. 247(2): pp. 170–7.

[34] Hughes, M.T., et al., Adaptation of influenza A viruses to cells expressing low levels of sialic acid leads to loss of neuraminidase activity. J Virol, 2001. 75(8): pp. 3766–70.

[35] Schild, G.C., et al., Evidence for host-cell selection of influenza virus antigenic variants. Nature, 1983. 303(5919): pp. 706–9.

[36] Laassri, M., et al., Deep sequencing for evaluation of genetic stability of influenza A/California/07/2009 (H1N1) vaccine viruses. PLoS One, 2015. 10(9): p. e0138650.

[37] Larder, B.A., et al., Quantitative detection of HIV-1 drug resistance mutations by automated DNA sequencing. Nature, 1993. 365(6447): pp. 671–3.

[38] Orita, M., et al., Detection of polymorphisms of human DNA by gel electrophoresis as single-strand conformation polymorphisms. Proc Natl Acad Sci U S A, 1989. 86(8): pp. 2766–70.

[39] Amexis, G., et al., Quantitative mutant analysis of viral quasispecies by chip-based matrix-assisted laser desorption/ionization time-of-flight mass spectrometry. Proc Natl Acad Sci U S A, 2001. 98(21): pp. 12097–102.

[40] Cherkasova, E., et al., Microarray analysis of evolution of RNA viruses: evidence of circulation of virulent highly divergent vaccine-derived polioviruses. Proc Natl Acad Sci U S A, 2003. 100(16): pp. 9398–403.

[41] Laassri, M., et al., Microarray techniques for evaluation of genetic stability of live viral vaccines, in Viral genomes – Molecular structure, diversity, gene expression mechanisms and host-virus interactions. Maria Laura Garcia Editor. 2012, InTech, pp. 181–94.

[42] Laassri, M., et al., Genomic analysis of vaccine-derived poliovirus strains in stool specimens by combination of full-length PCR and oligonucleotide microarray hybridization. J Clin Microbiol, 2005. 43(6): pp. 2886–94.

[43] Bidzhieva, B., M. Laassri, and K. Chumakov, Allele-specific PCR for quantitative analysis of mutants in live viral vaccines. J Virol Methods, 2014. 201: pp. 86–92.

[44] Shcherbik, S., et al., Application of real time RT-PCR for the genetic homogeneity and stability tests of the seed candidates for live attenuated influenza vaccine production. J Virol Methods, 2014. 195: pp. 18–25.

[45] Rogers, Y.H. and J.C. Venter, Genomics: massively parallel sequencing. Nature, 2005. 437(7057): pp. 326–7.

[46] Margulies, M., et al., Genome sequencing in microfabricated high-density picolitre reactors. Nature, 2005. 437(7057): pp. 376–80.

[47] Bentley, D.R., Whole-genome re-sequencing. Curr Opin Genet Dev, 2006. 16(6): pp. 545–52.

[48] Eid, J., et al., Real-time DNA sequencing from single polymerase molecules. Science, 2009. 323(5910): pp. 133–8.

[49] Victoria, J.G., et al., Metagenomic analyses of viruses in stool samples from children with acute flaccid paralysis. J Virol, 2009. 83(9): pp. 4642–51.

[50] Bainbridge, M.N., et al., Analysis of the prostate cancer cell line LNCaP transcriptome using a sequencing-by-synthesis approach. BMC Genomics, 2006. 7: p. 246.

[51] Cheval, J., et al., Evaluation of high-throughput sequencing for identifying known and unknown viruses in biological samples. J Clin Microbiol, 2011. 49(9): pp. 3268–75.

[52] Greninger, A.L., et al., A metagenomic analysis of pandemic influenza A (2009 H1N1) infection in patients from North America. PLoS One, 2010. 5(10): p. e13381.

[53] Kuroda, M., et al., Characterization of quasispecies of pandemic 2009 influenza A virus (A/H1N1/2009) by de novo sequencing using a next-generation DNA sequencer. PLoS One, 2010. 5(4): p. e10256.

[54] Nakamura, S., et al., Direct metagenomic detection of viral pathogens in nasal and fecal specimens using an unbiased high-throughput sequencing approach. PLoS One, 2009. 4(1): p. e4219.

[55] Pettersson, E., et al., Allelotyping by massively parallel pyrosequencing of SNP-carrying trinucleotide threads. Hum Mutat, 2008. 29(2): pp. 323–9.

[56] Satkoski, J.A., et al., Pyrosequencing as a method for SNP identification in the rhesus macaque (Macaca mulatta). BMC Genomics, 2008. 9: p. 256.

[57] Torres, T.T., et al., Gene expression profiling by massively parallel sequencing. Genome Res, 2008. 18(1): pp. 172–7.

[58] Wheeler, D.A., et al., The complete genome of an individual by massively parallel DNA sequencing. Nature, 2008. 452(7189): pp. 872–6.

[59] Neverov, A. and K. Chumakov, Massively parallel sequencing for monitoring genetic consistency and quality control of live viral vaccines. Proc Natl Acad Sci U S A, 2010. 107(46): pp. 20063–8.

[60] Bidzhieva, B., et al., Deep sequencing approach for genetic stability evaluation of influenza A viruses. J Virol Methods, 2014. 199: pp. 68–75.

[61] Seong, M.W., et al., Genotyping influenza virus by next-generation deep sequencing in clinical specimens. Ann Lab Med, 2016. 36(3): pp. 255–8.

[62] Kim, J.B., et al., Polony multiplex analysis of gene expression (PMAGE) in mouse hypertrophic cardiomyopathy. Science, 2007. 316(5830): pp. 1481–4.

[63] Leamon, J.H., et al., A massively parallel PicoTiterPlate based platform for discrete picoliter-scale polymerase chain reactions. Electrophoresis, 2003. 24(21): pp. 3769–77.

[64] Shendure, J., et al., Accurate multiplex polony sequencing of an evolved bacterial genome. Science, 2005. 309(5741): pp. 1728–32.

[65] Berka, J., et al., Bead emulsion nucleic acid amplification. 2005, Google Patents.

[66] Froehlich, T., D. Heindl, and A. Roesler, Miniaturized, high-throughput nucleic acid analysis. 2010, Google Patents.

[67] Simonyan, V. and R. Mazumder, High-performance integrated virtual environment (HIVE) tools and applications for big data analysis. Genes (Basel), 2014. 5(4): pp. 957–81.

[68] Wilson, C.A. and V. Simonyan, FDA's activities supporting regulatory application of "next gen" sequencing technologies. PDA J Pharm Sci Technol, 2014. 68(6): pp. 626–30.

[69] Shannon, C.E., A mathematical theory of communication. Bell Syst Technical J, 1948. 27(3): pp. 379–423.

[70] Lamb, R.A. and M.A. Krug, Orthomyxoviridae: the viruses and their replication, in Fields Virology, Howley P. M., Knipe D. M., Editor, 4th edition. 2007, Philadelphia: Lippincott Williams & Wilkins, pp. 1487–31.

[71] Steinhauer, D.A., E. Domingo, and J.J. Holland, Lack of evidence for proofreading mechanisms associated with an RNA virus polymerase. Gene, 1992. 122(2): pp. 281–8.

[72] Girard, M.P., et al., A review of vaccine research and development: human enteric infections. Vaccine, 2006. 24(15): pp. 2732–50.

[73] McCarthy, M.W. and D.R. Kockler, Trivalent intranasal influenza vaccine, live. Ann Pharmacother, 2004. 38(12): pp. 2086–93.

[74] Julian, T.R. and K.J. Schwab, Challenges in environmental detection of human viral pathogens. Curr Opin Virol, 2012. 2(1): pp. 78–83.

[75] Mokili, J.L., F. Rohwer, and B.E. Dutilh, Metagenomics and future perspectives in virus discovery. Curr Opin Virol, 2012. 2(1): pp. 63–77.

[76] Bhatt, S., E.C. Holmes, and O.G. Pybus, The genomic rate of molecular adaptation of the human influenza A virus. Mol Biol Evol, 2011. 28(9): pp. 2443–51.

[77] Tsai, K.N. and G.W. Chen, Influenza genome diversity and evolution. Microbes Infect, 2011. 13(5): pp. 479–88.

[78] Bourret, V., et al., Whole-genome, deep pyrosequencing analysis of a duck influenza A virus evolution in swine cells. Infect Genet Evol, 2013. 18: pp. 31–41.

[79] Crusat, M., et al., Changes in the hemagglutinin of H5N1 viruses during human infection--influence on receptor binding. Virology, 2013. 447(1–2): pp. 326–37.

[80] Hoper, D., et al., Highly pathogenic avian influenza virus subtype H5N1 escaping neutralization: more than HA variation. J Virol, 2012. 86(3): pp. 1394–404.

[81] Mertens, E., et al., Evaluation of phenotypic markers in full genome sequences of avian influenza isolates from California. Comp Immunol Microbiol Infect Dis, 2013. 36(5): pp. 521–36.

[82] Wilker, P.R., et al., Selection on haemagglutinin imposes a bottleneck during mammalian transmission of reassortant H5N1 influenza viruses. Nat Commun, 2013. 4: p. 2636.

[83] Waybright, N., et al., Detection of human virulence signatures in H5N1. J Virol Methods, 2008. 154(1–2): pp. 200–5.

[84] Deng, Y.M., N. Caldwell, and I.G. Barr, Rapid detection and subtyping of human influenza A viruses and reassortants by pyrosequencing. PLoS One, 2011. 6(8): p. e23400.

[85] Archer, J., et al., Analysis of high-depth sequence data for studying viral diversity: a comparison of next generation sequencing platforms using Segminator II. BMC Bioinformatics, 2012. 13: p. 47.

[86] Bartolini, B., et al., Assembly and characterization of pandemic influenza A H1N1 genome in nasopharyngeal swabs using high-throughput pyrosequencing. New Microbiol, 2011. 34(4): pp. 391–7.

[87] Deyde, V.M. and L.V. Gubareva, Influenza genome analysis using pyrosequencing method: current applications for a moving target. Expert Rev Mol Diagn, 2009. 9(5): pp. 493–509.

[88] Flaherty, P., et al., Ultrasensitive detection of rare mutations using next-generation targeted resequencing. Nucleic Acids Res, 2012. 40(1): p. e2.

[89] Hoper, D., B. Hoffmann, and M. Beer, Simple, sensitive, and swift sequencing of complete H5N1 avian influenza virus genomes. J Clin Microbiol, 2009. 47(3): pp. 674–9.

[90] Hoper, D., B. Hoffmann, and M. Beer, A comprehensive deep sequencing strategy for full-length genomes of influenza A. PLoS One, 2011. 6(4): p. e19075.

[91] Kampmann, M.L., et al., A simple method for the parallel deep sequencing of full influenza A genomes. J Virol Methods, 2011. 178(1–2): pp. 243–8.

[92] Levine, M., et al., Detection of hemagglutinin variants of the pandemic influenza A (H1N1) 2009 virus by pyrosequencing. J Clin Microbiol, 2011. 49(4): pp. 1307–12.

[93] Ren, X., et al., Full genome of influenza A (H7N9) virus derived by direct sequencing without culture. Emerg Infect Dis, 2013. 19(11): pp. 1881–4.

[94] Rutvisuttinunt, W., et al., Simultaneous and complete genome sequencing of influenza A and B with high coverage by Illumina MiSeq Platform. J Virol Methods, 2013. 193(2): pp. 394–404.

[95] Taubenberger, J.K., The virulence of the 1918 pandemic influenza virus: unraveling the enigma. Arch Virol Suppl, 2005(19): pp. 101–15.

[96] Taubenberger, J.K., et al., Characterization of the 1918 influenza virus polymerase genes. Nature, 2005. 437(7060): pp. 889–93.

[97] Tumpey, T.M., et al., Characterization of the reconstructed 1918 Spanish influenza pandemic virus. Science, 2005. 310(5745): pp. 77–80.

[98] Xiao, Y.L., et al., High-throughput RNA sequencing of a formalin-fixed, paraffin-embedded autopsy lung tissue sample from the 1918 influenza pandemic. J Pathol, 2013. 229(4): pp. 535–45.

[99] Clavijo, A., et al., Identification and analysis of the first 2009 pandemic H1N1 influenza virus from U.S. feral swine. Zoonoses Public Health, 2013. 60(5): pp. 327–35.

[100] Croville, G., et al., Field monitoring of avian influenza viruses: whole-genome sequencing and tracking of neuraminidase evolution using 454 pyrosequencing. J Clin Microbiol, 2012. 50(9): pp. 2881–7.

[101] Marchenko, V.Y., et al., Ecology of influenza virus in wild bird populations in Central Asia. Avian Dis, 2012. 56(1): pp. 234–7.

[102] Van Borm, S., et al., Phylogeographic analysis of avian influenza viruses isolated from Charadriiformes in Belgium confirms intercontinental reassortment in gulls. Arch Virol, 2012. 157(8): pp. 1509–22.

[103] Yu, X., et al., Influenza H7N9 and H9N2 viruses: coexistence in poultry linked to human H7N9 infection and genome characteristics. J Virol, 2014. 88(6): pp. 3423–31.

[104] Barrero, P.R., et al., Genetic and phylogenetic analyses of influenza A H1N1pdm virus in Buenos Aires, Argentina. J Virol, 2011. 85(2): pp. 1058–66.

[105] de la Rosa-Zamboni, D., et al., Molecular characterization of the predominant influenza A(H1N1)pdm09 virus in Mexico, December 2011-February 2012. PLoS One, 2012. 7(11): p. e50116.

[106] Lin, J., et al., Influenza seasonality and predominant subtypes of influenza virus in Guangdong, China, 2004-2012. J Thorac Dis, 2013. 5(Suppl 2): pp. S109–17.

[107] Church, J.D., et al., Sensitivity of the ViroSeq HIV-1 genotyping system for detection of the K103N resistance mutation in HIV-1 subtypes A, C, and D. J Mol Diagn, 2006. 8(4): pp. 430–2; quiz 527.

[108] Halvas, E.K., et al., Blinded, multicenter comparison of methods to detect a drug-resistant mutant of human immunodeficiency virus type 1 at low frequency. J Clin Microbiol, 2006. 44(7): pp. 2612–4.

[109] Leitner, T., et al., Analysis of heterogeneous viral populations by direct DNA sequencing. Biotechniques, 1993. 15(1): pp. 120–7.

[110] Archer, J., et al., Use of four next-generation sequencing platforms to determine HIV-1 coreceptor tropism. PLoS One, 2012. 7(11): p. e49602.

[111] Dudley, D.M., et al., Low-cost ultra-wide genotyping using Roche/454 pyrosequencing for surveillance of HIV drug resistance. PLoS One, 2012. 7(5): p. e36494.

[112] Fisher, R., et al., Deep sequencing reveals minor protease resistance mutations in patients failing a protease inhibitor regimen. J Virol, 2012. 86(11): pp. 6231–7.

[113] Gibson, R.M., et al., Sensitive deep-sequencing-based HIV-1 genotyping assay to simultaneously determine susceptibility to protease, reverse transcriptase, integrase, and maturation inhibitors, as well as HIV-1 coreceptor tropism. Antimicrob Agents Chemother, 2014. 58(4): pp. 2167–85.

[114] Shao, W., et al., Analysis of 454 sequencing error rate, error sources, and artifact recombination for detection of low-frequency drug resistance mutations in HIV-1 DNA. Retrovirology, 2013. 10: p. 18.

[115] Simen, B.B., et al., Low-abundance drug-resistant viral variants in chronically HIV-infected, antiretroviral treatment-naive patients significantly impact treatment outcomes. J Infect Dis, 2009. 199(5): pp. 693–701.

[116] Wang, C., et al., Characterization of mutation spectra with ultra-deep pyrosequencing: application to HIV-1 drug resistance. Genome Res, 2007. 17(8): pp. 1195–201.

[117] Arvia, R., et al., Monitoring the susceptibility to oseltamivir of Influenza A(H1N1) 2009 virus by nested-PCR and pyrosequencing during the pandemic and in the season 2010-2011. J Virol Methods, 2012. 184(1–2): pp. 113–6.

[118] Chen, L.F., et al., Cluster of oseltamivir-resistant 2009 pandemic influenza A (H1N1) virus infections on a hospital ward among immunocompromised patients--North Carolina, 2009. J Infect Dis, 2011. 203(6): pp. 838–46.

[119] Correia, V., et al., Antiviral drug profile of seasonal influenza viruses circulating in Portugal from 2004/2005 to 2008/2009 winter seasons. Antiviral Res, 2010. 86(2): pp. 128–36.

[120] Dharan, N.J., et al., Infections with oseltamivir-resistant influenza A(H1N1) virus in the United States. JAMA, 2009. 301(10): pp. 1034–41.

[121] Duwe, S.C., et al., Genotypic and phenotypic resistance of pandemic A/H1N1 influenza viruses circulating in Germany. Antiviral Res, 2011. 89(1): pp. 115–8.

[122] Pontoriero, A., et al., Virological surveillance and antiviral resistance of human influenza virus in Argentina, 2005-2008. Rev Panam Salud Publica, 2011. 30(6): pp. 634–40.

[123] Tellez-Sosa, J., et al., Using high-throughput sequencing to leverage surveillance of genetic diversity and oseltamivir resistance: a pilot study during the 2009 influenza A(H1N1) pandemic. PLoS One, 2013. 8(7): p. e67010.

[124] Bright, R.A., et al., Incidence of adamantane resistance among influenza A (H3N2) viruses isolated worldwide from 1994 to 2005: a cause for concern. Lancet, 2005. 366(9492): pp. 1175–81.

[125] Bright, R.A., et al., Adamantane resistance among influenza A viruses isolated early during the 2005-2006 influenza season in the United States. JAMA, 2006. 295(8): pp. 891–4.

[126] Deyde, V.M., et al., Surveillance of resistance to adamantanes among influenza A(H3N2) and A(H1N1) viruses isolated worldwide. J Infect Dis, 2007. 196(2): pp. 249–57.

[127] Higgins, R.R., et al., Differential patterns of amantadine-resistance in influenza A (H3N2) and (H1N1) isolates in Toronto, Canada. J Clin Virol, 2009. 44(1): pp. 91–3.

[128] Warren, S., et al., Extreme evolutionary conservation of functionally important regions in H1N1 influenza proteome. PLoS One, 2013. 8(11): p. e81027.

[129] Diaz, A., et al., Genome plasticity of triple-reassortant H1N1 influenza A virus during infection of vaccinated pigs. J Gen Virol, 2015. 96(10): pp. 2982–93.

[130] Robertson, J.S., et al., The development of vaccine viruses against pandemic A(H1N1) influenza. Vaccine, 2011. 29(9): pp. 1836–43.

[131] Connor, R.J., et al., Receptor specificity in human, avian, and equine H2 and H3 influenza virus isolates. Virology, 1994. 205(1): pp. 17–23.

[132] Matrosovich, M., et al., Early alterations of the receptor-binding properties of H1, H2, and H3 avian influenza virus hemagglutinins after their introduction into mammals. J Virol, 2000. 74(18): pp. 8502–12.

[133] Stevens, J., et al., Structure and receptor specificity of the hemagglutinin from an H5N1 influenza virus. Science, 2006. 312(5772): pp. 404–10.

[134] Varghese, J.N., et al., The structure of the complex between influenza virus neuraminidase and sialic acid, the viral receptor. Proteins, 1992. 14(3): pp. 327–32.

Chapter 3

Electrochemical Sensors for Detections of Influenza Viruses: Fundamentals and Applications

Hanna Radecka and Jerzy Radecki

Additional information is available at the end of the chapter

http://dx.doi.org/10.5772/64423

Abstract

Avian influenza viruses (AIVs) could cause severe diseases and, as the consequence, serious economic losses as well as a risk for potential transmission to humans. Therefore, the detection of viruses and their fragments or specific DNA sequences becomes an important approach in molecular diagnosis. Here, we present electrochemical genosensors devoted for detection of influenza virus H5N1 gene sequence. We focus our attention on ion-channel mechanism, E-DNA sensors, and genosensors based on redox-active layer. The novel dual DNA electrochemical sensor with "signal-off" and "signal-on" architecture for simultaneous detection of two different sequences of DNA derived from avian influenza virus type H5N1 by means of one electrode is presented. Immunosensors are also adequate analytical devices for detection of pathogens since antibodies are natural receptors responsible for binding of antigens. Thus, the binding selectivity and efficiency are naturally high. The immunosensors presented could be divided into two main groups: ion-channel mimetic and based on redox-active monolayer.

Keywords: Gold electrodes, Carbon electrodes, Electrochemical immunosensors, Genosensors, Influenza virus detection

1. Introduction

Infectious viral disease, which is spread among birds, in particular avian influenza (AI), could affect other animals, as well as humans [1].

The contact with infected live or dead poultry is the main source of risk of people's AI infection [2].

Controlling the AI in animals is the first step in decreasing risks to humans. Therefore, there is a high need for the development of the analytical methods allowing the fast and reliable AI virus detection.

The real-time polymerase chain reaction (PCR) [3], enzyme-linked immunoassay (ELISA) [4], and reverse transcription-polymerase chain reaction (RT-PCR) [5] are the most frequently used methods. Their main drawbacks are being time-consuming and demanding high-quality laboratories.

The biosensors are very good alternative. They are self-contained integrated analytical instruments which are capable of providing specific quantitative or semiquantitative analytical information applying a biological recognition element, which is indirect spatial contact with a transducer element. Main parameters describing the quality of biosensors are selectivity, sensitivity, reproducibility, and time of response.

Electrochemical biosensors belong to a subclass of biosensors, which contain an electrochemical transductor responsible for converting of energetic signal coming from an intermolecular recognition process into electrical on. Their main advantages are as follows: (1) the direct conversion of a biological event to an electronic signal, (2) excellent detection limits, (3) small analyte volumes in μl range, (4) ability to be used in turbid biofluids, (5) suitability for rapid measurements of analytes from human and animal samples, and (6) easy miniaturization.

The complete electrochemical biosensor should be cheap, small, portable, and capable of being used by semiskilled operators. In order to achieve this final goal, we have been working on several types of geno- and immunosensors.

In the ion-channel mimetic immunosensors and genosensors, the presence of redox marker in the sample solution is necessary. The antigen-antibody complex formation as well as hybridization process suppresses the accessibility of redox marker toward the electrode surface. This phenomenon, which is the base of analytical signal generation by ion-channel mimetic mode, was observed using the Osteryoung square-wave voltammetry (OSWV) or electrochemical impedance spectroscopy (EIS) in the presence of $[Fe(CN)_6]^{3-/4-}$ as an electroactive marker [6–14].

In the genosensors and immunosensors based on redox-active monolayer, the strategy for immobilization of the specific recognition elements involved their interactions with transition metal centers complexed on the electrode surface [15–19]. So, the presence of electroactive markers in the sample solution is not necessary. This is very important for analytical procedure involving naturally occurring molecules in which properties might be influenced by redox markers.

2. Electrochemical genosensors

In general, electrochemical genosensors monitor the DNA duplex formation at the surface of electrode through changes of current or potential values either using electrochemical labels or label-free system [20–25].

2.1. Methods for immobilization of recognition of ssDNA probe

The immobilization of single-stranded DNA (ssDNA) probe at the surface of electrode plays a crucial role for future genosensor analytical parameters. Various electrode materials such as gold, glassy carbon, carbon nanotubes, and graphene-modified electrodes have been applied for ssDNA immobilization. The physical adsorption, the simplest immobilization method, relies on the electrostatic interactions between ssDNA and surface of electrode. But such sensing layers are not stable. In addition, ssDNA strands are not well ordered, and because of this, they are not sufficiently accessible for target molecules.

The alternative method for immobilization of oligonucleotides on the electrode surface is their entrapping into polymer film deposited on the surface. The layer prepared according to this procedure is much more stable in comparison to the previous one. The weak point of this approach is the difficulty to control the flexibility of ssDNA probes and, as a consequence, their availability for target DNA.

The next method of DNA immobilization exploits the natural affinity of avidin to biotin. This method allows to create stable sensing layers with controlled density of ssDNA probes.

The most popular protocols of electrode modification are based on the formation of covalent bonds between the functional group introduced into ssDNA strand and functional group located at the surface of electrode. Therefore, the regulation of ssDNA probe density, as well as their stable (covalent) immobilization and proper orientation, is relatively easy to achieve.

2.2. Methods of hybridization process detection: selected examples of different types of genosensors

Different approaches for detection of the probe-analyte hybridization processes have been applied in various genosensors. One of them is based on changes of electrochemical activity of nucleobases upon the hybridization events. This concept has been proposed by Palecek and coworkers [26]. Oxidation of adenine (A) and guanine (G) can be readily observed using carbon electrodes or hanging mercury drop electrodes (HMDEs), which are suitable for investigation of reduction of nucleic acids. Their main drawback is background current at the relatively high potentials required for direct oxidation of DNA. In the case of reduction, the serious limitation is the necessity to use mercury electrode.

Another approach for voltammetric signal generation was presented by Umezawa and coworkers [6]. In their approach, the mechanism for generation of an analytical signal was connected with the binding event between target compound and recognition element immobilized at the electrode surface. Because of the creation of steric hindrance, as well as changing the surface charge, the accessibility of redox marker present in the sample solution toward the electrode is changed. Thus, creation of analyte-receptor supramolecular complex affected the electron transfer from marker to surface of electrode. The heterogeneous rate constant of electron transfer from marker to electrode surface became large or smaller; therefore, the redox current increased or decreased. The electrochemical sensors based on this mechanism are called ion-channel mimetic sensors.

Recently, in our laboratory, we have developed two genosensors working according to this mechanism based on the modified gold electrode intended for the detection of specific DNA sequence of avian influenza virus (AIV) H5N1 using NH_2-ssDNA or HS-ssDNA probes for the modification of gold electrode [11, 12].

NH_2-ssDNA probes were immobilized on the surface of mixed thioacid-thioalcohol monolayer via EDC/NHS coupling, whereas HS-ssDNA probes were immobilized directly to the gold surface via S-Au bonds. As marker ions in both cases, $[Fe(CN)_6]^{3-/4-}$ was employed. When SH-NC3 probe was used, detection limit in the 10 pM range was achieved. The much lower detection limit in fM range was recorded when NH_2-NC3 probe was applied. These data confirmed that the application of DNA probe with longer spacer part increased the hybridization signal. The better accessibility of target ssDNA toward more flexible DNA probe is the main reason of this phenomenon. But at the same time, the lower genosensor selectivity was observed. When SH-NC3 DNA probe with shorter spacer was applied, the sensor was able to distinguish between the PCR products with different positions of complementary parts, whereas the electrode modified with longer spacer molecules was not able to do this [11, 12].

Plaxo and coworkers [25] introduced another type of hybridization detection technique that exploits the difference in physical flexibility between single-stranded oligonucleotides and double-stranded ones. Upon hybridization, the physical changes in the probe structures, including the change in distances of the labeled electroactive moieties to the electrode surface, result in the switching "on/off" of the electrochemical signal.

The main advantages of E-DNA sensors are the conformational changes caused by hybridization, potential activation of redox label in the "safe" range separated from potential activation of majority of electroactive biomolecules present in the clinical and environmental samples, and detection limits in the picomoles of target DNA range.

The genosensors working on described mechanism belong to very wide "signal-off" mode family. It is worth to note that detection limit of E-DNA working according to "signal-off" mechanism is in the range of 10 pM. In case of genosensors that generated analytical signal according to "signal-on" mechanism, detection limit is around 200 pM [25].

The "signal-off" sensors have numerous advantages such as sequence specificity, reusability, and suitability for direct measurement in serum. But the suppression of signal generated after target binding is their main disadvantage, because only 100 % suppression of the original current could be detected. On the other hand, the "signal-on" sensors have a potential for great improvement of sensitivity, because the stimulation of these types of sensors with the target does not cause a limited increase of signal. A weak point of these types of E-DNA sensors is the use of rather complicated, but not very stable architectures. This approach does not work properly in the complex samples.

Today, more and more often, biosensor is required to be not only miniaturized and cost-effective but also capable of simultaneous detection of multiple analytes.

Recently, a novel dual E-DNA sensor working on "signal-off" and "signal-on" mode has been developed [20]. This sensor was suitable for simultaneous detection of two different oligonucleotide sequences present in avian influenza virus (AIV) type H5N1 with using one electrode. The ssDNA probe represented by hemagglutinin was functionalized with ferrocene (ssDNA-Fc). The functionalization with methylene blue (ssDNA-MB) was applied for sequence derived from neuraminidase. Both of them were covalently immobilized on the gold electrode surface. Hybridization process going at the electrode surface was controlled by the Osteryoung square-wave voltammetry. Detection limits determined by graphic method were 4.0 x 10^{-8} and 2.0 x 10^{-8} M, for simultaneous analysis of both sequences and for single one, respectively. These values, in particular the detection limits for parallel determinations of two sequences, are very promising from diagnosing point of view. The selectivity of duo-genosensor was similar for both targets. The limits of detection were in the range of 18–21 nM. The duo-genosensor was free from interferences. The presence of oligonucleotide sequences complementary to SH-ssDNA-Fc probe does not influence the function of the probe decorated with methylene blue and vice versa. The main advantage of duo-sensor is diminishing false-positive determinations which may appear in the case of non-perfect hybridization with component(s) present in non-infected host samples. The probability for existence in native samples of components efficiently interacting with two independent DNA probes is limited.

Recently, in our laboratory, we have developed the new group of electrochemical DNA sensors in which the analytical signal generation is based on the changes of accessibility of redox center attached directly to the analytical active layer or at the "foot" of the oligonucleotide probe, very close to the electrode surface [16, 17, 20–22]. Such localization exclude the changes of distance of redox marker from the electrode surface after hybridization. As a redox center, we have used the complexes of transition metals with dipyrromethene, porphyrin, and phenanthroline.

A novel mechanism of electrochemical signal generation based on changes of the ion-barrier energy "switch-off" system has been proposed. According to this mechanism, the proposed sensors generate an analytical signal because of changes in the environment surrounding the redox center occurring as a result of hybridization processes.

For the sensor based on the Cu(II) complex, during the redox cycle, Cu(II) is reduced to Cu(I). As a consequence, a single negative charge of the reduced form appears at the surface of the electrode. The precondition of redox reaction run is the compensation of this charge by ions from the supporting electrolyte, involving transport of cations. For the electrode modified with the Co(II) complex, an oxidation process is possible, which generates an extra positive charge of the oxidized form. For its neutralization, anions from the supporting electrolyte will be involved. The mechanism of analytical signal generation by this type of sensors relies on changes in accessibility of ions present in the supporting solution to the redox centers in order to neutralize the charge occurring as a result of oxidation/reduction processes. The good illustration of such sensors is genosensor intended for detection of the sequence specific of avian influenza virus type H5N1. A 20 mer probe (NH_2-NC3) was covalently attached to the gold electrode surface.

The detection limit of 1.39 pM for fully complementary single-stranded DNA target was achieved with genosensor based on (dipyrromethene)$_2$Cu(II) complex. A linear dynamic range was observed from 1 to 10 pM. The good discrimination between fully complementary, partially complementary (with only six complementary bases), and totally non-complementary to the probe was also recorded [16].

The Fe(III)-phenanthroline complex is the base of genosensor suitable for detection of target DNA as well as RNA. An efficient click reaction, carried out under mild conditions, between the NH_2-NC3 probe and the epoxy groups from Fe(III)-phenanthroline complex deposited on the gold electrode surface, has been successfully applied for the genosensor construction. The good detection limits of 73 and 0.87 pM for the 20 mer c-NC3 and the 283 mer RNA1, respectively, were achieved. The sensitivity of RNA sequence detection was about one hundred times better than the DNA sequence detection. The 20 mer nc-NC3 non-complementary to the probe generated a weak response. In the case of non-complementary to the probe 277 mer RNA3 fragment, even the opposite signal, an increase of the Fe(III)/Fe(II) peak currents was observed. These data confirmed the genosensor selectivity. The main advantage of genosensor based on Fe(III)-phenanthroline complex is its suitability for determination of RNA and distinguishing of the different positions of the complementary parts. Thus, it could be applied for the detection of the H5N1 genetic material [17].

3. Electrochemical immunosensors

3.1. Methods for immobilization of recognition element

The right immobilization of the proteins as the recognition elements on the transducer surface (e.g., gold, platinum, indium tin oxide, carbon materials) is a crucial factor to fully maintain their right conformation and activity.

Physical protein immobilization is based mainly on electrostatic forces and hydrophobic interactions. The entrapping of proteins into the polymer matrix, iridium oxide films [27], and nanotextured zinc oxide [28] belongs to this strategy.

The colloidal gold layers create friendly environment for proteins. Therefore, they are frequently used in immunosensor creation [7–10, 29–31].

In this approach, proteins are mainly immobilized on colloidal gold layers based on the electrostatic interactions, which could be enhanced by selecting the proper pH conditions. The drawbacks of this method are random orientation and rather weak attachment. In order to overcome these weak points, covalent antibody immobilization has been applied. Two polypeptide chains $F(ab')_2$ present in immunoglobulin molecule are responsible for antigen binding. Fc domain, which is not involved in this interaction, could be removed by enzyme digestions [32]. The presence of disulfide or thiol group allow the $F(ab')_2$ or F(ab') fragments to covalent self-assembling on the gold nanoparticle surface [33, 34]. This approach has been successfully applied for development of immunosensor destined for selective binding of antigen rSPI2-His_6 present in the sample solution by F(ab') fragment of antibody immobilized on a surface of the electrode using electrochemical impedance spectroscopy (EIS) and surface plasmon resonance (SPR) [30] as well as for selective detection of hemagglutinin from avian influenza virus H5N1 [9, 10]. The proteins A and G possessing high affinity toward the Fc part of immunoglobulins are frequently used for their covalent and oriented immobilization on the electrode surface [35]. The immunosensor based on glassy carbon electrode incorporating the protein A has been successfully applied to distinguish between sera of unvaccinated and vaccinated chickens against the avian influenza virus. Sensitivity of EIS immunosensor was almost 10^4 times much better than ELISA [8].

3.2. Methods of detection of immunoreaction: selected examples of different types of immunosensors

The majority of electrochemical immunosensors incorporate not only recognition element (antibody or antigen) but also secondary enzyme-labeled antibody, which follows the addition of proper enzymatic substrate. The antibody-antigen reaction is detected in no-direct manner but by electroactive molecules produced by enzymatic reaction [36, 37]. Such approach demands very precious labeled biological materials, which increase the cost of analysis. Also, it involved numerous modification steps. The no-direct detection of immunoreaction is the main drawback of sandwich type of immunoassays.

In order to overcome the above weak points, the immunosensors allowing the direct electrochemical detection of immunoreactions have been developed in our laboratories.

The whole antibodies or antibody-binding fragments (Fab′) have been immobilized on the surface of gold nanoparticle layers, which create friendly environment for proteins keeping their physiological activity. The formation of immunoreactions has been detected by the changes of accessibility of redox marker present in the sample solution to the electrode surface. The deposition of antibody-antigen complex on the electrode surface increases substantially the resistance of the analytical system, and as a consequence, faradaic current is very difficult to measure by voltammetric techniques. Therefore, electrochemical impedance spectroscopy (EIS) has been widely applied. EIS is an ac method that describes the response of an electrochemical cell to a small amplitude, sinusoidal voltage signal, and a function of frequency. The most popular mode for analyzing electrochemical impedance data is the plot of the imaginary impedance component versus real impedance component at each excitation frequency (the Nyquist plot). Numerous impedimetric immunosensors have been already reported [7, 30, 31, 38]. This approach has been successfully applied for detection of fragments of H5 hemagglutinin from avian influenza viruses [9, 10]. The antibody-binding fragments have been covalently attached to the gold nanoparticle layers. Application of 4,4′-thiobisbenzenethiol self-assembled monolayer [10] improved substantially immunosensor performance in the comparison to one incorporated 1,6-hexanedithiol [9]. Taking into account the immunosensor sensitivity with detection limit of 0.6 pg/mL and specificity (negative control H7 hemagglutinin generate negligible response), they could be recommended for direct electrochemical detection of H5 hemagglutinin from influenza virus in the field conditions.

Direct impedimetric immunosensor has been successfully applied for detection of antibodies generated against H5N1 virus [8]. The base of this immunosensor was glassy carbon electrode incorporated fragment of H5 hemagglutinin. The interaction with specific antibodies was detected electrochemically by changes of $[Fe(CN)_6]^{3-/4-}$ accessibility toward electrode surface.

The immunosensor was able to distinguish the sera from vaccinated and unvaccinated hen with sensitivity 10^4 better than ELISA.

In order to avoid the necessity of the redox marker present in the sample solution, the immunosensor-incorporated redox-active layer has been developed [39].

The Cu(II) complex with dipyrromethene deposited onto the gold electrode surface plays double roles. It is a site for covalent immobilization of the His-tagged fragment of H5 hemagglutinin, as well as redox centers for sensing the antigen-antibody interaction.

This type of immunosensor was also suitable for direct antibody detection in hen sera with 200 better sensitivity than ELISA.

4. Future perspective

The analytical chemists mainly search for improving sensitivity and selectivity of sensing devices. The intensive development of nanotechnology gives wide possibility of using nanomaterial labels for signal amplification generated upon immunoreaction [18, 19, 40–43]. Nanomaterials could be used for modification of electrochemical transducers in order to improve their electrochemical properties by lowering background current and signal to noise ratio, as well as increasing electron transfer rate.

The most frequently used nanomaterials are colloidal gold and silver, semiconductor quantum dots, carbon nanotubes, and graphene.

They are very promising in the development of ultrasensitive immunosensors. Could they be applied in point-of-care and clinical diagnoses? Taking into account so intensive effort done in this research area, the answer for this question is "yes."

5. Conclusions

The main advantage of ion-channel mimetic sensors is the possibility of their application for exploring the recognition processes occurring at the water/solid interface. It is very important from biological as well as medical point of view. The electrochemical sensors based on redox-active layer are new direction in sensing device development. Their main advantage is the lack of the necessity of using the external redox marker. The redox centers can simultaneously act as sites for host molecule immobilization and transducers.

Taking into account the following parameters of electrochemical biosensors presented such as very good sensitivity, very low sample consumption (in μl level), lack of matrix influence, simple operation, and reasonable cost, it might be concluded that they are analytical tools suitable for detection of viruses in the environmental sample.

http://dx.doi.org/10.5772/64423

Acknowledgements

This work was supported by a project from the National Centre for Research and Development No. PBS2/A7/14/2014 and Institute of Animal Reproduction and Food Research of Polish Academy of Sciences, Olsztyn, Poland.

Author details

Hanna Radecka* and Jerzy Radecki

*Address all correspondence to: h.radecka@pan.olsztyn.pl

Institute of Animal Reproduction and Food Research of Polish Academy of Sciences, Olsztyn, Poland

References

[1] http://www.who.int/influenza/human_animal_interface/en/

[2] Lopez-Martinez I, Balish A, Barrera-Badillo G, Jones J, Nuñez-García TE, Jang Y, Aparicio-Antonio R, Azziz-Baumgartner E, Belser JA, Ramirez-Gonzalez JE, Pedersen JC, Ortiz-Alcantara J, Gonzalez-Duran E, Shu B, Emery SL, Poh MK, Reyes-Teran G, Vazquez-Perez JA, Avila-Rios S, Uyeki T, Lindstrom S, Villanueva J, Tokars J, Ruiz-Matus C, Gonzalez-Roldan JF, Schmitt B, Klimov A, Cox N, Kuri-Morales P, Davis CT, Diaz-Quiñonez JA. Mint: Highly pathogenic avian influenza A(H7N3) virus in poultry workers, Mexico, 2012, Emerg Infect Dis. 2013;19(9):1531–1534

[3] Walker J, Rapley R. Molecular Biomethods Handbook, second ed., Humana Press, Totowa, NJ, 2008.

[4] Dowall SD, Richards KS, Graham VA, Chamberlain J, Hewson R. Mint: Development of an indirect ELISA method for the parallel measurement of IgG and IgM antibodies against Crimean-Congo haemorrhagic fever (CCHF) virus using recombinant nucleo-protein as antigen, J Virol Methods. 2012;179:335–341

[5] Majumder R,. Chowdhury EH, Parvin R, Begum JA, Giasuddin M, Islam, MR. Mint: Development of multiplex reverse transcription polymerase chain reaction (RT-PCR) for simultaneous detection of matrix, haemagglutinin and neuraminidase genes of H5N1 avian influenza virus, Bangladesh Vet. 2011;28:55–59

[6] Umezawa Y, Aoki H. Mint: Ion channel based on artificial receptors. Anal Chem. 2004;76:321A–326A

[7] Jarocka U, Wąsowicz M, Radecka H, Malinowski T, Michalczuk L, Radecki J. Mint: Impedimetric immunosensor for detection of plum pox virus in plant extract, Electroanalysis. 2011;23(9):2197–2204

[8] Jarocka U, Sawicka R, Góra-Sochacka A, Sirko A, Zagórski-Ostoja W, Radecka H, Radecki J. Mint: Electrochemical immunosensor for detection of antibodies against influenza A virus H5N1 in hen serum, Biosens Bioelectron. 2014;55:301–306

[9] Jarocka U, Sawicka R, Góra-Sochacka A, Sirko A, Zagórski-Ostoja W, Radecki J, Radecka H. Mint: An immunosensor based on antibody binding fragments attached to gold nanoparticles for the detection of peptides derived from avian influenza hemagglutinin H5, Sensors. 2014;14:15714–15728

[10] Jarocka U, Sawicka R, Góra-Sochacka A, Sirko A, Dehaen W, Radecki J, Radecka H. Mint: An electrochemical immunosensor based on a 4,4′-thiobisbenzenethiol self-assembled monolayer for the detection of hemagglutinin from avian influenza virus H5N1, Sens Actuator B Chem. 2016;228:25–30

[11] Malecka K, Grabowska I, Radecki J, Stachyra A, Góra-Spchacka A, Sirko A., Radecka H. Mint: Voltammetric detection of a specific DNA sequence of avian influenza virus H5N1 using HS-ssDNA probe deposited onto gold electrode, Electroanalysis. 2012;24(2):439–446

[12] Malecka K, Grabowska I, Radecki J, Stachyra A, Góra-Sochacka A, Sirko A, Radecka H. Mint: Electrochemical detection of avian influenza virus genotype using amino-ssDNA probe modified gold electrodes, Electroanalysis. 2013;25(8):1871–1878

[13] Malecka K, Michalczuk L, Radecka H, Radecki J. Mint: Ion-channel genosensor for the detection of specific DNA sequences derived from plum pox virus in plant extracts, Sensors. 2014;14:18611–18624

[14] Malecka K, Stachyra A, Góra-Sochacka A, Sirko A, Zagórski-Ostoja W, Radecka H, Radecki J.Mint: Electrochemical genosensor based on disc and screen printed gold electrodes for detection of specific DNA and RNA sequences derived from avian influenza virus H5N1, Sens Actuator B Chem. 2016;224:290–297

[15] Grabowska I, Malecka K, Jarocka U, Radecki J, Radecka H. Mint: Electrochemical biosensors for detection of avian influenza virus – current status and future trends, Acta Biochim Pol. 2014;61:471–478

[16] Kurzątkowska K, Sirko A, Zagórski-Ostoja W, Dehaen W, Radecka H, Radecki J. Mint: Electrochemical label-free and reagentless genosensors based on a ion barrier switch-off system for DNA sequence-specific detection of the avian influenza virus, Anal Chem. 2015;87:9702–9709

[17] Malecka K, Stachyra A, Góra-Sochacka A, Sirko A, Zagórski-Ostoja W, Dehaen W, Radecka H, Radecki J. Mint: New redox-active layer create via epoxy-amine reaction –

the base of genosensor for the detection of specific DNA and RNA sequences of avian influenza virus H5N1, Biosens Bioelectron. 2015;65:427–434

[18] Radecka H, Radecki J, Grabowska I, Kurzątkowska K. Electrochemical sensors and biosensors based on self-assembled monolayers: Application of nanoparticles for analytical signals amplification, in Maria Hepel and Chuan-Jian Zhong (Eds.), Functional Nanoparticles for Bioanalysis, Nanomedicine, and Bioelectronics Devices, Volume 1, American Chemical Society, Washington, DC, 2012, pp. 293–312. ISBN: 978-0-8412-2775-0-90000.

[19] Radecki J, Radecka H. Development of electrochemical sensors for DNA analysis, in: E. Stulz and G. H. Clever (Eds.), DNA in Supramolecular Chemistry and Nanotechnology, first edition, John Wiley & Sons, Ltd., The Atrium, Southern Gate, Chichester, West Sussex, PO19 8SQ, United Kingdom, 2015, pp. 139–157. ISBN: 978-1-118-69686-6

[20] Grabowska I, Malecka K, Stachyra A, Góra-Sochacka A, Sirko A, Zagórski-Ostoja W, Radecka H, Radecki J. Mint: Single electrode genosensor for simultaneous determination of sequences encoding hemagglutinin and neuraminidase of avian influenza virus type H5N1, Anal Chem. 2013;85:10167–10173

[21] Grabowska I, Stachyra A, Góra-Sochacka A, Sirko A, Olejniczak AB, Leśnikowski ZJ, Radecki J, Radecka H. Mint: DNA probe modified with 3-iron bis(dicarbollide) for electrochemical determination of DNA sequence of avian influenza virus H5N1, Biosens Bioelectron. 2014;51:170–176

[22] Grabowska I, Singleton DG, Stachyra A, Góra-Sochacka A, Sirko A, Zagórski-Ostoja W, Radecka H, Stulz E, Radecki J. Mint: A highly sensitive electrochemical genosensor based on co-porphyrin-labelled DNA, Chem Commun. 2014;50:4196–4199

[23] Nie J, Zhang D, Zhang F, Yuan F, Zhou Y, Zhang X. Mint: Highly sensitive surface plasmon resonance sensor for the detection of DNA and cancer cell by target-triggered multiple signal amplification strategy, Chem Commun. 2014;50:6211–6213

[24] Wang X, Nan F, Zhao J, Yang T, Ge T, Jiao K. Mint: A label-free ultrasensitive electrochemical DNA sensor based on thin-layer MoS2 nanosheets with high electrochemical activity, Biosens Bioelectron. 2015;64:386–391

[25] Xia F, White RJ, Zup X, Patterson A, Xiao Y, Kang D, Gong X, Plaxo KW, Heeger AJ. Mint: An electrochemical supersandwich assay for sensitive and selective DNA detection in complex matrices, J Am Chem Soc. 2010;132:14346–14348

[26] Palecek E, Bartosik M. Mint: Electrochemistry of nucleic acids, Chem Rev. 2012;112(6): 3427–3481

[27] Wilson MS, Rauh RD. Mint: Novel amperometric immunosensors based on iridium oxide matrices, Biosens Bioelectron. 2004;19:693–699

[28] Jacobs M, Muthukumar S, Selvam AP, Craven JE, Prasad S. Mint: Ultra-sensitive electrical immunoassay biosensors using nanotextured zinc oxide thin films on printed circuit board platforms, Biosens Bioelectron. 2014;55:7–13

[29] Pranjal C, Singh J, Singh A, Srivastava A, Goyal RN, Shim YB. Mint: Gold nanoparticles and nanocomposites in clinical diagnostics using electrochemical methods, J Nanopart. 2013: Article ID 535901, http://dx.doi.org/10.1155/2013/535901

[30] Wąsowicz M, Milner M, Radecka D, Grzelak K, Radecka H. Mint: Immunosensors incorporating anti-His (C-term) IgG F (ab`) fragments attached to gold nanorods for detection of His-tagged proteins in culture medium. Sensors. 2010;10:5409–5424

[31] Wąsowicz M, Subramanian V, Dvornyk A, Grzelak K, Kłudkiewicz B, Radecka H.Mint: Comparison of electrochemical immunosensors based on gold nano materials and immunoblot techniques for detection of histidine-tagged proteins in culture medium, Biosens Bioelectron. 2008;24:284–289

[32] Coleman L, Mahler S. Mint: Purification of fab fragments from a monoclonal antibody papain digest by Gradiflow electrophoresis. Protein Expr Purif. 2003;32:246–251

[33] Iwata R, Satoh R, Iwasaki Y, Akiyoshi K. Mint: Covalent immobilization of antibody fragments on well-defined polymer brushes via site-directed method. Colloids Surf B Biointerfaces. 2008;62:288–298

[34] Lee W, Oh BK, Lee WH, Choi JW. Mint: Immobilization of antibody fragment for immunosensor application based on surface plasmon resonance. Colloids Surf B Biointerfaces. 2005;40:143–148

[35] Liu X, Wang X, Zhang J, Feng H, Wong, DKY. Mint: Detection of estradiol at an electrochemical immunosensor with a Cu UPD|DTBP-Protein G scaffold, Biosens Bioelectron. 2012;35(1):56–62

[36] Pei X, Zhang BM, Tang J, Liu B, Lai W, Tang D. Mint: Sandwich-type immunosensors and immunoassays exploited nanostructure labels: A review. Anal Chim Acta. 2013;758:1–18

[37] Ricci R, Adornetto G, Palleschi G. Mint: A review of experimental aspects of electrochemical immunosensors. Elecrochim Acta.2012; 84:74–83

[38] Prodromidis M I. Mint: Impedimetric immunosensors—A review, Electrochim Acta. 2010; 55(14):4227–4233

[39] Jarocka U, Sawicka R, Stachyra A, Góra-Sochacka A, Sirko A, Zagórski-Ostoja W, Sączyńska V, Porębska A, Dehaen W, Radecki J, Radecka H. Mint: A biosensors based on electroactive dipyrromethene-Cu(II) layer deposited onto gold electrodes for the detection of antibodies against avian influenza virus type H5N1 in hen sera, Anal Bioanal Chem. 2015;407:7807–7814

[40] Liu G, Lin Y. Mint: Nanomaterial labels in electrochemical immunosensors and immunoassays, Talanta. 2007;74:308–317

[41] Rasheed PA, Andhyarani SN. Mint: A highly sensitive DNA sensor for attomolar detection of the BRCA1 gene: Signal amplification with gold nanoparticle clusters, Analyst. 2015;140:2713–2718

[42] Wan Y, Su Y, Zhu X, Liu G, Fan C. Mint: Development of electrochemical immunosensors towards point of care diagnostics. Biosens Bioelectron. 2013;47:1–11

[43] Wang X, Uchiyama S. State of the art in biosensors – general aspects, in Polymers for Biosensors Construction, Chapter 3 book edited by Toonika Rinken, ISBN 978-953-51-1004-0, Published: March 13, 2013 under CC BY 3.0 license. © The Author(s) http://dx.doi.org/10.5772/54428

Chapter 4

Biosensors for Rapid Detection of Avian Influenza

Ronghui Wang and Yanbin Li

Additional information is available at the end of the chapter

http://dx.doi.org/10.5772/64353

Abstract

The scope of this chapter was to review the advancements made in the area of biosensors for rapid detection of avian influenza viruses (AIVs). It is intended to provide general background about biosensor technology and to discuss important aspects for developing biosensors, such as selection of the suitable biological recognition elements (anti-AIV bioreceptors) as well as their immobilization strategies. A major concern of this chapter is also to critically review the biosensors' working principles and their applications in AIV detection. A table containing the types of biosensor, bioreceptors, target AIVs, methods, etc. is given in this chapter. A number of papers for the different types of biosensors give hints on the current trends in the field of biosensor research for its application on AIV detection. By discussing recent research and future trends based on many excellent publications and reviews, it is hoped to give the readers a comprehensive view on this fast-growing field.

Keywords: biosensor, avian influenza virus, rapid detection, bioreceptor, nanobiosensor

1. Introduction

Influenza viruses, which belong to the *Orthomyxoviridae* family, are classified as A, B, and C based on antigenic differences in their nucleoprotein (NP) and matrix (M_1) protein [1]. All avian influenza viruses (AIV) are classified as type A. Type A viruses are further subtyped on the basis of antigenic differences of the surface glycoproteins, the hemagglutinin (HA), and the neuraminidase (NA) proteins [2]. So far, seventeen HA (H1 through H17) and ten NA (N1 through N10) subtypes have been identified [3]. **Figure 1** presents a schematic diagram of influenza A virus, and **Figure 2** shows a transmission electron microscopy photograph. Influenza A virus is an enveloped RNA virus approximately 80–120 nm in diameter [1, 2]. There are two major surface glycoproteins (HA and NA) and a small number of M2 protein, which has ion channel activity. The ratio of HA and NA is approximately 4:1. The genome of type A virus consists of eight segments of negative-sense single-stranded RNA, which are associated with many NP and the transcriptase complex (RNA polymerase components PB1, PB2 and PA) to form ribonucleoproteins (RNPs). The matrix protein M1 has an interaction with the RNPs and is under the lipid bilayer. NS_1 is found only in infected cells and is not thought to be a structural component of the virus, but small amount of NS_2 are present in purified viruses.

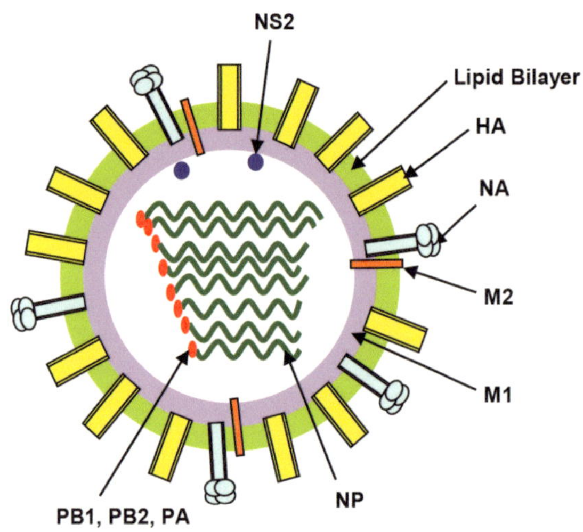

Figure 1. A schematic diagram of the structure of the influenza A virus particle.

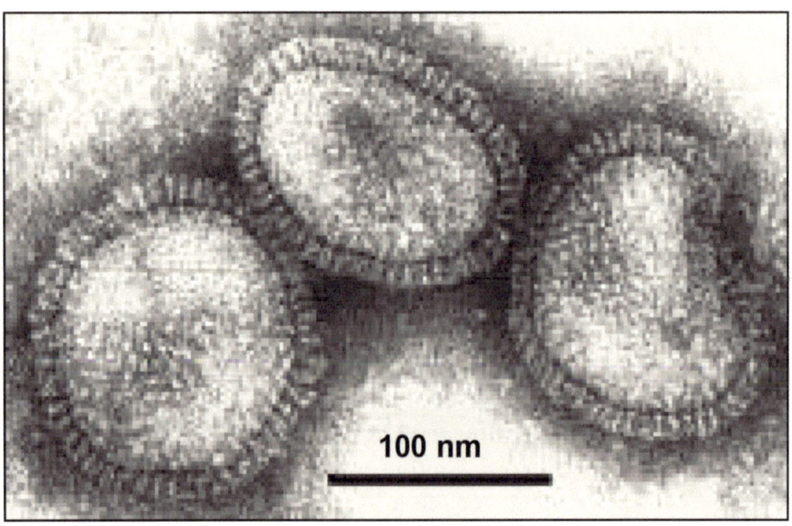

Figure 2. A transmission electron micrograph of influenza A virus particles.

AIVs have a large impact on the poultry each year and also represent a threat to human health. The highly pathogenic H5N1 avian influenza (HPAI H5N1), which originally emerged in Southeaster Asia in late 1990s, cost the poultry industry an estimated $10 billion between 1997 and 2008 [4]. HPAI H5N1 has also caused global concerns for public health and continues to spread throughout the world. Since 2003, a total of 62 countries (regions) have been affected by HPAI H5N1 and new human and animal cases are continuously being confirmed and reported [5]. The link between human and AI has raised concern among public health authorities and the scientific community about the prevalence and pandemic potential of AI virus. The H5N1 virus has caused 449 deaths of 846 people infected since 2003, according to the World Health Organization [5]. Therefore, advanced technologies for more rapid and sensitive AIV detection are needed for better surveillance and control of the outbreaks.

Current virus detection techniques are available, such as virus isolation, immunofluorescence antibody (FA) test, immunohistochemistry (IHC), and ELISA as well as rapid procedures based on molecular tools, such as polymerase chain reaction (PCR)-based assays, gene sequencing, and microarrays. Among these test methods, virus isolation has been the "gold standard" as its highest sensitivity and reliability, but it is a very time-consuming procedure (4–7 days). ELISA is a simple and rapid test in testing mass serum samples; thus, it is commonly used for serum antibody detection, but not used for virus detection in practice or diagnostics. Other immunoassays of FA or IHC can be used as a direct virus detection test from tissue specimens, but they either require labels or have limitations of low sensitivity and cross-reactions in certain circumstances. The molecular assays of RT-PCR and real-time RT-PCR methods have the advantages of high sensitivity and good specificity, but possess disadvantages of requiring expensive PCR equipment and reagents, and well-trained skillful technical personnel. Therefore, in order to minimize the social and economic costs, the development of rapid detection methods is essential. These rapid detection methods should meet the following requirements: (1) high throughput, (2) possibility of multiple target detection, (3) high sensitivity, (4) good specificity, (5) high speed, (6) simple operation, (7) suitability for on-site and/or in-field use, and (8) less cost. Biosensors have shown a great potential to meet such criteria.

The biosensor research began in the early 60 s of the twentieth century, when a glucose biosensor was proposed by Clark and Lyons [6] at Children's Hospital in Cincinnati. From then on, biosensor applications have expanded throughout the medical diagnosis field and also into the fields of environmental monitoring, agricultural production, food safety, pharmaceutical screening, and biodefense. A biosensor can be defined as a "compact analytical device or unit incorporating a biological or biologically derived sensitive recognition element integrated or associated with a physiochemical transducer" [7]. This device is composed of a biological recognition element (often called bioreceptor) and directly interfaced signal transducer (**Figure 3**). The selective and reversible process of interaction between the analyte and bioreceptor is transduced into a measurable signal, for example, electrical signal, which is proportional to the concentration or activity of an analyte in any type of samples. Biosensors can be classified based on the transduction element or the biological element. According to the basic principles of signal transduction, there are three main biosensor types, which have been studied for use in AIVs detection: piezoelectric, optical, and electrochemical biosensors. If we follow the types of biological element or bioreceptors, AIV biosensors can be classified into immunosensors, aptasensors, DNA or RNA-probe sensors, and more. In this chapter, we focus on these types of biosensors studied and developed recently for rapid detection of AIVs. It offers a survey of the principles, fabrication, operation, and the most popular types of biosensing devices in research or application today for AIVs detection. By discussing recent research and future trends based on many excellent publications and reviews, it is hoped to give the readers a comprehensive view on this fast-growing field.

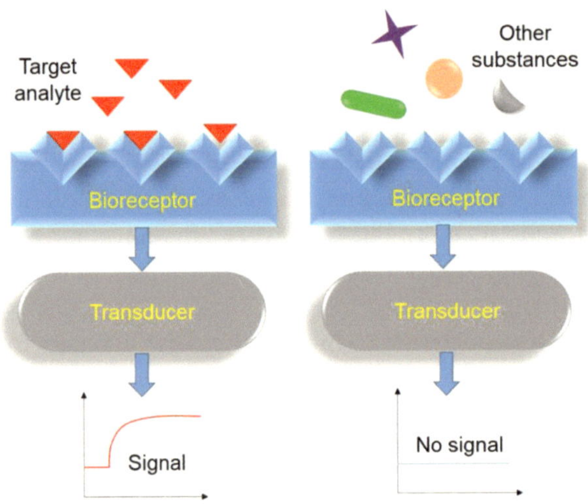

Figure 3. A schematic diagram of biorecognition and signal transduction in a typical biosensor.

2. Biosensors for detection of AIVs

As shown in **Figure 4**, the number of papers published in the field of biosensor research for detection of AI has kept increasing from year 2001 to 2015 based on PubMed. Biosensors offer the advantages of simple operation, rapid response, low cost, portability, automation, and easy to integrate with nanomaterials/nanostructure, Micro-Electro-Mechanical System(MEMS)/ Nano-Electro-Mechanical System(NEMS), biotechnology, Global Position System(GPS)/ wireless, and image technologies. One of the major requirements in developing a biosensor for AIVs is the need for a sensitive analytical device that can easily go down to very low detection levels without significant changes in selectivity. AIVs will spread rapidly through a community before any symptoms appear for the identification. A biosensor that can rapidly, sensitively and selectively detect target virus will be invaluable. In addition, a simple, robust, rapid, cost-effective, and potable biosensor, suitable for use in the field, is urgently needed. While a variety of biosensors have been developed for use in different applications, three types of biosensors have been mainly studied for AIV detection: piezoelectric, optical, and electrochemical biosensors.

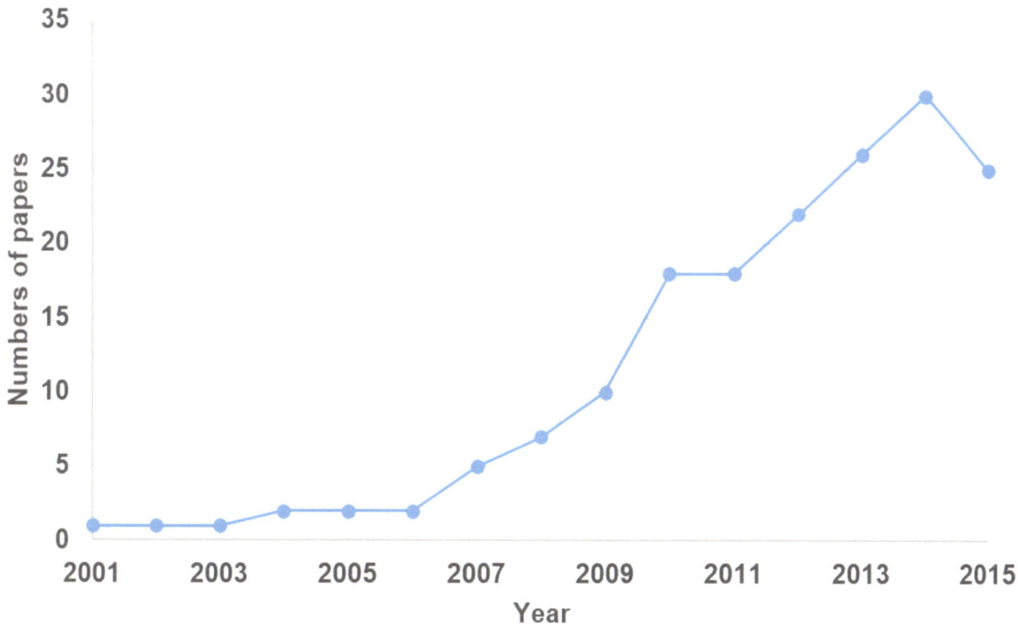

Figure 4. Numbers of papers published in the field of biosensor research for detection of AIVs between year 2001 and 2015.

2.1. Piezoelectric biosensors

Piezoelectric biosensors utilize crystals capable of generating a piezoelectric field to detect mass changes in the sensing environment [8]. The crystal is sandwiched between two excitation electrodes, which apply an electrical field that causes the crystal to undergo dimensional changes, or oscillations, at the crystals natural resonant frequency. An increase in the mass on the surface of the crystal, such as antibody immobilization or capture of antigen, decreases the resonant frequency. Piezoelectric biosensors are useful because they are low cost, label free, sensitive, and have extremely low detection levels [8]. The most intensively studied piezoelectric biosensor is the quartz crystal microbalance (QCM), which uses a thin wafer of quartz as the transducing crystal. Quartz crystals have the advantages of being widely available, relatively inexpensive, durable, direct detection, and real-time output. Other techniques are often coupled with QCM to increase the performance and capability of the biosensor. QCM biosensors have attracted interest in applications for AIVs detection. **Table 1** summarizes the main analytical features of QCM biosensors for detection of AIVs. Different studies used different concentration units for AIV. It would be helpful to know the comparable relationship between them. The common concentration units for AIV contain EID_{50} (50% egg infectious does), ELD_{50} (50% egg lethal does), PFU (plague-forming units), and HAU (hemagglutination unit). 1×10^3 EID_{50} ml^{-1} equals to ~0.0128 HAU/50 μl [9], $1 \times 10^{6.2}$ ELD_{50} ml^{-1} equals to 128 HAU/50 μl [10], and 1×10^5 PFU equals to 1 HAU [11].

Influenza subtype	Target	Bioreceptor	Sensitivity	Detection range	Detection time	Labelling method	Reference
H3N2	Virus	Antibody	4 virus particles/ml	0.02–3 HAU	–	Label-free	[12]
H1N1	Virus	Antibody	10^4 pfu/ml	10^3–10^7 pfu/ml	45 min	Label-free	[13]
			10^3 pfu/ml		105 min	Label with 13 nm gold nanoparticles	
H5N1	Virus	Antibody	0.0128 HAU	0.128–12.8 HAU	120 min	Label with 30 nm magnetic nanobeads	[14]
H5N1	Virus	Aptamer	1 HAU	1–4 HAU	60 min	Label with 30 nm magnetic nanobaeds	[22]
H5N1	Virus	Aptamer hydrogel	0.0128 HAU	0.0128–0.64 HAU	30 min	Label-free	[9]
H5N3	HA	Glycan	K_d 1.44 × 10^{-8} M	–	–	Label-free	[26]
H5N3	Virus	N-Acetylglucosamine (GlcNAc)	K_a 2.03 × 10^{10} M	–	–	Label-free	[27]
H5N1			K_a 4.35 × 10^{10} M				
H1N3			K_a 2.56 × 10^{12} M				

Table 1. QCM biosensors for detection of AIVs.

Antibodies are the most common bioreceptor of choice for sensing, and they are generated by immunizing an animal system with antigen. The interaction between antibody and antigen can be transduced into measurable signal changes. Early studies focused on the development of QCM immunosensor based on antibody-antigen interaction for influenza virus detection [12–14]. For example, the characterization of a QCM biosensor for the direct detection of influenza A viruses was reported by Owen et al. [12]. Self-assembled monolayers (SAMs) of mercaptoundecanoic acid (MUA) were formed on QCM gold electrodes for the immobilization of anti-influenza A antibodies, and the limit of detection was estimated to be 4 virus particles/ml. QCM immunosensor has been used also to detect avian influenza label free in nasal washings with a lower detection limit of 10^4 pfu/ml, although, with the addition of a gold nanoparticle conjugate, the detection limit was reduced to 10^3 pfu/ml, which is comparable to the sensitivity and specificity of viral isolation techniques [13]. Li et al. [14] reported a nanobeads amplified QCM immunosensor with polyclonal antibody as the recognition ligand for detection of AIV H5N1.

In recent years, aptamers have been investigated as an alternative of sensing elements, which have the potential to replace the antibodies. This is possible due to the unique features of aptamers (sensitivity, specificity, reusability, stability, nonimmunogenicity), which can be easily exploited in biosensor technology. Aptamers are single-stranded RNA or DNA oligonucleotides which rely on hydrogen bonding, electrostatic and hydrophobic interactions rather than Watson-Crick base pairing for recognition to their target. Aptamers can fold into distinct secondary and tertiary structures, bind to their targets with high affinity (dissociation constants on the order of nano- to picomolar), and recognize their targets with a specificity that challenges antibodies and other biological ligands. They are selected in vitro through systematic evolution of ligands by exponential enrichment (SELEX). The selection procedure involves the iterative isolation of ligands out of the random sequence pool with affinity for a defined target molecule and PCR-based amplification of the selected RNA or DNA oligonucleotides after each round of isolation. As biorecognition ligands, aptamers possess numerous advantages, including small size, rapid and reproducible synthesis, simple and controllable modification to fulfill different diagnostic and therapeutic purposes, slow degradation kinetics, nontoxicity, and a lack of immunogenicity.

The majority of aptamers developed for AIVs have focused on inhibition of the hemagglutinin protein preventing viral infection. For example, a DNA aptamer was developed by Jeon and co-workers [15]. RNA aptamers that inhibit membrane fusion of AIV H3N2 and influenza B virus hemagglutinin also were developed [16, 17]. DNA and RNA aptamers that target HA1 proteins of influenza virus hemagglutinin subtype H5 were investigated in two different studies [18, 19]. An aptamer that binds efficiently to the HA of highly pathogenic AIV H5N1 and H7N7 was studied by Suenaga and Kumar [20], which inhibits HA-glycan interactions. These aptamers were developed to inhibit function of the hemagglutinin protein and prevent or treat influenza infection. Based on the function and likely binding sites of these aptamers, it seems unlikely these aptamers would be optimal sequences to use in a biodetection assay. A DNA aptamer for avian influenza H5N1 was developed by Wang et al. [21] using a combination of protein and whole virus targets. It is unique in its binding affinity in that it specifically targets the H5N1 subtype, having no binding activity with other H5 or N1 subtype viruses. This suggests that the binding site be at an intersection of the H5 and N1 proteins.

Aptamer-based QCM biosensors, also called QCM aptasensors, have been developed for the detection of AIVs. Brockman et al. [22] studied a QCM aptasensor for detection of AIV H5N1 using magnetic nanobeads labels as mass amplifiers. The biosensor was found to have a lower detection limit of 1 HAU, although the detection time was reduced by half compared to a similar QCM biosensor using antibodies [14]. A hydrogel-based QCM aptasensor (**Figure 5**) was able to detect AIV H5N1 at 0.0128 HAU in 30 min [9]. The QCM aptasensor was based on swelling of the hydrogel after AIV H5N1 capture due to dissolution of the cross-linked aptamers and ssDNA in the hydrogel polymer. The developed aptasensor was both rapid and sensitive.

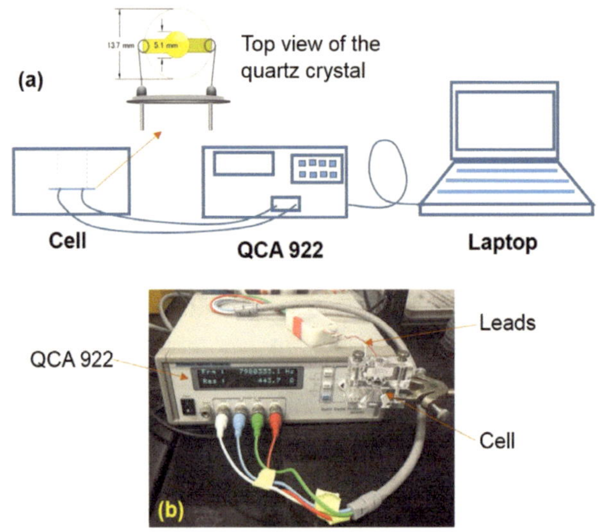

Figure 5. (a) Schematic of the QCM aptasensor; (b) a photograph of the QCM aptasensor setup. The aptamer hydrogel is immobilized on the gold electrode surface. The quartz in the electrode acts as a transducer, converting the mass and viscosity change to a frequency signal.

Influenza virus specificity for the host is mediated by the viral surface glycoprotein hemagglutinin (HA), which binds to receptors containing glycans with terminal sialic acids. This molecular recognition process leads to the host cell-virus adhesion stage [23]. The sialic acid receptor of various influenza virus strains differs in affinity to sialic acids terminally linked either in $\alpha(2,3)$ or $\alpha(2,6)$ position to the galactose (Gal) residues. Human influenza A viruses preferentially recognize the $\alpha(2,6)$-linkage, while avian viruses have preference for the $\alpha(2,3)$-linkage [24, 25]. Each monovalent sialic acid-binding site of HA is weak, with dissociation constants in the millimolar range, while the high virus-cell affinity is due to multivalency.

Takahashi and co-workers [26] demonstrated kinetics of HA binding to sulfatide and ganglioside GD1a by QCM analysis. QCM analysis showed that the HA bound with the K_d of 1.44×10^{-8} M to sulfatide immobilized on a sensor chip, which indicated that sulfatide directly binds to the ectodomain of HA with high affinity. N-Acetylglucosamine (GlcNAc) is a natural ligand and is part of the oligosaccharide ligand responsible for the influenza virus binding first step. In a report by Wangchareansak et al. [27], GlcNAc was employed as bioreceptor immobilized on QCM gold sensor surface for detection of influenza A virus (H5N3, H5N1, H1N3), which displayed high binding affinity with K_a values of 2.03×10^{10}, 4.35×10^{10}, and 2.56×10^{12} M, respectively.

QCM biosensor has advantages, such as simplicity, cost-effectiveness, real-time output, and direct detection. But there also exists some disadvantages, such as the lack of stability, difficulty with sensor surface regeneration, loss of the immobilized ligands after multiple washing and regeneration, nonspecific binding of other nontarget biomaterials, and relatively long incubation time. Further improvements are required to address these limitations before the QCM biosensor technology can be routinely employed for AIVs detection.

http://dx.doi.org/10.5772/64353

2.2. Optical biosensors

Optical biosensors rely on visual phenomena to detect the interaction between the biological element and the target analyte. Examples of optical biosensors include surface plasmon resonance (SPR), absorption, luminescence, and fluorescent sensors. Detection by optical biosensors can occur in two ways: by the analyte directly affecting the optical properties of the sensing environment, such as in SPR or absorption methods, or by the analyte being tagged with a label that produces an optical phenomenon, such as in fluorescence methods. Optical biosensors, which are sometimes referred to as "optodes," have received considerable interest in the detection of AIVs. The main analytical features of optical biosensors for detection of AIVs are summarized in **Table 2** [3, 28–38]. The target "virus" in **Table 2** is the entire virus particle and target "HA" is the HA protein or recombinant HA protein of virus.

Influenza subtype	Target	Bioreceptor	Sensitivity	Sensor	Labelling method	Reference
H1N1	Virus	Glycan	45.6×10^{-13} M	SPR	Label-free	[29]
H3N2	HA	Antibody	1 nM	Waveguide	Dye	[32]
H5N1	HA	Glycan	K_d 1.6×10^{-9} M	SPR	Label-free	[30]
H5N1	Virus	Aptamer	0.128 HAU	SPR	Label-free	[31]
H1N1	HA	Aptamer	K_d 67 fM	SPR	Label-free	[28]
H3N2	Virus	Antibody	0.2 HAU/ml	Prism-free SPR	Fluorescent	[33]
H3N2	Virus	Antibody	–	Waveguide	Gold nanoparticles	[3]
H9N2	Virus	Antibody	8.94 ng/ml	Nanobioprobe coupled with immunomagnetic beads, Fluorescent		[36]
H7 subtype	HA gene	Oligonucleotide probe	7 pM	Luminescence resonance energy transfer (LRET)		[37]
H1N1	Virus	Antibody	1.0×10^{-13} g/ml	Silver nanoparticles labeled antibodies with indirect fluorescence		[35]
H5N1	HA	Aptamer	2 ng/ml (buffer); 3.5 ng/ml (human serum)	Silver nanoparticles; Fluorescent		[34]
H1N1 H3N2	Virus	Antibody	0.1 pg/ml 50 pfu/ml	Gold nanoparticle-decorated carbon nanotubes; photoluminescence		[38]

Table 2. A list of optical biosensors reported for the detection of AIVs.

Various modes of optical measurement exist (i.e., absorption, reflection, fluorescence, chemiluminescence, and phosphorescence); however, biosensors based on surface plasmon resonance (SPR) and fluorescence principles are the most common and promising methods for AIVs detection.

The Kretschmann configuration [39] is the most popular optical setup for SPR applications. SPR biosensors measure the change in refractive index due to binding of biomolecules near the sensor surface. Refractive index is defined as the ratio of the speed of light in vacuum and the phase velocity of light in the medium. SPR is one of very few techniques that are able to provide noninvasive, real-time kinetic data on association, and dissociation rates, along with equilibrium binding constants for receptor or ligand systems. Estmer-Nilsson et al. [40] were able to utilize SPR to quantify influenza virus for vaccine production via an antibody inhibition assay using HA proteins immobilized on the sensor surface. Some research showed SPR biosensors for avian influenza DNA hybridization [41], adamantane binding sites in the influenza A M2 ion channel [42], influenza virus hemagglutinin monitoring [43], and binding kinetics study [44]. Studies by Gopinath et al. [28] revealed that SPR-based biosensor is a useful tool for detection of human and avian influenza viruses.

SPR-based Biacore technology has been designed to investigate biomolecular interactions, which was initiated in 1984. The commercial available systems include Biacore 1000, Biocore 3000, BIAlite, and Biacore T100. Biacore is the dominant SPR technique used for AIVs detection. The main advantage of this technology is its capacity to monitor weak macromolecular interactions that cannot be detected by other sensors and its subject ability to automation. SPR was used to evaluate the binding of influenza A virus H1N1 directly to a neomembrane of bovine brain lipid or an egg yolk lecithin fraction [29] and to monitor the interactions between influenza HA and glycan [30] or apatmers [28]. However, Biacore instruments are expensive and need proper maintenance. Bai and co-workers [31] have shown that a portable hand-held SPR-based biosensor (Spreeta™, Texas Instruments, Dallas, TX, USA) (**Figure 6**) can be employed for the detection of AIV H5N1. The fabrication of the SPR biosensor was based on the streptavidin-biotin binding. The streptavidin was directly adsorbed on the gold surface, and then, biotinylated ssDNA aptamers were immobilized. Target AIVs were captured by the immobilized aptamers and resulted in an increase in the refraction index. It was able to detect AIV H5N1 in poultry swab samples with a lower detection limit of 0.128 HAU in 1.5 h.

The working principle of a waveguide mode sensor is similar to that of a SPR sensor. The only difference is that the measurement is conducted using a waveguide mode rather than a surface mode [32]. Based on the properties of light-guiding and dimensions, there are two general classes, fiber optical waveguides and planar waveguides, which can be further divided into single mode and multimode [45]. Waveguide mode biosensors were developed using antibody as bioreceptor for the detection of HA from H3N2 [32] and H3N2 virus [3].

Of the optical methods requiring labels for detection, fluorescence is the most widely studied [34–36, 46, 47]. Fluorescence measurements are of particular interest in biosensor systems due to their high sensitivity. Commonly used labels in fluorescent biosensors are dyes, quantum dots (QDs), and fluorescent proteins, with the latter two becoming more popular as they are further researched [46]. A fluorescent aptasensor was developed by Pang and co-workers [34] for detection of AIV H5N1. The $Ag@SiO_2$ core-shell nanoparticles were coated with the anti-HA aptamers. The binding of aptamer-HA protein formed a G-quadruplex complex, which captured thiazole orange (TO) and reported the fluorescent signal of TO. Moreover, it caused a surface plasmon resonance enhancement and performed as a metal-enhanced fluorescence sensing. The detection of HA protein of the AIV H5N1 could be operated both in aqueous buffer and human serum with the detection limit of 2 and 3.5 ng/mL, respectively. The total detection time was only 30 min. Using antibodies as bioreceptors, Li et al. [35] developed a highly sensitive fluorescent immunosensor for detection of H1N1, which was based on Ag autocatalysis. It had a detection range of 1.0×10^{-12} to 1.0×10^{-8} g/ml with a detection limit of 10^{-13} g/ml.

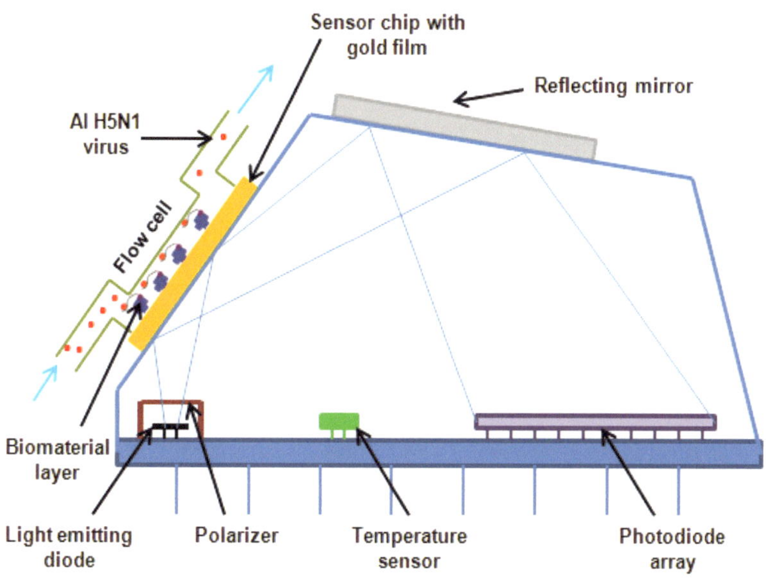

Figure 6. Configuration for measuring AIV H5N1using the portable SPR aptasensor (with permission from MDPI).

Fluorescence resonance energy transfer (FRET) is used in the design of a biosensor, which is based on the energy transfer between two light-sensitive molecules, a donor and an acceptor chromophore. In the nucleic acid-based FRET method, a reporter and a quencher are conjugated at the terminals of a nucleic acid probe. Without the target, the duplex is formed, bringing these two molecules in close proximity, which results in fluorescence quenching. The present of a target can cause the conformational change of the probe, which changes the position of the reporter and quencher and emits fluorescence. A QD-induced FRET system was developed by Chou and Huang [47] using two oligonucleotides. These two oligonucleotides were designed to specifically recognize two regions of the AIV H5 sequences and were employed as the capturing and reporter probes, respectively. They were conjugated to QD655 (donor) and Alexa Fluor 660 dye (acceptor), respectively. At target concentrations ranging from 0.5 nM to 1 μM, the QD emission decreased at 653 nm and dye emission increased at 690 nm. Another luminescence resonance energy transfer (LRET)-based biosensor was developed by Ye et al.

[37] for rapid and ultrasensitive detection of AIV H7 subtype. In this work, BaGdF5:Yb/Er upconversion nanoparticles (UCNPs) and gold nanoparticles (AuNPs) were used as the pair of donor and acceptor. The oligonucleotides with H7 HA gene sequence were conjugated with thiol and then were assembled on the AuNPs surfaces. The complementary sequence probes were modified with amino group and then were covalently bond to poly(ethylenimine) modified BaGdF5:Yb/Er UCNPs. The hybridization process brought these two molecules in close proximity, resulting in fluorescence quenching.

QDs are a type of semiconductor with a diameter typically between 2 and 10 nm whose excitons are confined in three spatial dimensions, giving them properties of both unconfined semiconductors and discrete molecules. In comparison with organic dyes and fluorescent proteins, QDs have unique optical and electronic properties including size-tunable light emission, improved signal brightness, high resistance against photobleaching, and simultaneous excitation of multiple fluorescence colors. QD-based bioconjugates used for optical sensing could dramatically increase the sensitivity that would permit simultaneous measurement of several targets. Lee and co-workers [38] developed a plasmon-assisted fluoro-immunosensor by the conjugation of antibody onto the surface of cadmium telluride QDs and the Au nanoparticle-decorated carbon nanotubes (AuCNTs) for the detection of H1N1 and H3N2. A detection limit of 0.1 pg/ml and 50 pfu/ml was obtained for H1N1 and H3N2, respectively.

Fluorescent biosensors are simple and show improved sensitivity and reduced detection time. But they have a drawback of requiring relatively expensive reagents. In order to apply the fluorescent biosensor for detection of real samples with complex background, such as tracheal and cloacal swabs from birds, further work would be required to combine an effective sample pretreatment method with the fluorescent biosensor for the detection of AIVs in the field.

2.3. Electrochemical biosensors

More than half of the biosensors used for the detection of AIVs are based on electrochemical transducers. Electrochemical biosensors use changes in the electrical properties caused by biochemical reactions to detect an analyte [48]. Electrochemical transducers offer several advantages: low cost, high sensitivity, ease of miniaturization, independence from solution turbidity, low power requirements, and simplicity of use [49]. These characteristics make electrochemical detection methods highly attractive for field monitoring of infectious diseases and biological warfare agents. Electrochemical biosensors can be divided by the electrical parameter that they measure: amperometric, potentiometric, conductimetric, and impedimetric. Amperometric biosensors work by applying a constant potential across an electrode and measuring the current associated with either the reduction or oxidation of an electroactive species created by the interaction of the biological element and the analyte. Amperometric biosensors are often used with an enzyme capable of catalyzing the production of an ionic product and increasing the selectivity and the sensitivity [50]. Potentiometric biosensors gather data by converting a biological reaction into a potential signal with the use of ion-selective electrodes [51]. Conductimetric biosensors simply measure the conductivity change in a medium caused by the analytes. Impedimetric biosensors measure a combination of the resistive and capacitive or inductive properties of a material in response to a small amplitude sinusoidal excitation signal [52].

A detailed review of the electrochemical biosensors for detection of AIVs before year 2014 can be found in the paper by Grabowska et al. [53], which covered the electrochemical genosensors and electrochemical immunosensors for detection of AIVs. A total of 69 references were cited in their review paper. Within the context of this chapter, the electrochemical biosensors reported prior to 2014 are referred to the review paper by Grabowska et al. and the electrochemical biosensors reported in the years 2014 and 2015 plus some impedance biosensors not mentioned by Grabowska et al. are reviewed in detail.

Impedance biosensors are a class of electrical biosensors that measure the electrical impedance of an interface in AC steady state with constant DC bias conditions. This is accomplished by imposing a sinusoidal voltage at a given frequency and measuring the current. This measurement can be done over a range of frequencies or at a given frequency [54]. Many impedance biosensors utilize a capture probe on the detecting surface to hold the target molecule, thereby stabilizing the point of detection. Due to the ease of miniaturization, low energy usage and relatively low cost, impedance biosensors show promise for AIVs applications. Impedance biosensors can use a variety of biological sensing elements but the most commonly used are antibodies. When using antibodies as the biological element the biosensor is often referred to as an impedance immunosensor. Impedance immunosensors rely on the interaction of the antibody and the antigen to generate a detectable signal for the transducing element. This allows the immunosensor to detect either indirect or direct impedance measurements. Direct impedance measurement, or label-free detection, is dependent on monitoring the changes in the electrical properties of the sensing environment caused by the antibody-antigen interaction. A label-free detection method has several advantages over an indirect detection method, including reduced detection time, lower cost, and simpler detection protocol.

There are two general classes of impedance biosensors, Faradic and non-Faradic impedance biosensor, which have been used for the detection of AIV H5N1 or subtype H5. A Faradic impedance biosensor was developed by Wang and co-workers [55] using an interdigitated array microelectrode. Polyclonal antibody against H5 was oriented immobilized on the gold surface through protein A to capture target virus, and red blood cells (RBCs) were used as biolabels for signal amplification. The biosensor had a lower detection limit of 10^3 EID_{50} ml^{-1}. Wang et al. [10] also reported a non-Faradic impedance biosensor for H5N2 avian influenza detection, which was based on the combination of an immunomagnetic nanobeads separation and a microfluidic chip with an interdigitated array microelectrode. A lower detection limit of 10^3 EID_{50} ml^{-1} was achieved with detection time less than 1 h. Then, Lum et al. [56] further improved the non-Faradic impedance biosensor for H5N1 detection by a combination of immunomagnetic nanoparticles, a microfluidic chip, an interdigitated array microelectrode, and RBCs for signal amplification. The specificity of the biosensor was improved due to the use of anti-H5 as a capture antibody and anti-N1 as a detection antibody.

A miniaturized biosensor was developed by Diouani et al. [57] for the detection of H7N1. Polyclonal antibodies against AIV H7N1 were attached to a gold electrode using a self-assembled monolayer. The impedance measurement was carried out in the presence of a redox probe and inside a Faraday cage. The lower detection limit of this biosensor was determined to be 5 μg/ml of specific antigen. Hassen et al. [58] developed an impedance biosensor capable of quantifying influenza A virus in a media comprised of numerous other proteins and viruses. The biosensor had a lower detection limit of 8 ng/ml, even in the presence of nonspecific viruses and proteins.

In **Table 3**, the electrochemical biosensors developed for the detection of AIVs in year 2014 and 2015 are summarized [59–79].

Influenza subtype	**Target**	**Bioreceptor**	**Sensitivity**	**Detection range**	**Reference**
H1N1	Virus	Antibody	1 pfu/ml	1–10^4 pfu/ml	[65]
H5N1	HA	Antibody	2.2 pg/ml	4–20 pg/ml	[66]
H1N1	PB1-F2 protein	Antibody	0.42 nM (monomeric); 16 nM (oligomeric)	5 nM–1.5 μM (monomeric); 5 nM–0.5 μM (oligomeric)	[60]
H5N1	Virus	Antibody	2^{-15} HAU/50 μl	2^{-15}–2^{-8} HAU/50 μl	[67]
H5N2, H7N1, H1N1	M1 protein	Antibody	20 pg/ml (80–100 virus/μl)	–	[59]
H1N1	PB1-F2 protein	Antibody	0.42 nM	5 nM–1.5 μM	[61]
H5N1	Antibody	HA	2.1 pg/ml	4–20 pg/ml	[63]
H5N1	Antibody	HA	2.4 pg/ml	4–100 pg/ml	[64]
H7N9	Virus	Antibody	6.8 pg/ml	0.01–20 ng/ml	[68]
H5N1	Virus	Antibody	2^{-1} HAU/50 μl	2^{-1}–2^{4} HAU/50 μl	[62]
H5N1	Complementary DNA (20-mer); RNA (280-mer)	Complementary sequences probe	73 pM (DNA 20-mer); 0.87 pM (RNA 280-mer)	–	[71]
H5N1	Full length H5 gene	DNA probe	fM level	–	[69]
H5N1	Full length H5 gene	DNA probe	0.03 fM (20-mer ssDNA); 0.08 fM (ds DNA)	–	[70]
H7N9	A fragment of the HA gene sequence	DNA probe	100 fM	–	[72]
H7N9	A fragment of the HA	Primer and DNAzyme	9.4 fM	50 fM–100 pM	[73]

Influenza subtype	Target	Bioreceptor	Sensitivity	Detection range	Reference
	gene sequence				
H5N1	Virus	Aptamer	8×10^{-4} HAU/ 200 μl	0.001–1 HAU	[74]
H5N1	Virus	Aptamer	0.0128 HAU	0.0128–12.8 HAU	[78]
H5N1	Viral proteins	Aptamer-antibody pair	100 fM	100 fM–10 pM	[75]
H5N1	Virus	Aptamer	2^{-9} HAU	0.001–4 HAU	[77]
H5N1	HA	Glycan	–	–	[76]
H5N1	HA	Glycan	aM level	140 aM–14 nM	[79]

Table 3. A list of electrochemical biosensors reported in 2014 and 2015 for the detection of AIVs.

For the past two years, the immunosensors have been the dominant electrochemical biosensors for detection of AIVs [59–68]. For example, universal anti-M1 antibodies, which allow detection of all serotypes of influenza A virus, were used for the development of an universal immunosensor for detection of the influenza A virus. It showed similar sensitivity (80–100 virus particles/μl) to molecular methods [59]. Miodek and co-workers [60, 61] developed an electrochemical immunosensor, which was based on conductive polypyrrole modified with ferrocenyl groups as a redox marker for the detection of PB1-F2, a nonstructural accessory protein of influenza A virus. Lin et al. [62] demonstrated that an impedance immunosensor, which was based on low-cost microelectrodes and specific monoclonal antibodies for rapid detection of AIV H5N1 in chicken swabs. Studies by Jarocka and co-workers [63, 64] revealed that the immobilization of the recombinant His-tagged HA was able to detect antibodies against AIV H5N1 in hen serum.

Although electrochemical biosensors for avian influenza detection have mostly been investigated for whole virus or virus protein detection, some groups have developed biosensors for the detection of avian influenza nucleic acid sequences [69–73]. These biosensors are based on the use of nucleic acid probes, which bind to specific sequence in the influenza genome. Several genosensors have been studied for the detection of the full length H5 gene of AIV H5N1. In the study of genosensors by Grabowska et al. [69, 70], redox active compounds (such as cobalt porphyrins or 3-iron bis(dicarbollide) were conjugated with the DNA probes, which were very close to the electrode surface. These developed genosensors showed a sensitivity in the fM range. Malecka and co-workers [71] reported an AET/Phen-Epoxy/Fe(III)/(Phen-Epoxy-NH2-NC3)2 genosensor, which has a working principle similar to this already reported by Grabowska et al. [69]. The hybridization process caused the formation of the duplex structure on the electrode surface, which resulted in the thickness changes of the double layer at the interface between the electrode and solution.

A new trend in the development of biosensors is the use of nanomaterials which exhibit unique and attractive chemical, physical, and electronic properties. Various nanomaterials have been used as an electrode platform in highly sophisticated electroanalytical biosensing devices. The working electrodes (actual physical transducers) upon modification with these materials gain large effective surface area, high catalytic capabilities, and high conductivity. Thus, these transducers could act as effective mediators and facilitate electron transfer between an active site on the receptor and the electrode surface. Nanoparticles [74, 75], carbon nanotubes [65], magnetic nanobeads [68, 74], or quantum dots [76] enhance sensitivity and selectivity of the electrochemical detection. Among the variety of metal nanoparticles, gold nanoparticles (GNPs) have been extensively utilized in recent years, mainly because of their nanoscopic size, good conductivity, and biocompatibility. One of the most commonly used is single-walled (SW) or multiwalled (MW) carbon nanotubes (CNTs) as well as graphene and graphene nanosheets. Thanks to their fast electron transfer ability, mechanical strength, chemical stability, catalysis effect, and thermal and electrical conductivity, they are attracting greater interest than other applied technologies.

A magnetic nanobeads-based impedance aptasensor was designed and developed by Fu and co-workers [74] (**Figure 7**). Briefly, H5N1 aptamers were coated on the magnetic nanobeads (MBs) for specifically capturing target AIV H5N1. Then, bionanocomposites (BNCs) were added using Au nanoparticles (AuNPs) as carriers, which were conjugated with concanavalin A (ConA) and glucose oxidase (GOx). The BNCs attached on the captured target virus through ConA-glycan interaction formed a sandwich complex. Finally, the sandwich complex was transferred to a glucose solution, resulting in an efficient enzymatic reaction and the impedance decreased correspondingly on a screen-printed interdigitated array electrode. This method took advantages of the high efficiency of enzymatic catalysis and the high susceptibility of electrochemical impedance on the ion strength and endowed the aptasensor with high sensitivity.

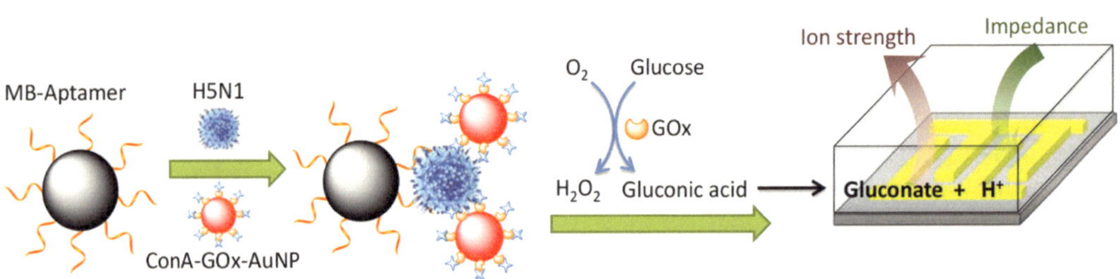

Figure 7. Illustration of the aptasensing mechanism and construction of the aptasensor (with permission from ACS).

Wang and co-workers [77] developed an aptamer-based bifunctional bionanogate, which could selectively respond to target molecules and control enzymatic reaction for electrochemical measurements (**Figure 8**). A nanoporous gold film with a pore size of ~20 nm was prepared by a metallic corrosion method and then was functionalized with two types of thiol-modified single-stranded oligos (SH-ssDNAs) by means of Au–thiolate bonding. The bases of the two immobilized SH-ssDNAs were selected to be partly complementary to that of the two ends of an aptamer, respectively. Then, aptamers were added and hybridized with the two immobilized SH-ssDNAs, resulting in the nanopore covered with aptamers, a "closed" bionanogate. Finally, the aptamer covered nanopore film was placed onto an enzyme precoated glassy carbon electrode to form an aptasensor. The working principle of the bionanogate-based aptasensor for detection of AIV H5N1 is illustrated in **Figure 8**. Initially, without the target AIV, the bionanogate was kept "closed," which isolated coenzymes and substrates in the testing solution from the enzymes immobilized on the electrode so that the enzymatic reaction was restricted (**Figure 8a**). Upon the target virus binding, the aptamers dissociated into solution from their ssDNAs and formed aptamer–virus complexes, which triggered the bionanogate "open" (**Figure 8b**). This "open" state allowed coenzymes and substrates to diffuse freely through the opened nanopore and to create contact with the immobilized enzymes, resulting in an efficient enzymatic reaction (**Figure 8c**).

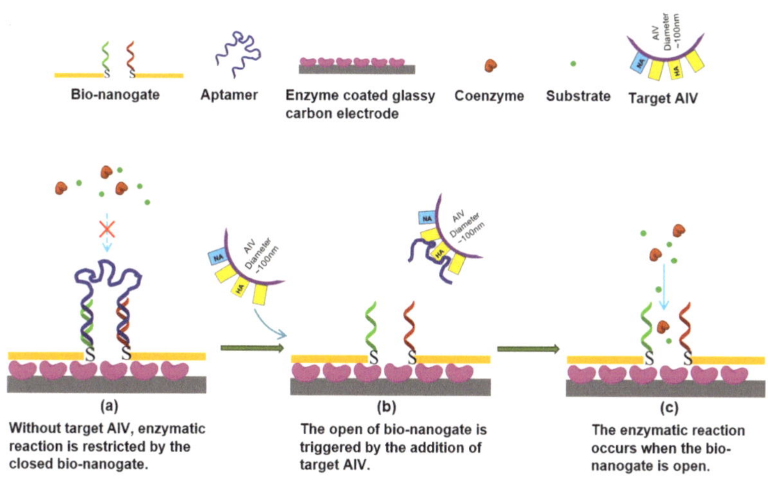

Figure 8. Principle of the bionanogate-based aptasensor for detection of AIV H5N1 (with permission from Elsevier).

Despite the remarkable sensitivity, rapid response, miniaturization capability, and low cost of the electrochemical biosensors for AIV detection, there are still problems with long-term stability and selectivity in real samples with complex background. Obviously, further work would be required to demonstrate that the electrochemical biosensors do not suffer from stability and selectivity problems when handling real samples in the field.

3. Conclusion

Biosensors have attracted tremendous interest in AIVs detection. They are characterized by good selectivity and sensitivity with a wide dynamic range from subfemtomolar to nanomolar, easy and rapid experimental protocol, reasonable cost, and usage of the sample volume in a μl range. Rapid development of nanotechnology has opened a new way for design and construction of biosensors with even better features. However, many contributions to the field of biosensors for AIVs detection still are at the "proof-of-concept" stage. Thus, authors hope that this chapter will promote lively and valuable discussions in order to generate new ideas and make new approaches toward the development of innovative biosensors for applications in AIVs detection.

Author details

Ronghui Wang[1,2] and Yanbin Li[1,2,3*]

*Address all correspondence to: yanbinli@uark.edu

1 College of Biosystems Engineering and Food Science, Zhejiang University, Hangzhou, China

2 Department of Biological and Agricultural Engineering, University of Arkansas, Fayetteville, AR, USA

3 Center of Excellence for Poultry Science, University of Arkansas, Fayetteville, AR, USA

References

[1] Murphy BR, Webster RG. Orthomyxoviruses. In: Fields, B.N., Knipe, D.M., Howley, P.M. editors. In Fields Virology. 3rd ed. Philadelphia, PA: Lippincott-Raven; 1996. p. 1397–1445.

[2] Lamb RA, Krug RM. Orthomyxoviridae. In: Knipe, D.M., Howley, P.M., editors. In Field Virology. Philadelphia, PA: Lippincott William & Wilkins Publisher; 2001. p. 1487–1531.

[3] Gopinath SC, Awazu K, Fujimaki M, Shimizu K. Evaluation of anti-A/Udorn/307/1972 antibody specificity to influenza A/H3N2 viruses using an evanescent-field coupled waveguide-mode sensor. PLoS One 2013;8(12):e81396. doi:10.1371/journal.pone.0081396

[4] Burns A, van der Mensbrugghe D, Timmer H. Evaluating the economic consequences of avian influenza. World Bank report [Internet]. 2008. Available from: http://siteresources.worldbank.org/EXTAVIANFLU/Resources/EvaluatingAHIeconomics_2008.pdf [Accessed: 2016-03-26]

[5] WHO. Cumulative number of confirmed human cases of avian influenza A (H5N1) reported to WHO, 2003–2015 [Internet]. 2016. Available from: http://www.who.int/influenza/human_animal_interface/2016_01_20_tableH5N1.pdf [Accessed: 2016-03-31]

[6] Clark LC, Jr., Lyons C. Electrode systems for continuous monitoring in cardiovascular surgery. Ann N Y Acad Sci 1962;102:29–45. doi:10.1111/j.1749-6632.1962.tb13623.x

[7] Turner AP. Biosensors-sense and sensitivity. Science 2000;290:1315–1317. doi:10.1126/science.290.5495.1315

[8] Amano Y, Cheng Q. Detection of influenza virus: traditional approaches and development of biosensors. Anal Bioanal Chem 2005;381(1):156–164. doi:10.1007/s00216-004-2927-0

[9] Wang R, Li Y. Hydrogel based QCM aptasensor for detection of avian influenza virus. Biosens Bioelectron 2013;42:148–155. doi:10.1016/j.bios.2012.10.038

[10] Wang R, Lin J, Lassiter K, Srinivasan B, Lin L, Lu H, Tung S, Hargis B, Bottje W, Berghman L, Li Y. Evaluation study of a portable impedance biosensor for detection of avian influenza virus. J Virol Methods 2011;178(1–2):52–58. doi:10.1016/j.jviromet.2011.08.011

[11] Jian YR, Chang SY, Lin PY, Yang YH, Chuang YH. Inactivated influenza virus vaccine is efficient and reduces IL-4 and IL-6 in allergic asthma mice. Influenza Other Respir Viruses 2013;7(6):1210–1217. doi:10.1111/irv.12150

[12] Owen TW, Al-Kaysi RO, Bardeen CJ, Cheng Q. Microgravimetric immunosensor for direct detection of aerosolized influenza A virus particles. Sens Actuators B Chem 2007;126:691–699. doi:10.1016/j.snb.2007.04.028

[13] Peduru-Hewa TM, Tannock GA, Mainwaring DE, Harrison S, Fecondo JV. The detection of influenza A and B viruses in clinical specimens using a quartz crystal microbalance. J Virol Methods 2009;162(1–2):14–21. doi:10.1016/j.jviromet.2009.07.001

[14] Li D, Wang J, Wang R, Li Y, Abi-Ghanem D, Berghman L, Hargis B, Lu H. A nanobeads amplified QCM immunosensor for the detection of avian influenza virus H5N1. Biosens Bioelectron 2011;26(10):4146–4154. doi:10.1016/j.bios.2011.04.010

[15] Jeon SH, Kayhan B, Ben-Yedidia T, Arnon R. A DNA aptamer prevents influenza infection by blocking the receptor binding region of the viral hemagglutinin. J Biol Chem 2004;279:48410–48419. doi:10.1074/jbc.M409059200

[16] Gopinath SC, Misono TS, Kawasaki K, Mizuno T, Imai M, Odagiri T, et al. An RNA aptamer that distinguishes between closely related human influenza viruses and inhibits haemagglutinin-mediated membrane fusion. J Gen Virol 2006;87(Pt 3):479–487. doi:10.1099/vir.0.81508-0

[17] Gopinath SC, Sakamaki Y, Kawasaki K, Kumar PK. An efficient RNA aptamer against human influenza B virus hemagglutinin. J Biochem 2006;139(5):837–846. doi:10.1093/jb/mvj095

[18] Cheng C, Dong J, Yao L, Chen A, Jia R, Huan L, et al. Potent inhibition of human influenza H5N1 virus by oligonucleotides derived by SELEX. Biochem Biophys Res Commun 2008;366(3):670–674. doi:10.1016/j.bbrc.2007.11.183

[19] Park SY, Kim S, Yoon H, Kim KB, Kalme SS, Oh S, et al. Selection of an antiviral RNA aptamer against hemagglutinin of the subtype H5 avian influenza virus. Nucleic Acid Ther 2011;21(6):395–402. doi:10.1089/nat.2011.0321

[20] Suenaga E, Kumar PK. An aptamer that binds efficiently to the hemagglutinins of highly pathogenic avian influenza viruses (H5N1 and H7N7) and inhibits hemagglutinin-glycan interactions. Acta Biomater 2014;10(3):1314–1323. doi:10.1016/j.actbio.2013.12.034

[21] Wang R, Zhao J, Jiang T, Kwon YM, Lu H, Jiao P, et al. Selection and characterization of DNA aptamers for use in detection of avian influenza virus H5N1. J Virol Methods 2013;189(2):362–369. doi:10.1016/j.jviromet.2013.03.006

[22] Brockman, L., Wang, R., Lum, L., Li, Y. QCM aptasensor for rapid and specific detection of avian influenza virus. O J Appl Biosens 2013;2:97–103. doi: 10.4236/ojab.2013.24013

[23] Paulson JC. The Receptors. In: Conn M., editor. Orlando, FL: Academic Press; 1985. p. 131–219.

[24] Rogers GN, Paulson JC, Daniels RS, Skehel JJ, Wilson IA, Wiley DC. Single amino acid substitutions in influenza haemagglutinin change receptor binding specificity. Nature 1983;304(5921):76–78. doi:10.1038/304076a0

[25] Rogers GN, Paulson JC. Receptor determinants of human and animal influenza virus isolates: differences in receptor specificity of the H3 hemagglutinin based on species of origin. Virology 1983;127(2):361–373. doi:10.1016/0042-6822(83)90150-2

[26] Takahashi T, Kawagishi S, Masuda M, Suzuki T. Binding kinetics of sulfatide with influenza A virus hemagglutinin. Glycoconj J 2013;30(7):709–716. doi:10.1007/s10719-013-9477-7

[27] Wangchareansak T, Sangma C, Ngernmeesri P, Thitithanyanont A, Lieberzeit PA. Self-assembled glucosamine monolayers as biomimetic receptors for detecting WGA lectin and influenza virus with a quartz crystal microbalance. Anal Bioanal Chem 2013;405(20):6471–6478. doi:10.1007/s00216-013-7057-0

[28] Gopinath SC, Kumar PK. Aptamers that bind to the hemagglutinin of the recent pandemic influenza virus H1N1 and efficiently inhibit agglutination. Acta Biomater 2013;9(11):8932–8941. doi:10.1016/j.actbio.2013.06.016

[29] Critchley P, Dimmock NJ. Binding of an influenza A virus to a neomembrane measured by surface plasmon resonance. Bioorg Med Chem 2004;12:2773–2780. doi:10.1016/j.bmc.2004.02.042

[30] Suenaga E, Mizuno H, Penmetcha KK. Monitoring influenza hemagglutinin and glycan interactions using surface plasmon resonance. Biosens Bioelectron 2012;32(1):195–201. doi:10.1016/j.bios.2011.12.003

[31] Bai H, Wang R, Hargis B, Lu H, Li Y. A SPR aptasensor for detection of avian influenza virus H5N1. Sensors (Basel) 2012;12(9):12506–12518. doi:10.3390/s120912506

[32] Gopinath SC, Awazu K, Fujimaki M. Detection of influenza viruses by a waveguide-mode sensor. Anal Methods 2010;2:1880–1884. doi:10.1039/C0AY00491J

[33] Nomura K, Gopinath SC, Lakshmipriya T, Fukuda N, Wang X, Fujimaki M. An angular fluidic channel for prism-free surface-plasmon-assisted fluorescence capturing. Nat Commun 2013;4:2855. doi:10.1038/ncomms3855

[34] Pang Y, Rong Z, Wang J, Xiao R, Wang S. A fluorescent aptasensor for H5N1 influenza virus detection based-on the core-shell nanoparticles metal-enhanced fluorescence (MEF). Biosens Bioelectron 2015;66:527–532. doi:10.1016/j.bios.2014.10.052

[35] Li Y, Hong M, Qiu B, Lin Z, Chen Y, Cai Z, et al. Highly sensitive fluorescent immunosensor for detection of influenza virus based on Ag autocatalysis. Biosens Bioelectron 2014;54:358–364. doi:10.1016/j.bios.2013.10.045

[36] Xiong LH, Cui R, Zhang ZL, Yu X, Xie Z, Shi YB, et al. Uniform fluorescent nanobioprobes for pathogen detection. ACS Nano 2014;8(5):5116–5124. doi:10.1021/nn501174g

[37] Ye WW, Tsang MK, Liu X, Yang M, Hao J. Upconversion luminescence resonance energy transfer (LRET)-based biosensor for rapid and ultrasensitive detection of avian influenza virus H7 subtype. Small 2014;10(12):2390–2397. doi:10.1002/smll.201303766

[38] Lee J, Ahmed SR, Oh S, Kim J, Suzuki T, Parmar K, Park SS, Lee J, Park EY. A plasmon-assisted fluoro-immunoassay using gold nanoparticle-decorated carbon nanotubes for monitoring the influenza virus. Biosens Bioelectron 2015;64:311–317. doi:10.1016/j.bios.2014.09.021

[39] Kretschmann E. The determination of the optical constants of metals by excitation of surface plasmons. Z Phys 1971;241:313–337.

[40] Estmer-Nilsson C, Abbas S, Bennemo M, Larsson A, Hämäläinen MD, Frostell-Karlsson Å. A novel assay for influenza virus quantification using surface plasmon resonance. Vaccine 2010;28:759–766. doi:10.1016/j.vaccine.2009

[41] Kim SA, Byun KM, Kim K, Jang SM, Ma K, Oh Y, et al. Surface-enhanced localized surface plasmon resonance biosensing of avian influenza DNA hybridization using subwavelength metallic nanoarrays. Nanotechnology 2010;21(35):355503. doi:10.1088/0957-4484/21/35/355503

[42] Rosenberg MR, Casarotto MG. Coexistence of two adamantane binding sites in the influenza A M2 ion channel. Proc Natl Acad Sci USA 2010;107(31):13866–13871. doi:10.1073/pnas.1002051107

[43] Mandenius CF, Wang R, Alden A, Bergstrom G, Thebault S, Lutsch C, et al. Monitoring of influenza virus hemagglutinin in process samples using weak affinity ligands and

surface plasmon resonance. Anal Chim Acta 2008;623(1):66–75. doi:10.1016/j.aca.2008.06.005

[44] Hidari KI, Shimada S, Suzuki Y, Suzuki T. Binding kinetics of influenza viruses to sialic acid-containing carbohydrates. Glycoconj J 2007;24(9):583–590. doi:10.1007/s10719-007-9055-y

[45] Schmitt K, Hoffmann C. Optical guided-wave chemical and biosensors I. In: Zourob, M., Lakhtakia, A., editors. Springer Series on Chemical Sensors and Biosensors. Berlin Heidelberg. Springer-Verlag; 2010. p. 21.

[46] Medintz IL, Uyeda HT, Goldman ER, Mattoussi H. Quantum dot bioconjugates for imaging, labelling and sensing. Nat Mater 2005;4(6):435–446. doi:10.1038/nmat1390

[47] Chou CC, Huang YH. Nucleic acid sandwich hybridization assay with quantum dot-induced fluorescence resonance energy transfer for pathogen detection. Sensors (Basel) 2012;12(12):16660–16672. doi:10.3390/s121216660

[48] Grieshaber D, MacKenzie R, Vörös J, Reimhult E. Electrochemical biosensors – sensor principles and architectures. Sensors 2008;8:1400–1458. doi:10.3390/s8031400

[49] Pejcic B, De Marco R, Parkinson G. The role of biosensors in the detection of emerging infectious diseases. Analyst 2006;131(10):1079–1090. doi:10.1039/b603402k

[50] Lojou E, Bianco P. Application of the electrochemical concepts and techniques to amperometric biosensor devices. J Electroceramics 2006;16:79–91. doi:10.1007/s10832-006-2365-9

[51] Koncki R. Recent developments in potentiometric biosensors for biomedical analysis. Anal Chim Acta 2007;599(1):7–15. doi:10.1016/j.aca.2007.08.003

[52] Varshney M, Li Y. Interdigitated array microelectrodes based impedance biosensors for detection of bacterial cells. Biosens Bioelectron 2009;24(10):2951–2960. doi:10.1016/j.bios.2008.10.001

[53] Grabowska I, Malecka K, Jarocka U, Radecki J, Radecka H. Electrochemical biosensors for detection of avian influenza virus-current status and future trends. Acta Biochim Pol 2014;61(3):471–478.

[54] Daniels JS, Pourmand N. Label-free impedance biosensors: opportunities and challenges. Electroanalysis 2007;19(12):1239–1257. doi:10.1002/elan.200603855

[55] Wang R, Wang Y, Lassiter K, Li Y, Hargis B, Tung S, et al. Interdigitated array microelectrode based impedance immunosensor for detection of avian influenza virus H5N1. Talanta 2009;79(2):159–164. doi:10.1016/j.talanta.2009.03.017

[56] Lum J, Wang R, Lassiter K, Srinivasan B, Abi-Ghanem D, Berghman L, et al. Rapid detection of avian influenza H5N1 virus using impedance measurement of immunoreaction coupled with RBC amplification. Biosens Bioelectron 2012;38(1):67–73. doi:10.1016/j.bios.2012.04.047

[57] Diouani MF, Helali S, Hafaid I, Hassen WM, Snoussi MA, Ghram A, Jaffrezic-Renault N, Abdelghani A. Miniaturized biosensor for avian influenza virus detection. Materials Sci Engr C 2008;28:580–583. doi:10.1016/j.msec.2007.10.043

[58] Hassen WM, Duplan V, Frost E, Dubowski JJ. Quantitation of influenza A virus in the presence of extraneous protein using electrochemical impedance spectroscopy. Electrochim Acta 2011;56:8325–8328. doi:10.1016/j.electacta.2011.07.009

[59] Nidzworski D, Pranszke P, Grudniewska M, Krol E, Gromadzka B. Universal biosensor for detection of influenza virus. Biosens Bioelectron 2014;59:239–242. doi:10.1016/j.bios.2014.03.050

[60] Miodek A, Vidic J, Sauriat-Dorizon H, Richard CA, Le Goffic R, Korri-Youssoufi H, et al. Electrochemical detection of the oligomerization of PB1-F2 influenza A virus protein in infected cells. Anal Chem 2014;86(18):9098–9105. doi:10.1021/ac5018056

[61] Miodek A, Sauriat-Dorizon H, Chevalier C, Delmas B, Vidic J, Korri-Youssoufi H. Direct electrochemical detection of PB1-F2 protein of influenza A virus in infected cells. Biosens Bioelectron 2014;59:6–13. doi:10.1016/j.bios.2014.02.037

[62] Lin J, Wang R, Jiao P, Li Y, Li Y, Liao M, et al. An impedance immunosensor based on low-cost microelectrodes and specific monoclonal antibodies for rapid detection of avian influenza virus H5N1 in chicken swabs. Biosens Bioelectron 2015;67:546–552. doi: 10.1016/j.bios.2014.09.037

[63] Jarocka U, Sawicka R, Góra-Sochacka A, Sirko A, Zagórski-Ostoja W, Radecki J, Radecka H. Electrochemical immunosensor for detection of antibodies against influenza A virus H5N1 in hen serum. Biosens Bioelectron 2014;55:301–306. doi: 10.1016/j.bios.2013.12.030

[64] Jarocka U, Sawicka R, Stachyra A, Gora-Sochacka A, Sirko A, Zagorski-Ostoja W, et al. A biosensor based on electroactive dipyrromethene-Cu(II) layer deposited onto gold electrodes for the detection of antibodies against avian influenza virus type H5N1 in hen sera. Anal Bioanal Chem 2015;407(25):7807–7814. doi:10.1007/s00216-015-8949-y

[65] Singh R, Sharma A, Hong S, Jang J. Electrical immunosensor based on dielectrophoretically-deposited carbon nanotubes for detection of influenza virus H1N1. Analyst 2014;139(21):5415–5421. doi:10.1039/c4an01335b

[66] Jarocka U, Sawicka R, Gora-Sochacka A, Sirko A, Zagorski-Ostoja W, Radecki J, et al. An immunosensor based on antibody binding fragments attached to gold nanoparticles for the detection of peptides derived from avian influenza hemagglutinin H5. Sensors (Basel) 2014;14(9):15714–15728. doi:10.3390/s140915714

[67] Xie Z, Huang J, Luo S, Xie Z, Xie L, Liu J, et al. Ultrasensitive electrochemical immunoassay for avian influenza subtype H5 using nanocomposite. PLoS One 2014;9(4):e94685. doi:10.1371/journal.pone.0094685

[68] Wu Z, Zhou CH, Chen JJ, Xiong C, Chen Z, Pang DW, Zhang ZL. Bifunctional magnetic nanobeads for sensitive detection of avian influenza A (H7N9) virus based on immu-

nomagnetic separation and enzyme-induced metallization. Biosens Bioelectron 2015;68:586–592. doi:10.1016/j.bios.2015.01.051

[69] Grabowska I, Singleton DG, Stachyra A, Gora-Sochacka A, Sirko A, Zagorski-Ostoja W, et al. A highly sensitive electrochemical genosensor based on Co-porphyrin-labelled DNA. Chem Commun (Camb) 2014;50(32):4196–4199. doi:10.1039/c4cc00172a

[70] Grabowska I, Stachyra A, Gora-Sochacka A, Sirko A, Olejniczak AB, Lesnikowski ZJ, et al. DNA probe modified with 3-iron bis(dicarbollide) for electrochemical determination of DNA sequence of Avian Influenza Virus H5N1. Biosens Bioelectron 2014;51:170–176. doi:10.1016/j.bios.2013.07.026

[71] Malecka K, Stachyra A, Gora-Sochacka A, Sirko A, Zagorski-Ostoja W, Dehaen W, et al. New redox-active layer create via epoxy-amine reaction—the base of genosensor for the detection of specific DNA and RNA sequences of avian influenza virus H5N1. Biosens Bioelectron 2014;65C:427–434. doi:10.1016/j.bios.2014.10.069

[72] Dong S, Zhao R, Zhu J, Lu X, Li Y, Qiu S, Jia L, Jiao X, Song S, Fan C, Hao R, Song H. Electrochemical DNA biosensor based on a tetrahedral nanostructure probe for the detection of avian influenza A (H7N9) virus. ACS Appl Mater Interfaces 2015;7(16): 8834–8842. doi:10.1021/acsami.5b01438

[73] Yu Y, Chen Z, Jian W, Sun D, Zhang B, Li X, Yao M. Ultrasensitive electrochemical detection of avian influenza A (H7N9) virus DNA based on isothermal exponential amplification coupled with hybridization chain reaction of DNAzyme nanowires. Biosens Bioelectron 2015;64:566–571. doi:10.1016/j.bios.2014.09.080

[74] Fu Y, Callaway Z, Lum J, Wang R, Lin J, Li Y. Exploiting enzyme catalysis in ultra-low ion strength media for impedance biosensing of avian influenza virus using a bare interdigitated electrode. Anal Chem 2014;86(4):1965–1971. doi:10.1021/ac402550f

[75] Diba FS, Kim S, Lee HJ. Amperometric bioaffinity sensing platform for avian influenza virus proteins with aptamer modified gold nanoparticles on carbon chips. Biosens Bioelectron 2015;72:355–361. doi:10.1016/j.bios.2015.05.020

[76] KrejcovaL,NejdlL,RodrigoMA,ZurekM,MatousekM,HynekD,etal.3Dprintedchipfor electrochemical detection of influenza virus labeled with CdS quantum dots. Biosens Bioelectron2014;54:421–427.doi:10.1016/j.bios.2013.10.031

[77] Wang R, Xu L, Li Y. Bio-nanogate controlled enzymatic reaction for virus sensing. Biosens Bioelectron 2015;67:400–407. doi:10.1016/j.bios.2014.08.071

[78] Lum J, Wang R, Hargis B, Tung S, Bottje W, Lu H, et al. An impedance aptasensor with microfluidic chips for specific detection of H5N1 avian influenza virus. Sensors (Basel) 2015;15(8):18565–18578.doi:10.3390/s150818565

[79] Hushegyi A, Bertok T, Damborsky P, Katrlik J, Tkac J. An ultrasensitive impedimetric glycan biosensor with controlled glycan density for detection of lectins and influenza hemagglutinins.ChemCommun(Camb)2015;51(35):7474–7477.doi:10.1039/c5cc00922g

Section 2

Vaccine Development

Chapter 5

Steps toward a Universal Influenza Vaccine: Research Models and Comparison of Current Approaches

Terianne Wong and Ted M. Ross

Additional information is available at the end of the chapter

http://dx.doi.org/10.5772/64369

Abstract

The ability of influenza virus to adapt to various species and evade natural immunity makes the ubiquitous pathogen particularly difficult to eradicate. Annual reformulation of influenza vaccines is costly and time-consuming and has varying efficacy against influenza virus strains. Therefore, worldwide efforts aim to develop a universal influenza vaccine to prevent potential healthcare emergencies such as pandemic influenza threats, such as the 1918 Spanish Flu and pandemic Swine Flu of 2009. Efficacy of a universal influenza vaccine must overcome current challenges with subtype diversity, antigenic drift, and adequately protect against emerging reassortants from both environmental and agricultural sources. Furthermore, the manufacturing and production of vaccines largely influence the effectiveness of a vaccine and technological advancements may soon rival current vaccine strategies. This review discusses the evolution and diversity of influenza viruses, how viral glycoprotein hemagglutinin plays a dominant role in influenza surveillance and assessment of protection and compares the methodologies of current and upcoming vaccine options. While the obstacles remain daunting, growing knowledge of influenza evolution and immunity may lead to more viable candidates that protect against broader varieties of influenza viruses and help prevent future international health crises.

Keywords: influenza, vaccine development, universal flu, flu strategies, immunology

1. Introduction

The World Health Organization (WHO) estimates 3–5 million cases of severe influenza worldwide will result between 250,000 and 500,000 deaths annually [1]. Within the United States, 24.7 million cases of seasonal influenza of various severities are predicted and an estimated

3,300–49,000 deaths occurred per year between 1979 and 2001 [2]. From 2013 to 2014, the hospitalization rate in the United States was 24.6 per 100,000 persons [3], although rates as high as 309 per 100,000 have been reported from 1993 to 2008, among elderly >65 years of age [4]. Including direct medical costs and loss of productivity and earnings associated with work absentness, seasonal influenza contributes an $87 billion burden on the US economy [5]. Furthermore, the spread of pandemic swine influenza virus from 2009 to 2010 attributed to 42–89 million cases of pandemic H1N1 (pdm H1N1) and an estimated 8870–18,300 deaths. Consequently, there is still a need to enhance our understanding of influenza virus evolution and manage the spread of pandemic influenza viruses.

Global influenza virus monitoring and surveillance systems track significant trends or real-time changes to influenza epidemiology and identify predominant viral subtypes during a particular season. Clinical symptoms include acute onset of cough, fever, and myalgia [6–9], and viral presence is confirmed by WHO-mandated laboratory standard operating procedures, such as immunostaining, cell culture growth, real-time polymerase chain reaction (RT-PCR), and detection of hemagglutination-inhibiting or viral neutralizing antibodies [10]. While viral culture in mammalian cells remains vital for characterization, RT-PCR remains the most rapid and sensitive diagnostic test available, with detection rates enhanced twofold over cell culture [8, 11, 12]. Alternatively, increases in hemagglutination-inhibiting antibody titers more than fourfold are counted as positive seroconversion and following viral infection or vaccination, which assists with monitoring immunogenicity. Collectively, data are shared through the WHO's Global Influenza Surveillance and Response System (GISRS), which includes 143 institutions in 113 WHO Member States [13], to help alert the emergence of antigenic variants or the beginning of a pandemic.

In April 2009, the Centers of Disease Control and Prevention (CDC) cited the first incidence of human-to-human transmission of pdmH1N1, also referred to as swine influenza A, which was antigenically distinct from other circulating human H1N1 [14]. As the first influenza pandemic of the twenty-first century, pandemic (pdm) H1N1 was not included in the annual trivalent vaccine regimen, leaving a large majority of the population unprotected from the newly emerging pathogen. In response to the increasing number of illnesses associated with pdm H1N1, satellite surveillance sites throughout the world rapidly collected clinical samples, surveyed seroconversion rates, and monitored the spread of the pandemic. Under the recommendation of WHO and CDC, the standard trivalent vaccine regimen of 2009–2010 [15] was reformulated to accommodate for the pdm H1N1 influenza strain (A/California/07/2009-like) [16, 17], and a median seroconversion rate of 59% was observed among healthy individuals ranging from 18 to 65 years of age [18]. During the 2010–2011 season, predicted efficacy in Sweden among individuals between 6 months and 64 years was between 63% and 80%, when 60% of the Swedish population received a monovalent AS03-adjuvanted vaccine against pdm H1N1 [19]; importantly, laboratory diagnosis of pdm09 H1N1 was utilized in this study. As of 2016, A/California/07/2009-like pdm H1N1 remains the predominant H1N1 strain circulating in the human population and remains a component in the annual trivalent or quadrivalent vaccine schedule. The remaining components of the annual vaccine, including prototype strains of Group B influenza strains and subtype H3N2, are frequently updated due to frequent antigenic changes to the hemagglutinins (HA). Ultimately, the WHO and CDC provide recommendations for vaccine formulation and identify what particular health concerns need to be address by the public, healthcare workers, and pharmaceutical/biomedical research industry.

2. Influenza diversity, tropism, and evolution

Currently, there are three types of influenza (A, B, and C), however, only types A and B infect humans. Influenza belongs to the family of Orthomyxoviridae and contains a negative sense, single segmented RNA genome. The influenza virion is pleomorphic or filamentous in shape, budding to approximately 80–120 nm in diameter, and attaches to sialic acid receptors found on numerous tissues in a diverse variety of hosts, including birds and mammals, such as swine, equine, canine, ferrets, and primates [20–23]. Upon budding from host cells, a lipid bilayer envelopes the viral ribonucleoprotein complex and presents surface viral glycoproteins, which are various combinations of hemagglutinins (HA, H1-H18) and neuraminidases (NA, N1-N11); the arrangement of HA and NA help distinguish the large diversity of influenza subtypes [24].

Avian influenza strains are ubiquitous in the wild; circulating in predominantly the wild ducks Anatidae bird populations [25–27] through an indirect fecal-oral transmission route and often results in little to no pathology [25, 28]. Replication of avian influenza virus (AIV) occurs in the intestinal tract of waterfowl and is shed in feces, such that contaminated waters infect other hosts; certain strains of AIV can persist in aquatic environments for 9 to 200 days, depending on salinity, pH, and temperature [29–31]. Consequently, poor water quality control and cohabitation of wild species increase the likelihood of AIV transmission into domestic birds markets [27, 32, 33] and livestock. Surveillance of live poultry markets in Asia indicate high prevalence of low pathogenic avian influenza strains, such as H3N2, H5N2, and H9N2 [32, 34–37]; isolates collected from poultry populations in Korea were used to experimentally infect mice and demonstrate zoonotic adaptation for mammalian hosts [38].

The human influenza virus threats are derived from avian [21, 39–42] or swine [14, 43] influenza predecessors, but these viruses have adapted to transmit and to replicate in the human host. Highly pathogenic avian influenza H5N1 (HPAIV H5N1) outbreaks during the end of the twentieth century led to lethal disease in domestic poultry and waterfowl, and eventually human intervention was needed to quarantine and cull millions of contaminated flocks worldwide [41, 44, 45]. Although most avian influenza strains typically do not cause disease in humans, HPAIV H5N1 was spread to humans in Hong Kong in 1997. From 2003 to January 2014, the WHO reported 386 human deaths out of the 650 confirmed H5N1 cases [46]. In February 2013, a novel avian influenza virus subtype, H7N9, was also detected in humans [47] and was thought to have arisen from nonpathogenic H7 strains.

In humans, influenza spreads through aerosolized respiratory droplet transmission and the virus attaches to primarily columnar epithelial cells lining the respiratory tract. Infection of influenza spreads to airway epithelial cells [48–50] and alveolar macrophages [51], although dendritic cells [52], natural killer cells [53], and mast cells are semi-permissive for influenza infection in vitro and in vivo. Typical incubation period for influenza virus is 1–4 days, in which an afflicted individual begins shedding virus and continues to shed up to 10 or more days after the onset of symptoms [9, 54]. Unlike human seasonal influenza, most AIV transmits directly from animal-to-human (zoonotic), but infrequently transmits between human hosts; however, since 1918, four influenza pandemics occurred after antigenic shift enabled human adaption and no prior immunity existed in the population. Since influenza hemagglutinin binds to sialic acid receptors that are on respiratory epithelial as well as erythrocytes, a rapid assay for sialic acid receptor binding is the red blood cell agglutination and hemagglutination inhibition (HAI) assays. Developed in the 1940s and based on the ability of influenza hemagglutinin to bind receptors of target cells and agglutinate red blood cells (RBCs), the HAI assay has become the standard serological assay for screening influenza hemagglutinin-reactive antibodies in sera [10]. Serial dilutions of heat-inactivated, receptor-destroying enzyme (RDE)-treated sera are incubated with a fixed amount of virus titrated in hemagglutination units and then RBCs are added to the virus-sera mixture to permit agglutination. The presence of influenza-specific, receptor-binding antibodies prevents RBC agglutination and potentially reduces infectivity. By standard, an antibody titer of >32, or most commonly 40, is correlated with up to 50% protection from influenza disease [14], and seroconversion is assumed when greater than fourfold increase is observed when comparing of pre- and post-vaccination HAI titers [13]. However, as important as the standard agglutination and HAI assays are for vaccine immunogenicity surveillance, new challenges arise when viruses have reduced species-specific RBC agglutination [55, 56] or when HAI titers do not correlate with protection [15]. Consequently, additional verification approaches are needed and applied to assess efficacy beyond immunogenicity of a vaccine candidate; the greatest obstacle, however, is overcoming the antigenic diversity in influenza strains and eliciting vaccine-induced protection prior to antigenic drifts or shifts.

Influenza glycoprotein hemagglutinin (HA) amino acid sequence variation fluctuates rapidly amidst cross-species infections, leading to shifts within HA subtypes. For example, the influenza viruses that spread internationally in 2009 were antigenically unique to seasonal H1N1 strains, but resembled the pandemic H1N1 strains isolated in 1918. The emergence of H1N1 into the human population in 1918 caused the first influenza pandemic of the twentieth century and caused ~50 million deaths worldwide [57]. Cross-reactive antibodies to the pdm H1N1 strains of 2009 were identified in the sera of older people [58] and therefore this implied that people infected with the 1918 H1N1 viruses elicited long-lasting antibodies that cross-reacted with the pdm H1N1 infecting people 90 year later. H3N2 influenza strains emerged in 1968 as a human pathogen after reassortment of HA & PB1 genes with avian source (1918 H1N1 (avian/human)→1957 H2N2 (avian)→1968 H3N2 (avian/human)) [43] leading to the loss of immune recognition among human hosts. The timeline in **Figure 1** illustrates the reassortment events that transitioned between avian influenza viruses into human pathogens and the emergence of pdm H1N1 or swine flu remained circulating in the swine population since early twentieth century and was reintroduced in the early 2000s.

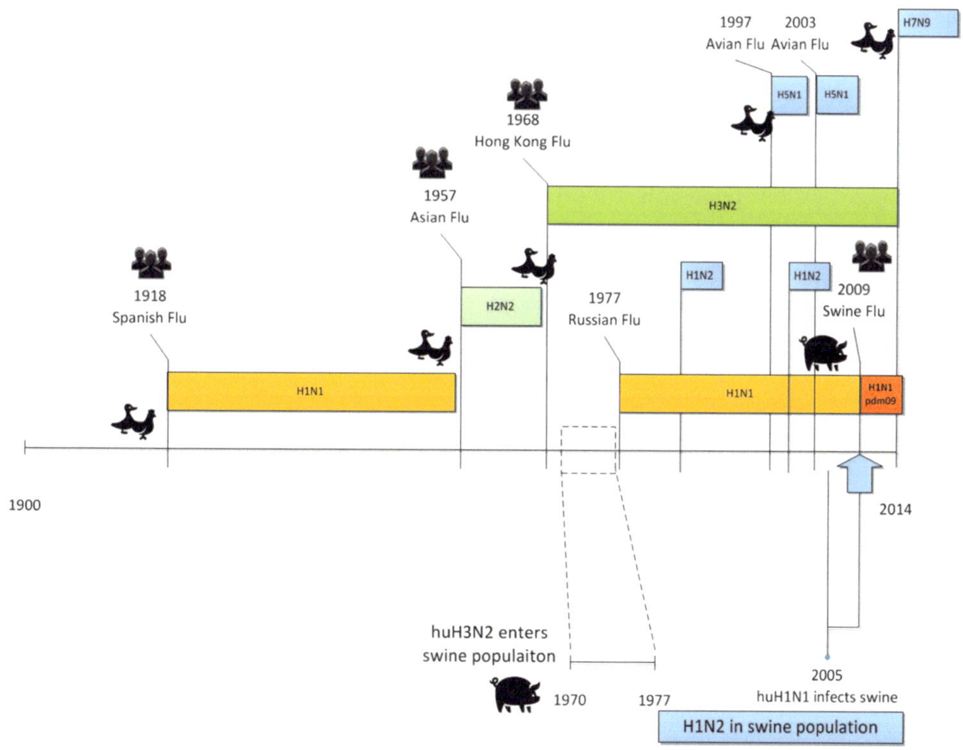

Figure 1. Timeline of influenza viruses and circulation among avian, swine and human populations.

The emergence of the 1918 Spanish Flu into the human population resulted from divergent reassortment of avian-like influenza and caused substantial morbidity and mortality worldwide. Further reassortment of the HA subsequently led to H2N2 and H3N2, which currently circulates abundantly in the human population. Introduction of H3N2 into the swine population during the 1970s and circulation of H1N2 permitted additional reassortment in the form of novel Swine Flu or pdm H1N1. The recent incidence of avian strains H5N1 and H7N1 is further evidence that zoonotic exchange of influenza viruses increases the likelihood of introduction to human populations.

Influenza HA mediates the binding to host cell surface receptors, dominantly sialic acid, which tends to be specific to species and tissue. HA proteins expressed by avian influenza strains preferentially bind to the sialic acids bound by an alpha 2-3 glycosidic bond, whereas an alpha 2-6 linkage is preferred by human adapted strains. Importantly, the upper human respiratory tract is lined with epithelial cells expressing sialic acids with alpha 2-6, whereas the lower respiratory tract contains sialic acids containing the alpha 2-3[41] potentially increasing susceptibility to lower respiratory tract infections by avian influenza viruses [42]; however, direct droplet transmission between humans is inefficient and remains limited.

In addition to receptor-binding specificity, the influenza HA sequence contains a critical cleavage site that is necessary for initiating pH-dependent fusion into the host cell. Influenza virus HA is synthesized as a precursor HA0, which is composed of a globular surface "head" HA1 and the stalk-like HA2. The HA2 portion contains a transmembrane domain spanning the viral membrane [23, 59, 60]. Within the HA1 subunit is the receptor-binding site (RBS) and a vestigial esterase domain that alters pH stability and ultimately, confers high or moderate pathogenicity [61, 62]. The exposure of the fusion peptide sequence is essential for conformational changes in the coiled-coil trimeric HA structure during a prefusion event, leading to extension of the HA, fold-back, hemifusion and eventual fusion of viral membrane to host membrane [63]. **Figure 2** is reprinted from a study [63] that analyzed the fusion event between influenza hemagglutinin and cell membrane of the infected cell, which utilizes a similar coiled-coil hemifusion state as other viral pathogens, such as HIV, respiratory syncytial virus, and Ebola virus [64].

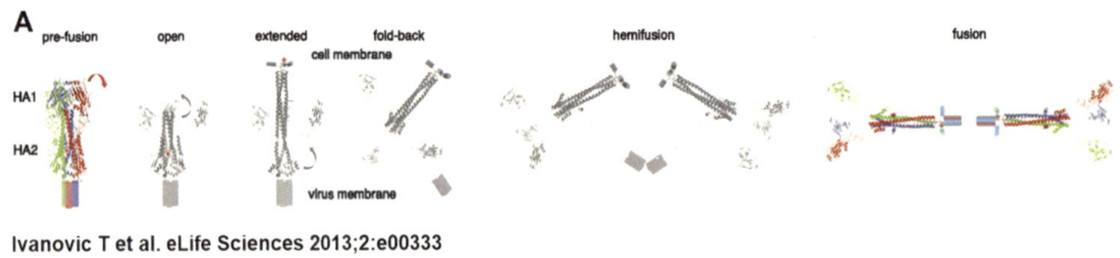

Figure 2. Fusion event of influenza hemagglutinin on host cell. Adapted from Ivanovic et al. [63].

Utilizing the coiled-coil motif to extend into a host cell, the hemagglutinin fusion peptide serves as an anchoring "hook" to attach to the cell membrane; through pH-mediated hairpin folding, the hemifusion event occurs, followed by complete fusion of the two membranes and release of viral components into the host cytoplasm.

The majority of low pathogenic influenza strains have HA0 containing a monobasic arginine residue that is cleaved by extracellular enzymes; within the human respiratory tract, the transmembrane protease, serine 2 (TMPRSS2) and human airway trypsin-like protease (HAT) are capable of mediating mono-basic cleavage to yield disulfide-bonded HA1 and HA2 subunits [65]. Several highly pathogenic avian influenza strains (H1N1v, H5 and H7) contain multi-arginine motifs that are cleaved by subtilisin-like cellular proteases and are often present in the intestinal and respiratory tracts of birds and mammals; cleavage by host proteinases, such as furin and PC6, occurs intracelluarly upon exit of the endoplasmic reticulum, and proteolysis is blocked by inhibitors of serine proteases, such as aprotinin [50, 66]. Interestingly, within a human large intestine carcinoma cell line Caco-1, aprotinin treatment and disruption of the late Golgi transport mechanisms by brefeldin A inhibit cleavage of HA0, regardless whether the influenza strain contains mono- or multi-basic proteolytic sites [66]. **Figure 3** illustrates the domains HA1 and HA2 in a homotrimer of HA from A/Fujian/411/2002-H3N2 influenza predicted using SWISS-MODEL service [67–70], with antigenic sites highlighted. Sites in H3 HA have been best characterized, with antigenic epitopes defined as A, B, C, D, and E [71–73]. Alternatively, H1 contains five antigenic sites, Cb, Sa, Sb, Ca1, and Ca2, that were originally modeled from H3 structure [74].

http://dx.doi.org/10.5772/64369

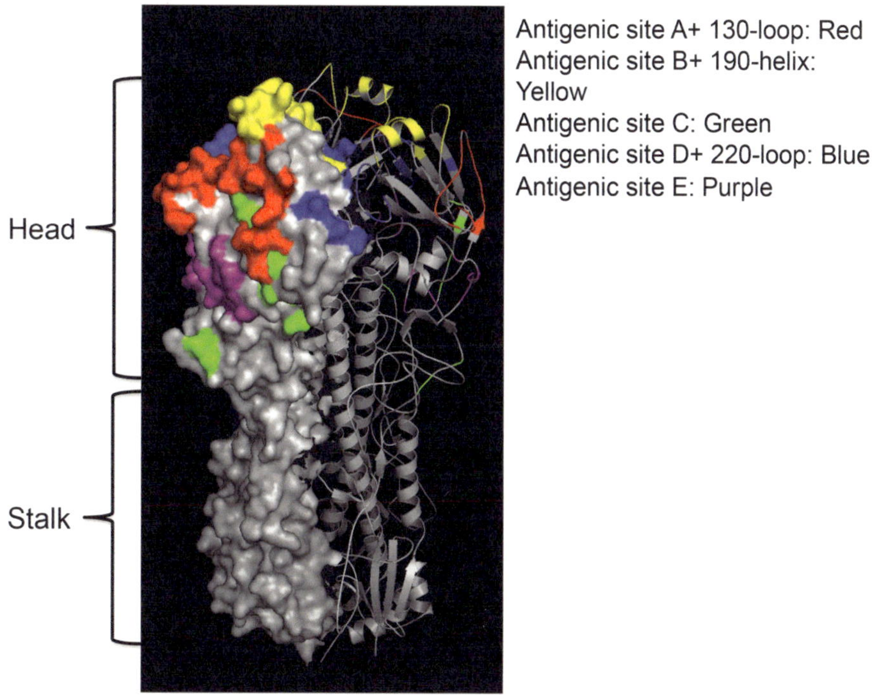

Figure 3. Structure of influenza hemagglutinin with antigenic sites and domains highlighted.

Influenza hemagglutinin is a homotrimer of a globular head and stalk domains. The HA of A/Fujian/411/2002-H3N2 influenza was modeled to PDB 2yp2.1.a using structure homology software SWISS-MODEL and further manipulated with PyMol. One monomer is shown with surface, whereas the remaining two monomers illustrated in ribbon-cartoon form. Highlighted antigenic sites A (red), B (yellow), C (green), D (blue), and E (purple) are present in H3 HA (shown), whereas Cb, Sa, Sb, Ca1, and Ca2 are the known antigenic epitopes in H1 influenza subtypes. Sites used were derived from 73.

Incomplete cleavage of HA0 yields lower viral titers [50, 65, 75] and virions incapable of HA0 cleavage are less infectious upon subsequent replication cycles, with more than 4 log-units lower than cleaved HA [50, 76]. Current cell-based approaches to influenza propagation using Madin-Darby canine kidney (MDCK) cells require artificial addition of trypsin or serine protease treatment to yield appreciable viral titers, but native enzymes in egg-based culture sufficiently cleave HA; therefore, no addition treatment is required [77, 78]; consequently, post-translational HA processing is substantially different between the two standard methods [79]. Recent human isolates, particularly H3N2 subtype, are difficult to propagate in conventional egg or MDCK cell lines; advancements in stable-overexpression of α2–6 sialic acids on the MDCK cell line (MDCK-SIAT1) have improved virus isolation rates[56] and typically retains HA sequence identity better than the aforementioned egg or MDCK approaches. These characteristic of HA and sialic acid binding affinity determine species- and tissue-specificity, and further complicate the likelihood of zoonotic diseases and transmission among humans.

Fears of an avian HA and NA reassortment with a human seasonal influenza virus are well justified given the emergence of avian-to-human and human-to-human transmissible HPAI H5N1 [45, 80] and subsequent fatality rates averaging 56% [81]. Human infection with H7N9 [47, 82–85] and H10N8 [86, 87] is high risks to individuals working or residing near live poultry markets, and mammalian receptor adaptation remains a significant concern for health officials. While H10N8 does not immediately appear to pose an imminent threat to global health, there are at least 450 confirmed cases of H7N9 by June 2014 since its initial emergence in China in March 2013. Historically associated with a highly pathogenic avian influenza strain, the H7 subtype strains, such as H7N2, H7N3, and H7N7 [47, 88, 89], have the preferential binding to α2–6-linked sialic acids, which increase their affinity to human upper respiratory epithelial cells [88, 90]; however, incidence of H7 avian and rare human infections remained isolated [91]. Experimental aerosol transmission studies in 2012 [92, 93] and 2013 [94, 95] using viruses in subtypes H5 and H7 showed that, similar HPAI H5N1, the H7N9 viruses potentially poses greater threat to humans since it has a limited capacity to transmit through aerosol droplets (REFS) and therefore further investigations are needed to elucidate H7 pathogenesis and HA evolution.

3. Challenges of generating a universal influenza vaccine

The diversity of influenza virus strains and subtypes exacerbates the challenge for generating a universal vaccine against influenza. The WHO makes recommendations for influenza vaccine composition for each flu season based on international surveillance systems and compares the ability of monovalent vaccine prototypes to elicit cross-reactive antibodies against prevalent circulating strains [16, 96, 97]. Unfortunately, delays in surveillance and the generation and evaluation of serology data hinder the selection of the optimal candidates and seasonal efficacy depends on prompt production by vaccine manufacturers and subsequent distribution. Moreover, the emergence of antigenic drift variants after selection of vaccine candidates may result in poor efficacy and wasted production time and resources [98]. Consequently, there is a demand for a universal, or more broadly reactive, vaccine against influenza virus. Utilizing various manufacturing platforms, adjuvants, and targets, researchers worldwide are currently seeking ways to improve current influenza vaccination strategies [99]. The following traits are desired in an ideal universal vaccine candidate: [1] recognition of antigenic drift variants; [2] elicitation of long-lasting memory responses; and [3] minimal manufacturing lag time between vaccine formulations. Additional desirable features may include cost-efficient production methods, predictive measures to protect against future antigenic variants, and efficacy among immunocompromised target populations, infants and elderly over the age of 65. Despite nearly a century of research, human influenza vaccine production is largely based on the traditional technologies. The rapid emergence of antigenically unique subtypes continues to challenge the current pace of diagnosis, prototype selection, and egg-based vaccine distribution. Furthermore, the importance of pre-existing immunity determines the level of protection from novel strains and depends on the presence of circulating cross-reactive antibodies. For example, individuals born prior to 1957 reportedly had fewer complications associated with pdm H1N1 than the younger, naïve population potentially because the elderly population encountered similar historical H1N1 strains during their lifetime and therefore had pre-existing neutralizing antibodies to antigenically similar strains [100].

Common name	Distributor	Inactivation	Detergent	Platform	Derived from:	Ref
Inactivated influenza, Trivalent (IIV3) or Quadrivalent (IIV4), intramuscular						
Afluria®	CSL Limited	beta-propiolactone	sodium taurodeoxycholate	Split virus	Embroynated chicken eggs	[110]
Fluarix®	GlaxoSmithKline	formaldehyde	sodium deoxycholate	Split virus	Embroynated chicken eggs	[111]
FluLaval®	ID Biomedical Corporation of Quebec (GSK)	UV, formaldehyde	sodium deoxycholate	Split virus	Embroynated chicken eggs	[112]
Fluvirin®	CSL Limited (Formerly Novartis Vaccines)	beta-propiolactone	nonylphenol ethoxylate	Subunit	Embroynated chicken eggs	[114]
Fluzone®	Sanofi Pasteur	formaldehyde	Triton X-100	Split virus	Embroynated chicken eggs	
Flucelvax®	CSL Limited (Formerly Novartis Vaccines)	beta-propiolactone	Cetyltrimethylammonium bromide	Subunit	MDCK mammalian cells	[115]
Inactivated influenza, Trivalent (IIV3) or Quadrivalent (IIV4), intradermal						
Fluzone®	Sanofi Pasteur	formaldehyde	Triton X-100	Split virus	Embroynated chicken eggs	[116]
Live, Trivalent (LAIV3) or Quadrivalent (LAIV4), intranasal						
FluMist®	MedImmune	N/A-cold-adapted, temperaturesensitive, or attenuated		Live reassortant	Embroynated chicken eggs	[117]
Recombinant Influenza Vaccine, Trivalent (RIV3)						
FluBlok®	Protein Sciences	none-purified HA	Triton X-100	Recombinant HA	expresSF+ insect cells	[118]
Trivalent, inactivated with adjuvant						
FLUAD™	Seqirus™ (CSL Limited)	formaldehyde	Cetyltrimethylammonium bromide	Split virus, MF59C.1	Embroynated chicken eggs	

Table 1. A list of FDA-approved influenza vaccines in US market as of March 2016.

In contrast, recent evidence suggests that sequential exposure to seasonal strains confers greater protection against novel antigenic drift variants; consequently, the question remains whether the existence of protective neutralizing antibodies in the elderly is due to immunological recall, or rather, enhanced broadly reactive response due to immunological boosts of heterologous strains over a lifetime. This has since been modeled in the ferret animal models and, without prior exposure to the pdm H1N1, ferrets sequentially challenged with seasonal H1N1 [101, 102] or immunized with inactivated seasonal vaccine [103] strains mount protective responses to pdm H1N1. In summary, seroprotection against influenza may also depend on the individual's pre-existing immunity, as well as the platform and strategy implemented.

Current 2016–2017 influenza vaccines recommended by the WHO are available as an inactivated trivalent or quadrivalent formulation delivered intramuscularly or as live attenuated mixture of influenza strains (LAIV) administered through intranasal route [104]. The various doses and formulations may or may not contain ovalbumin or mercury, and eligibility for some formulations is age restricted. Vaccine manufacturers have proprietary methods for virus propagation and inactivation, which often alters the antigenic properties of the vaccine candidate. Vaccine antigens may be prepared as whole virus, detergent or solvent disrupted split virions [105, 106], or subunit vaccines [107–109]. **Table 1** displays the 2016–2017 FDA-approved influenza vaccines used in the United States and exhibits formulation differences as described in the package inserts of each product [110–118]. Essentially, all current formulations aim to elicit protective antibody responses, predominantly against HA, and therefore protect against antigenically similar viral strains to the vaccine strain. Since the vaccine is often generated as a reassortant (6:2) vaccine strain from a high yield genetic backbone A/Puerto Rico/8/34 (H1N1), the HA and NA selected as a seasonal vaccine recommendation must be reformulated each season and validated for cross-reactivity to antigenically similar strains using HAI assay [98].

Adverse reactogenicity remains a safety concern for the young, immunocompromised, and elderly, therefore split or subunit vaccines are preferred over live or whole inactivated virus, despite enhanced humoral responses elicited by whole virus preparations [119]. Efforts to reduce the risks associated with LAIV are particularly important since humoral and cross-reactive T-cell responses are superior to that of inactivated vaccines in experimental swine and ferret studies [120–122]; among children, LAIV, but not inactivated vaccine, led to enhanced CD4+, CD8+, and γδ T-cell responses [123]. In contrast to inactivated vaccines that require reformulation each year, there is evidence that LAIV induces cross-reactivity with heterologous strains. This cross-reactivity phenomenon makes LAIV a promising candidate for the development of a universal vaccine platform. The route of administration, absence of active viral replication, and process of inactivation are different between influenza vaccine formulations. Further studies are needed to understand the mechanisms that promote influenza-specific T-cell responses upon LAIV immunization.

The WHO recommends propagating influenza viruses in embryonic chicken eggs, and this methodology is predominant source of high yield vaccine strains [124]. A list of FDA-approved influenza vaccines, majority of which are derived from embryonated chicken eggs, is provided in **Table 1**.

Table 1 shows differences in inactivation, detergents, and platforms used in the current vaccine market.

Despite the frequent use of the relatively inexpensive but highly productive virus production egg-based platform, some challenges are arising. Spontaneous mutations due to egg adaptation were recognized as early as 1951 [125] and, as a recent vaccine efficacy (VE) study showed, may present unanticipated challenges to vaccine development. In the 2012–2013 influenza season, MDCK-grown prototypes were selected for vaccine production and classical reassortant methodology was performed; in brief, co-culture of high-yield A/Puerto Rico/8/34 (H1N1) reassortant (6:2) with the HA and NA gene products from A/Victoria/361/2011 (H3N2) in the presence of antiserum to A/Puerto Rico/8/34 yielded reassortant A/Victoria/361/2011(H3N2)-IVR-165 [126]. During vaccine production, the high growth strain acquired several substitutions within the antigenic site B, which reduced reactogenicity against the original prototype A/Victoria/361/2011 and antigenically similar circulating field strains, resulting in a disappointing 39% (95% CI, 29%–47%) rate in humans vaccinated with the 2012–2013 egg-based preparations [127]. Consequently, the low VE for the 2012–2013 H3N2 season is attributed to changes in the HA due to vaccine manufacturing, not antigenic drift. In contrast, growth in mammalian cell lines results in fewer mutations than in eggs, with up to two mutations in the hemagglutinin of H3N2 strains after three passages in MDCK [128–130] or MDCK-SIAT1 [56] but no genotypic changes reported after 10 passages of avian influenza using human colorectal adenocarcinoma cell line, Caco-2 [131]. These examples suggest that alternative methods for influenza propagation are expanding and optimization could ensure more consistency and efficacy.

In 2013, the FDA approved the first MDCK cell-culture influenza vaccine (CCIV) called Flucelvax®, originally developed by Novartis Vaccines and Diagnostics, Inc., Cambridge, MA, USA [115] but acquired by CSL Limited, Melbourne, Australia, as of December 2015 [132], which is tolerable and safe, and demonstrates comparable, if not greater, protection to that of traditional egg-based technologies [133–137]. Furthermore, trials involving trivalent preparation of influenza viruses through growth in green monkey kidney cell line, Vero, is another new alternative to egg-based propagation [138]. Although not yet FDA approved in the United States, the Vero cell-based technology licensed as Vepacel® from Baxter AG, Vienna, Austria, is a pre-pandemic whole, inactivated virus H5N1 vaccine designed to elicit strong immunological responses in healthy, as well as immunocompromised populations [139]. Also in 2013, the FDA approved a recombinant HA (rHA) only influenza vaccine (Flubok®) from Protein Sciences Corporation, Meriden, CT, USA [118]. Flubok is generated from insect cells using a baculovirus expression system to produce high yield rHA vaccine against each seasonal influenza subtype. Further studies are still needed to assess cost-effectiveness in transitioning the current platforms of egg-derived influenza virus to mammalian cell culture. Modifications to standard method of virus propagation have economical and practical challenges, but federal initiatives suggest divergence from traditional egg-based approaches.

4. Alternatives to current influenza vaccine strategies

A disadvantage of mammalian cell culture is the need for regulated growth conditions and reagents, which hinder immediate production and increase cost; however, advancements in high-throughput bioreactors are ongoing [140]. However, the same types of technologies involved in mammalian cell culture virus propagation may further advance novel alternatives to eggs. Virus-like particles (VLPs) are non-replicating, self-assembling nanostructures that mimic virus surface protein presentation and are synthesized through co-expression of recombinant DNA in insect or mammalian cell culture [141–147]. Multiple advantages are associated with VLP over standard methods [141], including [1] they are non-infectious material and therefore not a biohazard risk and inactivation is not required, [2] VLPs self-assemble into proper conformation and multivalency, and [3] influenza VLPs have enhanced stability and HA potency up to 12 months with no degradation [148]. Several investigators have utilized this platform for evaluating immunogenicity of influenza HA [149–151], NA [144], M2 [152], and combinations of viral proteins. A mammalian VLP derived in Vero cells, H5N1-VLP (RG-14) [153], was composed of four influenza virus structural proteins and protected against a lethal H5N1 challenge in mice, yielding H5-specific IgG1 antibodies with a dose as low as 2.5 μg in a prime-boost regimen. Similarly, baculovirus-derived VLPs expressing H3N2 protected against a lethal challenge of mouse-adapted influenza H3N2 A/Hong Kong/68 [149], with intranasal instillation providing the greatest HA-specific antibody titers and protection as compared to intramuscular administration or two doses of sublethal intranasal challenges. The baculovirus/insect cell expression systems generate high yields of VLPs, and trivalent vaccine preclinical studies in mice and ferrets demonstrate the baculovirus-derived VLPs effectively elicit serum HAI antibodies against H1N1, H3N2, and influenza B, although cross-reactivity to heterologous strains was poor [154]. Importantly, side-by-side comparison of baculovirus-derived VLPs versus whole virion vaccine or recombinant HA suggests VLPs elicit comparable, if not higher, IgG titers, but also yielded antibodies that cross-react to a broader panel of non-homologous influenza viruses [146]. The baculovirus-derived VLPs have been fully characterized by Novavax , Inc. from Rockville, MD, USA, for the HA content, NA activity, stability, and VLP purity [155], and safety and reactogenicity were evaluated in two clinical trials with H5N1 and H1N1 baculovirus-derived VLPs [156, 157].

Proprietary application of recombinant RNA bacteriophage Qbeta by Cytos Biotechnology Ltd., Switzerland, offers an alternative strategy for conformational antigen presentation on the surface of Qbeta-derived virus-like particles through covalent chemical linkage [158]. Since presentation on Qbeta-derived VLPs does not involve post-translational modifications from the VLP-producing cell, potential cell type-specific alterations to the viral surface glycoprotein are avoided [159]; moreover, chemical linkage of antigens to Qbeta-derived VLPs overcomes the steric hindrance associated with masked immunodominant epitopes and efficiently elicits B cell responses in the absence of an adjuvant [160]. Importantly, specific sites or domains can be exclusively presented on the Qbeta-VLPs, such as the globular head of influenza hemagglutinin to induce hemagglutination inhibiting antibodies [161]. Consequently, this approach advanced to Phase I clinical trial in Singapore through sponsorship of the manufacturer Cytos

Biotechnology; the findings suggest that the Qbeta-VLP is tolerable and elicits HAI-specific antibodies comparable to the standard influenza vaccines [162]. However, as with any new approach, insect-, mammalian-, or Qbeta-VLP manufacturing processes still need to undergo more thorough safety evaluation and quality control; therefore, marketing and production are still a few years away.

Modern recombinant technology offers alternatives to live virus preparation. Synthetic or subunit viral peptide vaccines stimulate the immune response in similar mechanism as split inactivated vaccines and may be formulated with pattern recognition receptor agonists or emulsions to enhance adjuvant activity. Plasmid DNA encoding an immunogenic viral protein can be electroporated [163], administered intranasally in conjugation with nanoparticles [164], or delivered with a biolistic system. Particle-mediated epidermal delivery of DNA encoding influenza HA was recently optimized in an experimental ferret model and, when administered to the abdomen or tongue, yielded HAI titers greater than 1:40 [165]; sublingual route of vaccine administration has potential to elicit mucosal immunity and mount protective secretory immunoglobulin A (sIgA) [166, 167]. Previously in preclinical studies, delivery of recombinant IgA protects against infection in the experimental animal influenza model [168] while elicitation of IgG controls disease severity, thus elicitation of IgA by any universal vaccine candidate would be highly beneficial. In the effort to reduce infant morbidity associated with influenza infections, ongoing studies will test the safety, efficacy, and tolerability of vaccination of pregnant mothers and their newborns [169–171]; subsequent protection through maternal IgG and sIgA lasting up to 6 months could reduce infection within influenza virus [172].

In addition to the HA, DNA vaccination of the neuraminidase N1 from H1N1, A/New Caledonia/20/99, also partially protects against heterologous challenge with H5N1, A/Vietnam/1203/04, in the mouse model; similarly, passive immunization of heterologous anti-N1 sera in naïve mice provided modest protection against H5N1 challenge [173]. NA-DNA vaccination also conferred crossprotection against heterologous H3N2 strains in a lethal H3N2 influenza challenge [174], further suggesting neuraminidase may be an additional target for eliciting protection against drift variants within a influenza subtype. In addition to the neuraminidase, viral targets such as the nucleoprotein (NP), matrix 1 and 2 (M1 and M2), and polymerase (PB1) are different immunogens for vaccine candidates, resulting in varied immunological responses. Internal NP is the predominant target antigen for cytotoxic T lymphocyte (CTL) activity and is well conserved among influenza A viruses; peptide-based and DNA vaccination strategies have demonstrated promising protection against homologous and heterologous challenge with influenza A viruses. However, as with epitope-specific T cell responses, binding and affinity between epitope and human leukocyte antigen (HLA) could be restricted to highly polymorphic HLA alleles and could reduce efficacy among particular populations [175]. Consequently, promiscuous T cell epitopes that bind sufficiently to a wide range of HLA alleles remain to be identified. Recent studies also suggest cooperative T helper cell assistance to mount B cell immunological responses to promiscuous epitopes on the ectodomain of M2 protein, M2e [176]. Modified M2e, termed M2e multiple antigenic peptides (M2e-MAPs), appears to protect against influenza challenges among mice of various genetic background, providing proof of concept that M2e-MAPs are not necessarily MHC allele-restricted. Multiple efforts remain ongoing to test the feasibility of M2e-MAP-based vaccine strategies against influenza.

Clinical Trials	Immunogen	Principle	Immune response target	Phase	ClinicalTrials.gov ID	Sponsor	Route	Ref
VAX102	Adjuvanted recombinant antigen	M2e fused to TLR5 ligand S. typhimurium flagellin	M2e	1, 2	NCT00603811 ; NCT00921947	VaxInnate Corporation	I.M. & S.C.	
MVA-NP+M1	Viral Vector	Attenuated vaccina virus prime-boost regimen	NP and M1	1	NCT00993083 ; NCT00942071	University of Oxford	I.D.	[177]
MVA-NP+M1 and ChAdOx1 NP+M1	Viral vector	Attenuated adenoviral and vaccinia virus prime-boost regimen	NP and M1	1	NCT01818362	University of Oxford	I.M & I.M.	
FLU-v	Synthetic polypeptides	Lyophilized polypeptides T- cell epitopes	M1, M2, NP and PB1	1	NCT01181336	PepTcell Limited	S.C	
ACAM FLU-A	Recombinant antigen	Recombinant M2e	M2e	1	NCT00819013	Sanofi	I.M.	
NIBRG-14	Reassortant, inactivated influenza virosome	A/Vietnam/1194/2004 (H5N1) and A/Puerto Rico/8/34 (H1N1) (PR8) with alum or ISCOM-like Matrix M™ adjuvant	HA (Head/Stalk)	1, 2	NCT00660257 ; NCT00535665	Sinovac Biotech Co., Ltd	I.M.	[150], [151]
H5N1 VLP-1	Baculovirus VLP	A/Indonesia/05/2005 VLP	HA, NA, and M1	1,2	NCT00519389	Novavax	I.M.	[157]
H1N1 VLP	Baculovirus VLP	A/California/07/2009 VLP	HA, NA, and M2	1,2		Novavax	I.M.	[158]
gH1-Qbeta	Qbeta VLPs	A/California/07/2009 VLP	HA	1	CIRB Ref: 2012/906/E	Cytos Biotech.	I.M.	[163]

Table 2. Clinical trials ongoing the US testing novel influenza vaccine or antiviral approaches.

Since monovalent HA reactivity is thought to limit broad use of an influenza vaccine, alternative strategies aimed at less conventional tactics aside from full-length, wild-type HA. Directed reactogencity to either the globular head or stalk have been examined in mice, ferrets, and human clinical studies [150, 151, 156]. Broad protection against heterologous influenza virus strains is thought to rely on elicitation of well-conserved, HA2, stalk- or stem-specific antibodies [177]. Cross-protection against heterologous strains and crossreactivity to various subtypes appears the most rational direction toward a universal influenza vaccine. Immunization with recombinant HA2 construct that maintains a neutral pH conformation conferred protection against homologous H3-type virus strains, such as A/Philadelphia/2/82 and A/HK/68, but not heterologous H1-type viruses [178]. Importantly, prime-boost immunization of chimeric hemagglutinin expressing mismatched globular HA heads on homologous HA stalk (cH6/1, cH9/1, and cH5/1) elicited stalk-reactive, neutralizing antibodies and conferred protection against lethal H1N1challenge [179]. Protection, however, remained limited within a particular influenza group; therefore, further investigation remains to overcome such large diversity of influenza viruses. In an attempt to address the vast diversity of globular HA, computationally optimized broadly reactive antigens (COBRA) have been utilized in mammalian VLP platforms against H5N1 infection in mice, ferrets, and nonhuman primates [180–182]. Through multiple layers of consensus sequences of influenza hemagglutinin, COBRA methodology avoids database input bias associated with influenza surveillance systems; constructs generated have been validated to stimulate greater immunological breadth than monovalent vaccine strategies while successfully eliciting seroconversion, yielding hemagglutination-inhibiting antibody titers more than fourfold. **Table 2** is a summary of several clinical trials that investigated novel influenza vaccine strategies with various targets and approaches for eliciting protective immunity. In conclusion, the efficacy of the immunogen, route of administration, and types of immune responses elicited will further determine whether novel approaches could replace current vaccination methods.

The ClinicalTrial.gov database provides latest information regarding past and current clinical trials and the status toward future applications. Unlike the conventional influenza vaccines that dominant to HA-mediated immune responses, recent clinical trials test antiviral therapies targeting influenza matrix (M and M2e, matrix ectodomain) or highly conserved nucleoprotein (NP). These strategies come from various technologies, including virus-like particles (VLPs) and platforms, which do not rely on the egg-based vaccine manufacturing processes. The routes of delivery also vary, including intramuscular (IM), intradermal (ID), and subcutaneous (SC).

5. Concluding remarks

The pursuit of a universal vaccine against influenza is a constant battle between influenza virus evolution and current technologies. Since influenza infections remain ubiquitous among humans, as well as wildlife and domestic livestock, reassortment of genomic segments can still yield combinations that the human species has not previously encountered; alternatively, gradual antigenic variation of the hemagglutinin also results in poor cross-reactivity and protection against heterologous strains. As such, protective measures such as effective vaccination and more thorough understanding of HA evolution are needed to prevent forthcoming pandemics. Current practices rely on relatively traditional technologies for vaccine selection and manufacturing, and as witnessed during the pandemic H1N1 outbreak of 2009, it took months to identify and manufacture a new vaccine [183, 184]. In addition, inadequate quality control led to sterility breaches of millions of doses Fluvirin®, which at-time was manufactured by Chiron, acquired first by Novartis Vaccines and Diagnostics Limited, Speke, Liverpool, UK [185, 186] but now recently under Seqirus™, a CSL Limited company. During such shortages, it was evident that influenza vaccine resources were insufficient given the substantial health risks. To minimize future damages, both in morbidity and economical losses, the international community must disseminate new findings rapidly and cooperatively strive for more effective and readily available preventative actions.

In addition to the current vaccine approaches, innovative strategies are being tested for feasibility, safety, and the elicitation of broad immunogenicity to influenza strains and subtypes. Overcoming the antigenic diversity remains the greatest challenge to the efforts of designing a universal influenza vaccine. Moreover, changes in manufacturing and rapid implementation are critical for vaccine efficacy and may require divergence from the currently accepted methodologies. The recombinant technology and nonconventional vaccine platforms aforementioned demonstrate potential and may rival the current standard of care. As our understanding of immune responses to influenza and antigenic variability furthers, improvements to influenza vaccine strategies are expected to prevent significant morbidity and unnecessary disease through preventative measures.

Author details

Terianne Wong and Ted M. Ross*

*Address all correspondence to: tedross@uga.edu

Department of Infectious Diseases, College of Veterinary Medicine, University of Georgia, Athens, GA, United States

References

[1] Ross T, Zimmer S, Burke D, Crevar C, Carter D, Stark J, et al. Seroprevalence following the second wave of pandemic 2009 H1N1 influenza. PLoS Currents. 2010;2:RRN1148.

[2] Zimmer SM, Crevar CJ, Carter DM, Stark JH, Giles BM, Zimmerman RK, et al. Seroprevalence following the second wave of Pandemic 2009 H1N1 influenza in Pittsburgh, PA, USA. PLoS One. 2010;5(7):e11601.

[3] Arriola CS, Brammer L, Epperson S, Blanton L, Kniss K, Mustaquim D, et al. Update: influenza activity - United States, September 29, 2013-February 8, 2014. Morbidity and Mortality Weekly Report. 2014;63(7):148-154.

[4] Zhou H, Thompson WW, Viboud CG, Ringholz CM, Cheng PY, Steiner C, et al. Hospitalizations associated with influenza and respiratory syncytial virus in the United States, 1993-2008. Clinical Infectious Diseases. 2012;54(10):1427-1436.

[5] Molinari N-AM, Ortega-Sanchez IR, Messonnier ML, Thompson WW, Wortley PM, Weintraub E, et al. The annual impact of seasonal influenza in the US: Measuring disease burden and costs. Vaccine. 2007;25(27):5086-5096.

[6] Ebell MH, Afonso A. A systematic review of clinical decision rules for the diagnosis of influenza. Annals of Family Medicine. 2011;9(1):69-77.

[7] Ebell MH, Afonso AM, Gonzales R, Stein J, Genton B, Senn N. Development and validation of a clinical decision rule for the diagnosis of influenza. Journal of the American Board of Family Medicine: JABFM. 2012;25(1):55-62.

[8] Zambon M, Hays J, Webster A, Newman R, Keene O. Diagnosis of influenza in the community: relationship of clinical diagnosis to confirmed virological, serologic, or molecular detection of influenza. Archives of Internal Medicine. 2001;161(17): 2116-2122.

[9] van Elden LJ, van Essen GA, Boucher CA, van Loon AM, Nijhuis M, Schipper P, et al. Clinical diagnosis of influenza virus infection: evaluation of diagnostic tools in general practice. The British Journal of General Practice : The Journal of the Royal College of General Practitioners. 2001;51(469):630-634.

[10] Hirst GK. The quantitative determination of influenza virus and antibodies by means of red cell agglutination. Journal of Experimental Medicine. 1942;75(1):49-64.

[11] Weinberg GA, Erdman DD, Edwards KM, Hall CB, Walker FJ, Griffin MR, et al. Superiority of reverse-transcription polymerase chain reaction to conventional viral culture in the diagnosis of acute respiratory tract infections in children. The Journal of Infectious Diseases. 2004;189(4):706-710.

[12] Storch GA. Rapid diagnostic tests for influenza. Current Opinion in Pediatrics. 2003;15(1):77-84.

[13] Hannoun C, Megas F, Piercy J. Immunogenicity and protective efficacy of influenza vaccination. Virus Research. 2004;103(1-2):133-138.

[14] Potter CW, Oxford JS. Determinants of immunity to influenza infection in man. British Medicine Bulletin. 1979;35(1):69-75.

[15] Ohmit SE, Petrie JG, Cross RT, Johnson E, Monto AS. Influenza hemagglutination-inhibition antibody titer as a correlate of vaccine-induced protection. The Journal of Infectious Diseases. 2011;204(12):1879-1885.

[16] Barr IG. WHO recommendations for the viruses used in the 2013–2014 Northern Hemisphere influenza vaccine: Epidemiology, antigenic and genetic characteristics of influenza A(H1N1)pdm09, A(H3N2) and B influenza viruses collected from October 2012 to January 2013. Vaccine.

[17] Recommended composition of influenza virus vaccines for use in the 2010 southern hemisphere influenza season. World Health Organization, 23 September 2009 (Rev. 8 October 2009). Report No.

[18] Osterholm MT, Kelley NS, Sommer A, Belongia EA. Efficacy and effectiveness of influenza vaccines: a systematic review and meta-analysis. The Lancet Infectious Diseases. 2012;12(1):36-44.

[19] Widgren K, Magnusson M, Hagstam P, Widerstrom M, Ortqvist A, Einemo IM, et al. Prevailing effectiveness of the 2009 influenza A(H1N1)pdm09 vaccine during the 2010/11 season in Sweden. Euro surveillance: bulletin Europeen sur les maladies transmissibles = European Communicable Disease Bulletin. 2013;18(15):20447.

[20] Carroll S, Higa H, Paulson J. Different cell-surface receptor determinants of antigenically similar influenza virus hemagglutinins. Journal of Biological Chemistry. 1981;256(16):8357-8363.

[21] Connor R, Kawaoka Y, Webster R, Paulson J. Receptor specificity in human, avian and equine H2 and H3 influenza virus isolates. Virology. 1994;205:17 - 23.

[22] Ito T, Suzuki Y, Mitnaul L, Vines A, Kida H, Kawaoka Y. Receptor specificity of influenza A viruses correlates with the agglutination of erythrocytes from different animal species. Virology. 1997;227:493-499.

[23] Mair CM, Ludwig K, Herrmann A, Sieben C. Receptor binding and pH stability - How influenza A virus hemagglutinin affects host-specific virus infection. Biochimica et Biophysica Acta. 2013.

[24] A revision of the system of nomenclature for influenza viruses: a WHO memorandum. Bulletin of the World Health Organization. 1980;58(4):585-591.

[25] Brown JD, Poulson R, Stallknecht DE. Wild bird surveillance for avian influenza virus. Methods in Molecular Biology (Clifton, NJ). 2014;1161:69-81.

[26] Kaleta EF, Hergarten G, Yilmaz A. Avian influenza A viruses in birds—an ecological, ornithological and virological view. DTW Deutsche tierarztliche Wochenschrift. 2005;112(12):448-456.

[27] Stallknecht DE, Shane SM, Zwank PJ, Senne DA, Kearney MT. Avian influenza viruses from migratory and resident ducks of coastal Louisiana. Avian Diseases. 1990;34(2): 398-405.

[28] Hinshaw VS, Wood JM, Webster RG, Deibel R, Turner B. Circulation of influenza viruses and paramyxoviruses in waterfowl originating from two different areas of North America. Bulletin of the World Health Organization. 1985;63(4):711-719.

[29] Brown JD, Goekjian G, Poulson R, Valeika S, Stallknecht DE. Avian influenza virus in water: infectivity is dependent on pH, salinity and temperature. Veterinary Microbiology. 2009;136(1-2):20-26.

[30] Stallknecht DE, Kearney MT, Shane SM, Zwank PJ. Effects of pH, temperature, and salinity on persistence of avian influenza viruses in water. Avian Diseases. 1990;34(2): 412-418.

[31] Stallknecht DE, Shane SM, Kearney MT, Zwank PJ. Persistence of avian influenza viruses in water. Avian Diseases. 1990;34(2):406-411.

[32] Abao LN, Jamsransuren D, Bui VN, Ngo LH, Trinh DQ, Yamaguchi E, et al. Surveillance and characterization of avian influenza viruses from migratory water birds in eastern Hokkaido, the northern part of Japan, 2009-2010. Virus Genes. 2013;46(2):323-329.

[33] Fournie G, Guitian J, Desvaux S, Cuong VC, Dung do H, Pfeiffer DU, et al. Interventions for avian influenza A (H5N1) risk management in live bird market networks. Proceedings of the National Academy of Sciences of the United States of America. 2013;110(22): 9177-9182.

[34] Baek YH, Pascua PN, Song MS, Park KJ, Kwon HI, Lee JH, et al. Surveillance and characterization of low pathogenic H5 avian influenza viruses isolated from wild migratory birds in Korea. Virus Research. 2010;150(1-2):119-128.

[35] Jadhao SJ, Nguyen DC, Uyeki TM, Shaw M, Maines T, Rowe T, et al. Genetic analysis of avian influenza A viruses isolated from domestic waterfowl in live-bird markets of Hanoi, Vietnam, preceding fatal H5N1 human infections in 2004. Archives of Virology. 2009;154(8):1249-1261.

[36] Liu M, He S, Walker D, Zhou N, Perez DR, Mo B, et al. The influenza virus gene pool in a poultry market in south central China. Virology. 2003;305(2):267-275.

[37] Choi YK, Heui Seo S, Kim JA, Webby RJ, Webster RG. Avian influenza viruses in Korean live poultry markets and their pathogenic potential. Virology. 2005;332(2):529-537.

[38] Song M-S, Oh T-K, Moon HJ, Yoo D-W, Lee EH, Lee J-S, et al. Ecology of H3 avian influenza viruses in Korea and assessment of their pathogenic potentials. Journal of General Virology. 2008;89(4):949-957.

[39] Cong Y, Wang G, Guan Z, Chang S, Zhang Q, Yang G, et al. Reassortant between human-like H3N2 and Avian H5 subtype influenza a viruses in pigs: a potential public health risk. PLoS One. 2010;5(9):e12591.

[40] Matrosovich M, Gambaryan A, Teneberg S, Piskarev V, Yamnikova S, Lvov D, et al. Avian influenza A viruses differ from human viruses by recognition of sialyloligosac-

charides and gangliosides and by a higher conservation of the HA receptor-binding site. Virology. 1997;233(1):224 - 234.

[41] Nicholls JM, Chan MC, Chan WY, Wong HK, Cheung CY, Kwong DL, et al. Tropism of avian influenza A (H5N1) in the upper and lower respiratory tract. Nature Medicine. 2007;13(2):147-149.

[42] Shinya K, Ebina M, Yamada S, Ono M, Kasai N, Kawaoka Y. Avian flu: influenza virus receptors in the human airway. Nature. 2006;440(7083):435-436.

[43] Komadina N, McVernon J, Hall R, Leder K. A historical perspective of influenza A(H1N2) virus. Emerging Infectious Diseases. 2014;20(1):6-12.

[44] Cauthen AN, Swayne DE, Schultz-Cherry S, Perdue ML, Suarez DL. Continued circulation in China of highly pathogenic avian influenza viruses encoding the hemagglutinin gene associated with the 1997 H5N1 outbreak in poultry and humans. Journal of Virology. 2000;74(14):6592-6599.

[45] Shortridge KF, Zhou NN, Guan Y, Gao P, Ito T, Kawaoka Y, et al. Characterization of avian H5N1 influenza viruses from poultry in Hong Kong. Virology. 1998;252(2): 331-342.

[46] Shi X-W, Liu Y, Lewandowski AT, Wu L-Q, Wu H-C, Ghodssi R, et al. Chitosan biotinylation and electrodeposition for selective protein assembly. Macromolecular Bioscience. 2008;8(5):451-457.

[47] Xie L, Ding H, Kao QJ, Yang XH, Wen YY, Lv HK, et al. Clinical and epidemiological survey and analysis of the first case of human infection with avian influenza A(H7N9) virus in Hangzhou, China. European Journal of Clinical Microbiology & Infectious Diseases: Official Publication of the European Society of Clinical Microbiology. 2013;32(12):1617-1620.

[48] Bateman AC, Karasin AI, Olsen CW. Differentiated swine airway epithelial cell cultures for the investigation of influenza A virus infection and replication. Influenza and Other Respiratory Viruses. 2013;7(2):139-150.

[49] Punyadarsaniya D, Liang CH, Winter C, Petersen H, Rautenschlein S, Hennig-Pauka I, et al. Infection of differentiated porcine airway epithelial cells by influenza virus: differential susceptibility to infection by porcine and avian viruses. PLoS One. 2011;6(12):e28429.

[50] Zhirnov OP, Ikizler MR, Wright PF. Cleavage of influenza A virus hemagglutinin in human respiratory epithelium is cell associated and sensitive to exogenous antiproteases. Journal of Virology. 2002;76(17):8682-8689.

[51] Hoeve MA, Nash AA, Jackson D, Randall RE, Dransfield I. Influenza virus A infection of human monocyte and macrophage subpopulations reveals increased susceptibility associated with cell differentiation. PLoS One. 2012;7(1):e29443.

[52] Smed-Sörensen A, Chalouni C, Chatterjee B, Cohn L, Blattmann P, Nakamura N, et al. Influenza A virus infection of human primary dendritic cells impairs their ability to cross-present antigen to CD8 T cells. PLoS Pathogens. 2012;8(3):e1002572.

[53] Mao H, Tu W, Qin G, Law HKW, Sia SF, Chan P-L, et al. Influenza virus directly infects human natural killer cells and induces cell apoptosis. Journal of Virology. 2009;83(18): 9215-9222.

[54] Meschi S, Selleri M, Lalle E, Bordi L, Valli MB, Ferraro F, et al. Duration of viral shedding in hospitalized patients infected with pandemic H1N1. BMC Infectious Diseases. 2011;11:140.

[55] Skowronski DM, Janjua NZ, De Serres G, Dickinson JA, Winter AL, Mahmud SM, et al. Interim estimates of influenza vaccine effectiveness in 2012/13 from Canada's sentinel surveillance network, January 2013. Euro surveillance: bulletin Europeen sur les maladies transmissibles = European Communicable Disease Bulletin. 2013;18(5).

[56] Oh DY, Barr IG, Mosse JA, Laurie KL. MDCK-SIAT1 cells show improved isolation rates for recent human influenza viruses compared to conventional MDCK cells. Journal of Clinical Microbiology. 2008;46(7):2189-2194.

[57] Taubenberger JK, Morens DM. 1918 Influenza: the mother of all pandemics. Revista Biomedica 2006;17:69-79.

[58] Khurana S, Verma N, Talaat KR, Karron RA, Golding H. Immune response following H1N1pdm09 vaccination: differences in antibody repertoire and avidity in young adults and elderly populations stratified by age and gender. The Journal of Infectious Diseases. 2012;205(4):610-620.

[59] Kumari K, Gulati S, Smith D, Gulati U, Cummings R, Air G. Receptor binding specificity of recent human H3N2 influenza viruses. Virology Journal. 2007;4(1):42.

[60] Stevens J, Blixt O, Tumpey T, Taubenberger J, Paulson J, Wilson I. Structure and receptor specificity of the hemagglutinin from an H5N1 influenza virus. Science. 2006;312(5772): 404 - 410.

[61] DuBois RM, Zaraket H, Reddivari M, Heath RJ, White SW, Russell CJ. Acid stability of the hemagglutinin protein regulates H5N1 influenza virus pathogenicity. PLoS Pathogens. 2011;7(12):e1002398.

[62] Fereidouni SR, Harder TC, Starick E. Rapid pathotyping of recent H5N1 highly pathogenic avian influenza viruses and of H5 viruses with low pathogenicity by RT-PCR and restriction enzyme cleavage pattern (RECP). Journal of Virological Methods. 2008;154(1-2):14-19.

[63] Ivanovic T, Choi JL, Whelan SP, van Oijen AM, Harrison SC, Brunger AT. Influenza-virus membrane fusion by cooperative fold-back of stochastically induced hemagglutinin intermediates. eLife. 2013;2.

[64] Singh M, Berger B, Kim PS. LearnCoil-VMF: computational evidence for coiled-coil-like motifs in many viral membrane-fusion proteins. Journal of Molecular Biology. 1999;290(5):1031-1041.

[65] Bottcher E, Matrosovich T, Beyerle M, Klenk HD, Garten W, Matrosovich M. Proteolytic activation of influenza viruses by serine proteases TMPRSS2 and HAT from human airway epithelium. Journal of Virology. 2006;80(19):9896-9898.

[66] Zhirnov OP, Vorobjeva IV, Ovcharenko AV, Klenk HD. Intracellular cleavage of human influenza A virus hemagglutinin and its inhibition. Biochemistry (Moscow). 2003;68(9): 1020-1026.

[67] Arnold K, Bordoli L, Kopp J, Schwede T. The SWISS-MODEL workspace: a web-based environment for protein structure homology modelling. Bioinformatics. 2006;22(2): 195-201.

[68] Biasini M, Bienert S, Waterhouse A, Arnold K, Studer G, Schmidt T, et al. SWISS-MODEL: modelling protein tertiary and quaternary structure using evolutionary information. Nucleic Acids Research 2014;42(Web Server issue):W252-W258.

[69] Guex N, Peitsch MC, Schwede T. Automated comparative protein structure modeling with SWISS-MODEL and Swiss-PdbViewer: a historical perspective. Electrophoresis. 2009;30 Suppl 1:S162-S173.

[70] Kiefer F, Arnold K, Kunzli M, Bordoli L, Schwede T. The SWISS-MODEL Repository and associated resources. Nucleic Acids Research. 2009;37(Database issue):D387-D392.

[71] Tharakaraman K, Raman R, Stebbins NW, Viswanathan K, Sasisekharan V, Sasisekharan R. Antigenically intact hemagglutinin in circulating avian and swine influenza viruses and potential for H3N2 pandemic. Scientific Reports 2013;3.

[72] Wiley DC, Wilson IA, Skehel JJ. Structural identification of the antibody-binding sites of Hong Kong influenza haemagglutinin and their involvement in antigenic variation. Nature. 1981;289(5796):373-378.

[73] Stray S, Pittman L. Subtype- and antigenic site-specific differences in biophysical influences on evolution of influenza virus hemagglutinin. Virology Journal. 2012;9(1): 91.

[74] Caton AJ, Brownlee GG, Yewdell JW, Gerhard W. The antigenic structure of the influenza virus A/PR/8/34 hemagglutinin (H1 subtype). Cell. 1982;31(2 Pt 1):417-427.

[75] Chaipan C, Kobasa D, Bertram S, Glowacka I, Steffen I, Solomon Tsegaye T, et al. Proteolytic activation of the 1918 influenza virus hemagglutinin. Journal of Virology. 2009;83(7):3200-3211.

[76] Zhirnov OP, Ovcharenko AV, Bukrinskaya AG. A modified plaque assay method for accurate analysis of infectivity of influenza viruses with uncleaved hemagglutinin. Archives of Virology. 1982;71(2):177-183.

[77] WHO Global Influenza Surveillance Network. Manual for the Laboratory Diagnosis and Virological Surveillance of Influenza. World Health Organization; 2011.

[78] Webster RG, Krauss S. WHO manual on animal influenza diagnosis and surveillance. World Health Organization,Department of Communicable Disease Surveillance and Response; 2002.

[79] Cottey R, Rowe CA, Bender BS. Influenza Virus. Current Protocols in Immunology. John Wiley & Sons, Inc.; 2001.

[80] Li KS, Guan Y, Wang J, Smith GJ, Xu KM, Duan L, et al. Genesis of a highly pathogenic and potentially pandemic H5N1 influenza virus in eastern Asia. Nature. 2004;430(6996):209-213.

[81] Fiebig L, Soyka J, Buda S, Buchholz U, Dehnert M, Haas W. Avian influenza A(H5N1) in humans: new insights from a line list of World Health Organization confirmed cases, September 2006 to August 2010. Euro surveillance : bulletin Europeen sur les maladies transmissibles = European communicable disease bulletin. 2011;16(32).

[82] Poovorawan Y. Epidemic of avian influenza A (H7N9) virus in China. Pathogens and Global Health. 2014;108(4):169-170.

[83] Wang D, Yang L, Gao R, Zhang X, Tan Y, Wu A, et al. Genetic tuning of the novel avian influenza A(H7N9) virus during interspecies transmission, China, 2013. Euro surveillance : bulletin Europeen sur les maladies transmissibles = European Communicable Disease Bulletin. 2014;19(25).

[84] Yum J, Park EH, Ku KB, Kim JA, Oh SK, Kim HS, et al. Low infectivity of a novel avian-origin H7N9 influenza virus in pigs. Archives of Virology. 2014.

[85] Liu D, Gao GF. The new emerging H7N9 influenza virus indicates poultry as new mixing vessels. Science China Life Sciences. 2014;57(7):731-732.

[86] Su S, Qi W, Zhou P, Xiao C, Yan Z, Cui J, et al. First evidence of H10N8 Avian influenza virus infections among feral dogs in live poultry markets in Guangdong Province, China. Clinical Infectious Diseases: An Official Publication of the Infectious Diseases Society of America. 2014.

[87] Qi W, Zhou X, Shi W, Huang L, Xia W, Liu D, et al. Genesis of the novel human-infecting influenza A(H10N8) virus and potential genetic diversity of the virus in poultry, China. Euro surveillance: bulletin Europeen sur les maladies transmissibles = European Communicable Disease Bulletin. 2014;19(25).

[88] Banks J, Plowright L. Additional glycosylation at the receptor binding site of the hemagglutinin (HA) for H5 and H7 viruses may be an adaptation to poultry hosts, but does it influence pathogenicity? Avian Diseases. 2003;47(3 Suppl):942-950.

[89] Kobayashi Y, Horimoto T, Kawaoka Y, Alexander DJ, Itakura C. Pathological studies of chickens experimentally infected with two highly pathogenic avian influenza viruses. Avian Pathology: Journal of the WVPA. 1996;25(2):285-304.

[90] Belser JA, Blixt O, Chen LM, Pappas C, Maines TR, Van Hoeven N, et al. Contemporary North American influenza H7 viruses possess human receptor specificity: Implications for virus transmissibility. Proceedings of the National Academy of Sciences of the United States of America. 2008;105(21):7558-7563.

[91] Belser JA, Bridges CB, Katz JM, Tumpey TM. Past, present, and possible future human infection with influenza virus A subtype H7. Emerging Infectious Diseases. 2009;15(6): 859-865.

[92] Imai M, Watanabe T, Hatta M, Das SC, Ozawa M, Shinya K, et al. Experimental adaptation of an influenza H5 HA confers respiratory droplet transmission to a reassortant H5 HA/H1N1 virus in ferrets. Nature. 2012;486(7403):420-428.

[93] Herfst S, Schrauwen EJ, Linster M, Chutinimitkul S, de Wit E, Munster VJ, et al. Airborne transmission of influenza A/H5N1 virus between ferrets. Science. 2012;336(6088):1534-1541.

[94] Richard M, Schrauwen EJ, de Graaf M, Bestebroer TM, Spronken MI, van Boheemen S, et al. Limited airborne transmission of H7N9 influenza A virus between ferrets. Nature. 2013;501(7468):560-563.

[95] Belser JA, Gustin KM, Pearce MB, Maines TR, Zeng H, Pappas C, et al. Pathogenesis and transmission of avian influenza A (H7N9) virus in ferrets and mice. Nature. 2013;501(7468):556-559.

[96] WHO guidelines on the use of vaccines and antivirals during influenza pandemics. Releve epidemiologique hebdomadaire/Section d'hygiene du Secretariat de la Societe des Nations = Weekly Epidemiological Record/Health Section of the Secretariat of the League of Nations. 2002;77(47):394-404.

[97] WHO guidelines on the use of vaccines and antivirals during influenza pandemics. Global Health Security. 2004; Epidemic Alert & Response:51.

[98] Stohr K, Bucher D, Colgate T, Wood J. Influenza virus surveillance, vaccine strain selection, and manufacture. Methods in Molecular Biology (Clifton, NJ). 2012;865:147-162.

[99] Osterholm MT, Kelley NS, Manske JM, Ballering KS, Leighton TR, Moore KA. The Compelling Need for Game-Changing Influenza Vaccines: An analysis of the influenza vaccine enterprise and recommendations for the future. Center for Infectious Disease Research & Policy (University of Minnesota). Executive Summary.

[100] Greenbaum JA, Kotturi MF, Kim Y, Oseroff C, Vaughan K, Salimi N, et al. Pre-existing immunity against swine-origin H1N1 influenza viruses in the general human population. Proceedings of the National Academy of Sciences. 2009;106(48):20365-20370.

[101] Laurie KL, Carolan LA, Middleton D, Lowther S, Kelso A, Barr IG. Multiple infections with seasonal influenza A virus induce cross-protective immunity against A(H1N1) pandemic influenza virus in a ferret model. Journal of Infectious Diseases. 2010;202(7): 1011-1020.

[102] Carter DM, Bloom CE, Nascimento EJ, Marques ET, Craigo JK, Cherry JL, et al. Sequential seasonal H1N1 influenza virus infections protect ferrets against novel 2009 H1N1 influenza virus. Journal of Virology. 2013;87(3):1400-1410.

[103] Pearce MB, Belser JA, Gustin KM, Pappas C, Houser KV, Sun X, et al. Seasonal trivalent inactivated influenza vaccine protects against 1918 Spanish influenza virus infection in ferrets. Journal of Virology. 2012;86(13):7118-7125.

[104] Macdonald NE, Hall CB, Suffin SC, Alexson C, Harris PJ, Manning JA. Respiratory syncytial viral-infection in infants with congenital heart-disease. New England Journal of Medicine. 1982;307(7):397-400.

[105] Bresson JL, Perronne C, Launay O, Gerdil C, Saville M, Wood J, et al. Safety and immunogenicity of an inactivated split-virion influenza A/Vietnam/ 1194/2004 (H5N1) vaccine: phase I randomised trial. Lancet. 2006;367(9523): 1657-1664.

[106] Jackson LA, Gaglani MJ, Keyserling HL, Balser J, Bouveret N, Fries L, et al. Safety, efficacy, and immunogenicity of an inactivated influenza vaccine in healthy adults: a randomized, placebo-controlled trial over two influenza seasons. BMC Infectious Diseases 2010;10:71.

[107] Giezeman KM, Nauta J, de Bruijn IA, Palache AM. Trivalent inactivated subunit influenza vaccine Influvac®: 25-Year experience of safety and immunogenicity. Vaccine. 2009;27(18):2414-2417.

[108] van de Witte SV, Nauta J, Giezeman-Smits KM, de Voogd JM. Trivalent inactivated subunit influenza vaccine Influvac®: 30-year experience of safety and immunogenicity. Trials in Vaccinology. 2012;1(0):42-48.

[109] Krammer F, Hai R, Yondola M, Tan GS, Leyva-Grado V, Ryder AB, et al. Assessment of influenza virus hemagglutinin stalk-based immunity in ferrets. Journal of Virology. 2014.

[110] Haynes LM, Tonkin J, Anderson LJ, Tripp RA. Neutralizing anti-F glycoprotein and anti-substance P antibody treatment effectively reduces infection and inflammation associated with respiratory syncytial virus infection. Journal of Virology. 2002;76(14):6873-6881.

[111] Behera AK, Matsuse H, Kumar M, Kong X, Lockey RF, Mohapatra SS. Blocking intercellular adhesion molecule-1 on human epithelial cells decreases respiratory syncytial virus infection. Biochemical and Biophysical Research Communications. 2001;280(1):188-195.

[112] Charles CH, Luo GX, Kohlstaedt LA, Morantte IG, Gorfain E, Cao L, et al. Prevention of human rhinovirus infection by multivalent fab molecules directed against ICAM-1. Antimicrobial Agents and Chemotherapy. 2003;47(5):1503-1508.

[113] Welch K, Franke J, Kohler M, Macara IG. RanBP3 contains an unusual nuclear localization signal that is imported preferentially by importin-alpha 3. Molecular and Cellular Biology. 1999;19(12):8400-8411.

[114] Choudhary S, Boldogh S, Garofalo R, Jamaluddin M, Brasier AR. Respiratory Syncytial Virus Influences NF-{kappa}B-Dependent Gene Expression through a Novel Pathway Involving MAP3K14/NIK Expression and Nuclear Complex Formation with NF-{kappa}B2. Journal of Virology. 2005;79(14):8948-8959.

[115] Kosugi S, Hasebe M, Entani T, Takayama S, Tomita M, Yanagawa H. Design of peptide inhibitors for the importin alpha/beta nuclear import pathway by activity-based profiling. Chemistry Biology. 2008;15(9):940-949.

[116] Krishnan B, Szymanska A, Gierasch LM. Site-specific fluorescent labeling of poly-histidine sequences using a metal-chelating cysteine. Chemical Biology & Drug Design. 2007;69(1):31-40.

[117] Soh N. Selective chemical labeling of proteins with small fluorescent molecules based on metal-chelation methodology. Sensors. 2008;8(2):1004-1024.

[118] Lakowicz JR. Principles of fluorescence spectroscopy. New York: Plenum Press; 1983. xiv, 496 p.

[119] Okamoto S, Matsuoka S, Takenaka N, Haredy AM, Tanimoto T, Gomi Y, et al. Intranasal immunization with a formalin-inactivated human influenza A virus whole-virion vaccine alone and intranasal immunization with a split-virion vaccine with mucosal adjuvants show similar levels of cross-protection. Clinical and Vaccine Immunology: CVI. 2012;19(7):979-990.

[120] Huber VC, McCullers JA. Live attenuated influenza vaccine is safe and immunogenic in immunocompromised ferrets. Journal of Infectious Diseases. 2006;193(5):677-684.

[121] Sandbulte MR, Platt R, Roth JA, Henningson JN, Gibson KA, Rajao DS, et al. Divergent immune responses and disease outcomes in piglets immunized with inactivated and attenuated H3N2 swine influenza vaccines in the presence of maternally-derived antibodies. Virology. 2014;464-465C:45-54.

[122] Vincent AL, Ma W, Lager KM, Richt JA, Janke BH, Sandbulte MR, et al. Live attenuated influenza vaccine provides superior protection from heterologous infection in pigs with maternal antibodies without inducing vaccine-associated enhanced respiratory disease. Journal of Virology. 2012;86(19):10597-10605.

[123] Hoft DF, Babusis E, Worku S, Spencer CT, Lottenbach K, Truscott SM, et al. Live and inactivated influenza vaccines induce similar humoral responses, but only live vaccines

induce diverse T-cell responses in young children. The Journal of Infectious Diseases. 2011;204(6):845-853.

[124] Gerdil C. The annual production cycle for influenza vaccine. Vaccine. 2003;21(16): 1776-1779.

[125] Smith W, Westwood MA, Westwood JC, Belyavin G. Spontaneous mutation of influenza virus A during routine egg passage. British Journal of Experimental Pathology. 1951;32(5):422-432.

[126] National Institute for Biological Standards and Control. Influenza Virus Infectious IVR-165; NIBSC code: 11/220 (Ver. 1.0). WHO International Laboratory for Biological Standards,UK Official Medicines Control Laboratory.

[127] Skowronski DM, Janjua NZ, De Serres G, Sabaiduc S, Eshaghi A, Dickinson JA, et al. Low 2012–2013 influenza vaccine effectiveness associated with mutation in the egg-adapted H3N2 vaccine strain not antigenic drift in circulating viruses. PLoS One. 2014;9(3):e92153.

[128] Donis RO. Performance characteristics of qualified cell lines for isolation and propagation of influenza viruses for vaccine manufacturing. Vaccine.

[129] Hussain AI, Cordeiro M, Sevilla E, Liu J. Comparison of egg and high yielding MDCK cell-derived live attenuated influenza virus for commercial production of trivalent influenza vaccine: in vitro cell susceptibility and influenza virus replication kinetics in permissive and semi-permissive cells. Vaccine. 2010;28(22):3848-3855.

[130] Mochalova L, Gambaryan A, Romanova J, Tuzikov A, Chinarev A, Katinger D, et al. Receptor-binding properties of modern human influenza viruses primarily isolated in Vero and MDCK cells and chicken embryonated eggs. Virology. 2003;313(2):473-480.

[131] Jahangir A, Ruenphet S, Hara K, Shoham D, Sultana N, Okamura M, et al. Evaluation of human intestinal epithelial differentiated cells (Caco-2) for replication, plaque formation and isolation of avian influenza viruses. Journal of Virological Methods. 2010;169(1):232-238.

[132] Update on Novartis influenza vaccines acquisition [press release]. Melbourne, Australia, July 31, 2015.

[133] Vesikari T, Block SL, Guerra F, Lattanzi M, Holmes S, Izu A, et al. Immunogenicity, safety and reactogenicity of a mammalian cell-culture-derived influenza vaccine in healthy children and adolescents three to seventeen years of age. The Pediatric Infectious Disease Journal. 2012;31(5):494-500.

[134] Groth N, Montomoli E, Gentile C, Manini I, Bugarini R, Podda A. Safety, tolerability and immunogenicity of a mammalian cell-culture-derived influenza vaccine: a sequential Phase I and Phase II clinical trial. Vaccine. 2009;27(5): 786-791.

[135] Novartis Vaccines and Diagnositics I. FLUCELVAX [package insert]. 2013 (Cambridge, MA).

[136] Administration USFaD. FDA approves first seasonal influenza vaccine manufactured using cell culture technology [news release]. 2013.

[137] Doroshenko A, Halperin SA. Trivalent MDCK cell culture-derived influenza vaccine Optaflu (Novartis Vaccines). Expert Review of Vaccines. 2009;8(6):679-688.

[138] Chan CY, Tambyah PA. Preflucel(R): a Vero-cell culture-derived trivalent influenza vaccine. Expert Review of Vaccines. 2012;11(7):759-773.

[139] Plosker GL. A/H5N1 prepandemic influenza vaccine (whole virion, vero cell-derived, inactivated) [Vepacel(R)]. Drugs. 2012;72(11):1543-1557.

[140] Genzel Y, Rodig J, Rapp E, Reichl U. Vaccine production: upstream processing with adherent or suspension cell lines. Methods in Molecular Biology (Clifton, NJ). 2014;1104:371-393.

[141] Thompson C, Petiot E, Lennaertz A, Henry O, Kamen A. Analytical technologies for influenza virus-like particle candidate vaccines: challenges and emerging approaches. Virology Journal. 2013;10(1):141.

[142] Quan F, Steinhauer D, Huang C, Ross T, Compans R, Kang S-M. A bivalent influenza VLP vaccine confers complete inhibition of virus replication in lungs. Vaccine. 2008;26:3352-3361.

[143] Mahmood K, Bright R, Mytle N, Carter D, Crevar C, Achenbach J, et al. H5N1 VLP vaccine induced protection in ferrets against lethal challenge with highly pathogenic H5N1 influenza viruses. Vaccine. 2008;26:5393-5399.

[144] Wu C-Y, Yeh Y-C, Chan J-T, Yang Y-C, Yang J-R, Liu M-T, et al. A VLP vaccine induces broad-spectrum cross-protective antibody immunity against H5N1 and H1N1 subtypes of influenza A virus. PLoS One. 2012;7:e42363.

[145] Tang X-C, Lu H-R, Ross T. Baculovirus-produced influenza virus-like particles in mammalian cells protect mice from lethal influenza challenge. Viral Immunology 2011;24:311-319.

[146] Bright R, Carter D, Daniluk S, Toapanta F, Ahmad A, Gavrilov V, et al. Influenza virus-like particles elicit broader immune responses than whole virion inactivated influenza virus or recombinant hemagglutinin. Vaccine. 2007;25:3871-3878.

[147] Schneider-Ohrum K, Ross TM. Virus-like particles for antigen delivery at mucosal surfaces. Current Topics in Microbiology and Immunology. 2012;354:53-73.

[148] Pincus S BS, Li J, Sadowski T, Pincus BS. Release and stability testing programs for a novel virus-like particle vaccine. BioPharm International. 26-34.

[149] Galarza JM, Latham T, Cupo A. Virus-like particle (VLP) vaccine conferred complete protection against a lethal influenza virus challenge. Viral Immunology. 2005;18(1):244-251.

[150] Cox RJ, Pedersen G, Madhun AS, Svindland S, Saevik M, Breakwell L, et al. Evaluation of a virosomal H5N1 vaccine formulated with Matrix M adjuvant in a phase I clinical trial. Vaccine. 2011;29(45):8049-8059.

[151] Nachbagauer R, Wohlbold TJ, Hirsh A, Hai R, Sjursen H, Palese P, et al. Induction of broadly-reactive anti-hemagglutinin stalk antibodies by an H5N1 vaccine in humans. Journal of Virology. 2014.

[152] Kim MC, Lee YN, Hwang HS, Lee YT, Ko EJ, Jung YJ, et al. Influenza M2 virus-like particles confer a broader range of cross protection to the strain-specific pre-existing immunity. Vaccine. 2014.

[153] Wu CY, Yeh YC, Yang YC, Chou C, Liu MT, Wu HS, et al. Mammalian expression of virus-like particles for advanced mimicry of authentic influenza virus. PLoS One. 2010;5(3):e9784.

[154] Ross TM, Mahmood K, Crevar CJ, Schneider-Ohrum K, Heaton PM, Bright RA. A trivalent virus-like particle vaccine elicits protective immune responses against seasonal influenza strains in mice and ferrets. PLoS One. 2009;4(6):e6032.

[155] Pincus S, Boddapati S, Li J, Sadowski T, Pincus B. Release and stability testing programs for a novel virus-like particle vaccine. BioPharm International 2010: 26-34.

[156] Khurana S, Wu J, Verma N, Verma S, Raghunandan R, Manischewitz J, et al. H5N1 virus-like particle vaccine elicits cross-reactive neutralizing antibodies that preferentially bind to the oligomeric form of influenza virus hemagglutinin in humans. Journal of Virology. 2011;85(21):10945-10954.

[157] Lopez-Macias C, Ferat-Osorio E, Tenorio-Calvo A, Isibasi A, Talavera J, Arteaga-Ruiz O, et al. Safety and immunogenicity of a virus-like particle pandemic influenza A (H1N1) 2009 vaccine in a blinded, randomized, placebo-controlled trial of adults in Mexico. Vaccine. 2011;29(44):7826-7834.

[158] Vasiljeva I, Kozlovska T, Cielens I, Strelnikova A, Kazaks A, Ose V, et al. Mosaic Qbeta coats as a new presentation model. FEBS Letters. 1998;431(1):7-11.

[159] Fang NX, Frazer IH, Fernando GJ. Differences in the post-translational modifications of human papillomavirus type 6b major capsid protein expressed from a baculovirus system compared with a vaccinia virus system. Biotechnology and Applied Biochemistry. 2000;32 (Pt 1):27-33.

[160] Jegerlehner A, Tissot A, Lechner F, Sebbel P, Erdmann I, Kundig T, et al. A molecular assembly system that renders antigens of choice highly repetitive for induction of protective B cell responses. Vaccine. 2002;20(25-26):3104-3112.

[161] Jegerlehner A, Zabel F, Langer A, Dietmeier K, Jennings GT, Saudan P, et al. Bacterially produced recombinant influenza vaccines based on virus-like particles. PLoS One. 2013;8(11):e78947.

[162] Low JG, Lee LS, Ooi EE, Ethirajulu K, Yeo P, Matter A, et al. Safety and immunogenicity of a virus-like particle pandemic influenza A (H1N1) 2009 vaccine: Results from a double-blinded, randomized Phase I clinical trial in healthy Asian volunteers. Vaccine. 2014;32(39):5041-5048.

[163] Ogunremi O, Pasick J, Kobinger GP, Hannaman D, Berhane Y, Clavijo A, et al. A single electroporation delivery of a DNA vaccine containing the hemagglutinin gene of Asian H5N1 avian influenza virus generated a protective antibody response in chickens against a North American virus strain. Clinical and Vaccine Immunology: CVI. 2013;20(4):491-500.

[164] Sawaengsak C, Mori Y, Yamanishi K, Srimanote P, Chaicumpa W, Mitrevej A, et al. Intranasal chitosan-DNA vaccines that protect across influenza virus subtypes. International Journal of Pharmaceutics. 2014;473(1-2):113-125.

[165] Yager EJ, Stagnar C, Gopalakrishnan R, Fuller JT, Fuller DH. Optimizing particle-mediated epidermal delivery of an influenza DNA vaccine in ferrets. Methods in Molecular Biology (Clifton, NJ). 2013;940:223-237.

[166] Shim BS, Choi JA, Song HH, Park SM, Cheon IS, Jang JE, et al. Sublingual administration of bacteria-expressed influenza virus hemagglutinin 1 (HA1) induces protection against infection with 2009 pandemic H1N1 influenza virus. Journal of Microbiology (Seoul, Korea). 2013;51(1):130-135.

[167] Song JH, Nguyen HH, Cuburu N, Horimoto T, Ko SY, Park SH, et al. Sublingual vaccination with influenza virus protects mice against lethal viral infection. Proceedings of the National Academy of Sciences of the United States of America. 2008;105(5): 1644-1649.

[168] Seibert CW, Rahmat S, Krause JC, Eggink D, Albrecht RA, Goff PH, et al. Recombinant IgA is sufficient to prevent influenza virus transmission in guinea pigs. Journal of Virology. 2013;87(14):7793-7804.

[169] Christian LM. Optimizing benefits of influenza virus vaccination during pregnancy: potential behavioral risk factors and interventions. Vaccine. 2014;32(25):2958-2964.

[170] Eichner M, Schwehm M, Hain J, Uphoff H, Salzberger B, Knuf M, et al. 4Flu - an individual based simulation tool to study the effects of quadrivalent vaccination on seasonal influenza in Germany. BMC Infectious Diseases. 2014;14:365.

[171] O'Grady KA, McHugh L, Nolan T, Richmond P, Wood N, Marshall HS, et al. FluMum: a prospective cohort study of mother-infant pairs assessing the effectiveness of maternal influenza vaccination in prevention of influenza in early infancy. BMJ open. 2014;4(6):e005676.

[172] Blanchard-Rohner G, Meier S, Bel M, Combescure C, Othenin-Girard V, Swali RA, et al. Influenza vaccination given at least 2 weeks before delivery to pregnant women facilitates transmission of seroprotective influenza-specific antibodies to the newborn. The Pediatric Infectious Disease Journal. 2013;32(12):1374-1380.

[173] Sandbulte MR, Jimenez GS, Boon AC, Smith LR, Treanor JJ, Webby RJ. Cross-reactive neuraminidase antibodies afford partial protection against H5N1 in mice and are present in unexposed humans. PLoS Medicine. 2007;4(2):e59.

[174] Chen Z, Kadowaki S, Hagiwara Y, Yoshikawa T, Matsuo K, Kurata T, et al. Cross-protection against a lethal influenza virus infection by DNA vaccine to neuraminidase. Vaccine. 2000;18(28):3214-3222.

[175] Jameson J, Cruz J, Ennis FA. Human cytotoxic T-lymphocyte repertoire to influenza A viruses. Journal of Virology. 1998;72(11):8682-8689.

[176] Antrobus RD, Berthoud TK, Mullarkey CE, Hoschler K, Coughlan L, Zambon M, et al. Coadministration of seasonal influenza vaccine and MVA-NP+M1 simultaneously achieves potent humoral and cell-mediated responses. Molecular Therapy: the Journal of the American Society of Gene Therapy. 2014;22(1):233-238.

[177] Khanna M, Sharma S, Kumar B, Rajput R. Protective immunity based on the conserved hemagglutinin stalk domain and its prospects for universal influenza vaccine development. BioMed Research International. 2014;2014:546274.

[178] Bommakanti G, Citron MP, Hepler RW, Callahan C, Heidecker GJ, Najar TA, et al. Design of an HA2-based Escherichia coli expressed influenza immunogen that protects mice from pathogenic challenge. Proceedings of the National Academy of Sciences. 2010;107(31):13701-13706.

[179] Krammer F, Pica N, Hai R, Margine I, Palese P. Chimeric hemagglutinin influenza virus vaccine constructs elicit broadly protective stalk-specific antibodies. Journal of Virology. 2013;87(12):6542-6550.

[180] Giles BM, Bissel SJ, Dealmeida DR, Wiley CA, Ross TM. Antibody breadth and protective efficacy are increased by vaccination with computationally optimized hemagglutinin but not with polyvalent hemagglutinin-based H5N1 virus-like particle vaccines. Clinical and VaccineI: CVI. 2012;19(2):128-139.

[181] Giles BM, Ross TM. A computationally optimized broadly reactive antigen (COBRA) based H5N1 VLP vaccine elicits broadly reactive antibodies in mice and ferrets. Vaccine. 2011;29(16):3043-3054.

[182] Giles BM, Crevar CJ, Carter DM, Bissel SJ, Schultz-Cherry S, Wiley CA, et al. A computationally optimized hemagglutinin virus-like particle vaccine elicits broadly reactive antibodies that protect nonhuman primates from H5N1 infection. Journal of Infectious Diseases. 2012;205(10):1562-1570.

[183] Kempe A, Daley MF, Stokley S, Crane LA, Beaty BL, Barrow J, et al. Impact of a severe influenza vaccine shortage on primary care practice. American Journal of Preventive Medicine. 2007;33(6):486-491.

[184] McQuillan L, Daley MF, Stokley S, Crane LA, Beaty BL, Barrow J, et al. Impact of the 2004-2005 influenza vaccine shortage on pediatric practice: a national survey. Pediatrics. 2009;123(2):e186-e192.

[185] Singer E. Chiron flu flap suggests vaccine industry needs shot in the arm. Nature Medicine. 2004;10(11):1148.

[186] Sheridan C. Chiron's manufacturing misfortunes boost competitors. Nat Biotechonology. 2005;23(10):1191.

Chapter 6

Influenza Inactive Virus Vaccine with the Fusion Peptide (rTα1-BP5) Enhances Protection Against Influenza Through Humoral and Cell-Mediated Immunity

Chen Wang, Chengshui Liao, Wufan Zhang,
Deyuan Li and Puyan Chen

Additional information is available at the end of the chapter

http://dx.doi.org/10.5772/64403

Abstract

Thymosin $\alpha 1$ (Tα1) and Bursopentin (BP5) are both immunopotentiators. To explore whether the thymosin α1-Bursopentin (rTα1-BP5) is an adjuvant or not, we cloned the gene of Tα1-BP5 and provided evidence that the gene of Tα1-BP5 in a recombinant prokaryotic expression plasmid was successfully expressed in *Escherichia coli* BL21. To evaluate the immune adjuvant properties of rTα1-BP5, chickens were immunized with rTα1-BP5 combined with H9N2 avian influenza whole-inactivated virus (WIV). The titers of HI antibody, antigen-specific antibodies, Avian influenza virus (AIV)-neutralizing antibodies, levels of Th1-type cytokines (gamma interferon (IFN-γ)) and Th2-type cytokines (interleukin 4 (IL-4)), and lymphocyte proliferation responses were determined. We found that rTα1-BP5 enhanced HI antibody and antigen-specific immunoglobulin G (IgG) antibodies titers, increased the level of AIV-neutralizing antibodies, induced the secretion of Th1- and Th2-type cytokines, and promoted the proliferation of T and B lymphocyte. Furthermore, virus challenge experiments confirmed that rTα1-BP5 contributed to the inhibition replication of the virus (H9N2 AIV (A/chicken/Jiangsu/NJ07/05) from chicken lungs. Altogether, these findings suggest that rTα1-BP5 is a novel adjuvant suitable for H9N2 avian influenza vaccine.

Keywords: thymosin α1 (Tα1), Bursopentin (BP5), fusion peptide, avian influenza vaccine, adjuvant

1. Introduction

Avian influenza virus (AIV) is an enveloped virus that belongs to the *Orthomyxoviridae* family and has an eight-segmented, single-stranded, negative-sense RNA genome. Among the proteins encoded by the genome, there are two surface glycoproteins, hemagglutinin (HA) and neuraminidase (NA) [1]. AIVs are classified into subtypes according to the combination of 16 HA and nine NA molecules. Among the many subtypes of AIV, H9N2 is thought to have originated from shorebirds and gulls, and has rapidly spread to become one of the most prevalent diseases in domestic poultry worldwide. It also causes serious economic loss in the poultry industry [2] (see **Table 1**).

Abbreviation	Full name
Tα1	Thymosin α1
BP5	Bursopentin
rTα1-BP5	Thymosin α1-Bursopentin
WIV	Whole-inactivated virus
AIV	Avian influenza virus
HA	Hemagglutinin
NA	Neuraminidase
BRM	Biological response modifier
MIF	Macrophage migration inhibitory factor
BF	Bursa of Fabricius
BLP	Bursin-like epitope peptide
HI	Hemagglutination inhibition assay
IFN-γ	Interferon-γ
IL-4	Interleukin-4
TNF-α	Tumor necrosis factor-α
Th	T-helper type
Th1	T-helper type 1
Th2	T-helper type 2
MDCK	Madin-Darby canine kidney
FBS	Fetal bovine serum
MTT	3-(4,5-dimethylthiazol-2-yl)2,5-diphenyltetrazolium bromide
IPTG	Isopropyl-β-D-thiogalactoside
ConA	Concanavalin A
PMA	Phorbol-12-myristate-13-acetate

http://dx.doi.org/10.5772/64403

Abbreviation	Full name
TMB	Tetramethyl benzidine
HRP	Horseradish peroxidase
SPF	Specific pathogen-free
SOE-PCR	Splicing overlap extension PCR method
TRX	Thioredoxin
$TCID_{50}$	50% tissue culture infective dose
PBS	phosphate-buffered saline
pfu	Plaque-forming unit
OD	Optical density
IgG	Immunoglobulin G
ELISA	Enzyme-linked immunosorbent assay
$PRNT_{50}$	50% plaque-reducing neutralizing titer

Table 1. Abbreviations for full name.

In domestic avian species in North America, H9N2 influenza viruses occur primarily in turkeys, occasionally in quail, and rarely if ever in chickens. The H9N2 virus subtype was first isolated from turkeys in 1966 [3], when the virus was associated with mild respiratory disease. In Asia, long-term surveillance in live poultry markets in Hong Kong from 1975 to 1985 detected H9N2 influenza viruses in apparently healthy ducks but not in chickens [4]. Since the early 1990s, H9N2 influenza viruses have become widespread in domestic chickens in Asia [5]. Among the avian influenza A virus subtypes, H9N2 viruses have the potential to cause an influenza pandemic because they are widely prevalent in avian species in Asia and have demonstrated the ability to infect humans [6]. In April 1999, two World Health Organization reference laboratories independently confirmed the isolation of avian influenza A (H9N2) viruses for the first time in humans [7].

The best protection against influenza virus infection remains effective vaccination [8]. Inactivated vaccines have been undergoing clinical trials as pandemic vaccine candidates, and it has been shown that inactivated vaccines elicit strong humoral responses; however, it is commonly accepted that no adequate mucosal or cellular immunity is achieved [9]. Adjuvants are able to improve the quantity and quality of innate immune responses by enhancing their speed and duration, and by inducing adequate adaptive immunity [10]. To improve methods for influenza vaccine production, the current strategy of many investigators is to increase the efficacy of pandemic influenza vaccines by the addition of adjuvants to boost immune responses, such as aluminum salts, MF59, IC31®, and chitosan [11–14].

A defined peptide sequence able to stimulate specific immune cell subsets has the potential to act as an adjuvant for a variety of immunogens. The thymus is an important central immune organ for T-lymphocyte differentiation and maturation [15]. It is capable of secreting many peptides with the functions of regulating the development of different phenotypic markers and lymphocyte [16]. Thymosin alpha 1 (Tα1), an immunomodulatory peptide consisting of 28 amino acid residues, was isolated originally from calf thymus [17]. As a biological response modifier (BRM), Tα1 has multiple biological activities in the immune system. It can promote specific lymphocyte functions, stimulate the production of lymphokines such as gamma interferon (IFN-γ), tumor necrosis factor-α (TNF-α), interleukin 2 (IL-2), macrophage migration inhibitory factor (MIF), and precursor stem cell into the CD4+/CD8+ T cells, increase T-cell proliferation, differentiation and maturation, and so on [18, 19]. Furthermore, it has the activities of antitumor and protection against oxidative damage [20]. Consequently, Tα1 is widely used in clinic treating various diseases including immunodeficiency diseases, severe sepsis, and systemic infectious disorder [21].

The bursa of Fabricius (BF) is a primary humoral immune organ unique to birds and is the site of B-lymphocyte development and differentiation. The tripeptidebursin (LysHisGlyNH2) has been described as an endogenous B-cell stimulant or differentiation factor [22]. BS and bursin-like peptide T-X-N-L-K-H-G significantly enhance the JEV subtype vaccine-induced immune response in immunized mice [23]. Bursin-like epitope peptide (BLP) is one of bursin-like peptides and enhances immune responses in mice immunized with inactivated H9N2 avian influenza vaccine [24]. Our previous study has been reported that Bursopentin (BP5) is a small peptide separated from BF, which amino acid sequence is CKDVY. We found that BP5 not only promotes T-cell and B-cell proliferation, enhances humoral immunity and cellular immunity but also balances Th1 and Th2 immune responses [25, 26].

Although both Tα1 and BP5 have the potent adjuvant effects, this study designed and synthesized Tα1-BP5 fusion gene according to the preferential codons of *Escherichia coli*, fused with prokaryotic expression vector pET-32a, and then transferred into *E. coli* BL21 to induce its expression. Then, we tested whether rTα1-BP5 could enhance immune responses in chicken upon vaccination with H9N2 avian influenza whole-inactivated virus (WIV).

2. Materials and methods

2.1. Plasmid, viruses, and reagents

pET-32a (+), *E. coli* DH5α, *E. coli* BL21 (DE3), pET32a (+)-BP5, and avian influenza virus A/Chicken/Jiangsu/JS-1/2002(H9N2) were maintained in our laboratory. Avian influenza virus A/Chicken/Jiangsu/NJ08/05(H9N2) was kindly provided by Dr. Qi-Sheng Zheng. Virus titers were determined in MDCK cells. H9N2 avian influenza whole-inactivated virus (WIV) was prepared by diluting the virus 1:4000 (v/v) in formalin [27, 28]. All restriction enzymes and *Taq* polymerase were purchased from TakaRa Biotechnology (Dalian, China). RPMI 1640 medium and fetal bovine serum (FBS) were purchased from Gibco (New York, NY, USA). Isopropyl-β-D-thiogalactoside (IPTG), 3-(4,5-dimethylthiazol-2-yl)2,5-diphenyltetrazolium bromide (MTT), TEMED, dNTP, Concanavalin A (ConA), Phorbol-12-myristate-13-acetate (PMA), and tetramethylbenzidine (TMB) were purchased from Jiu Shi Corporation (Zhengzhou, China). Horseradish peroxidase (HRP)-conjugated goat anti-mice IgG was obtained from Boshide Corporation (Wuhan, China). Control Standard Tα1 and BP5 peptides were synthesized by

Shanghai Science Peptide Biological Technology Co., Ltd. (Shanghai, China), and the purity was over 95%.

2.2. Chicken embryos, animals, and vaccines

Specific pathogen-free (SPF) Roman chicken and chicken embryos were obtained from the Henan Experimental Animal Research Center. Avian influenza virus A/Chicken/Jiangsu/NJ08/05(H9N2) (10^7 $TCID_{50}$/0.1 mL) was inoculated into the allantoic cavities of 10-day-old SPF chicken embryos; the embryos that died within 24 h were discarded, and the allantoic fluids were harvested from the infected embryos at 48 h postinfection and inactivated by treatment with 0.2% formalin. The inactivated virus was emulsified with mineral oil to make an oil-formulated inactivated H9N2 AIV vaccine. One dose of the vaccine contained 10^7 $TCID_{50}$/0.1 mL, which was equal to it before inactivation. Procedure and test of inactivated vaccine were described according to OIE Terrestrial Manual 2012 [29].

2.3. Gene cloning and expression of the recombinant fusion peptide Tα1-BP5

Gene of the recombinant fusion peptide thymosin α1-Bursopentin (Tα1-BP5) was designed according to the preferential codons of *E. coli* and amplified by splicing overlap extension polymerase chain reaction (SOE-PCR) method [30]. Sequences of the primers used for the synthetic Tα1-BP5 are as follows: F1: 5′-CCG GAA TTC AGC GAC GCT GCT GTT GAC ACT AGC AGC GAA ATC ACT ACTA AAG ACT TG-3′; F2: 5′-GTT CGG GGT GCTG CCG CCG CCG CCG TTT TCA GCT TCT TCA ACA ACT TCT TTT TTT TCT TTC AAG TCT TTA GTA GT-3′; and F3: 5′-GGC GGC GGC GGC AGC TGC AAA AAT GTG TAT TAA GTC GAC TCG-3′, with *EcoR* I and *Sal* I site (underlined). The genes of Tα1 and BP5 were connected with the gene of the GGGGS linker to form the Tα1-BP5 fusion gene. And then, the amplified DNA fragment was digested by *EcoR* I and *Sal* I, and then ligated into the expression vector pET32a. The ligation mix was transformed into competent DH5α cells and the single bacterial colony was selected by overnight growth on Luria broth (LB) agar plates containing 100-μg/mL ampicillin. The obtained recombinant plasmid pET32a-Tα1-BP5 was confirmed by restriction endonuclease digestion and DNA sequencing. The pET32a-Tα1-BP5 plasmid was transformed into *E. coli* BL21 (DE3) for inducing expression. The expression products were examined by sodium dodecyl sulfate-polyacrylamide gel electrophoresis (SDS-PAGE). And the recombinant proteins were purified on a Ni-affinity chromatography column (Amersham Bioscience HiTrap chelating HP 5 mL × one column) following the manufacturer's instructions.

2.4. Activity testing of fusion peptide Tα1-BP5 (rTα1-BP5) in vitro

Thymus and spleens from 4 to 6-week-BALB/c mice with (20 ± 2) g were collected aseptically, put them at 200-mesh stainless screen mesh cells, and gently minced into single cell suspension with a syringe followed by adding Hank's solution. The red blood cells were removed by centrifugation at 500 rpm for 5 min. The supernatant was centrifuged at 500 rpm for 5 min. The obtained pellet was washed with Hank's solution twice. The density of lymphocytes was adjusted to around 5×10^6 cells/mL using RPMI-1640 medium containing 10% FBS. ConA and PMA were added into thymic lymphocytes and splenic lymphocytes to make the concentrations reach 5 μg/mL and 300 ng/mL, respectively. The two kinds of solutions were subpackaged into a 96-well plate with 100 μL/well, respectively, and three parallel samples were set for each well. The plates were incubated in CO_2 incubator at 37°C for 6 h, followed by adding 100-μL/well rTα1-BP5 (affinity chromatography purified through Ni column) with different concentrations (1.25, 2.5, 5.0, 10.0, and 20.0 μg/mL) and continued culturing for 72 h. Control groups (phosphate-buffered saline (PBS), 10.0 μg/mL thioredoxin, 10.0 μg/mL Tα1, and 10.0 μg/mL BP5) were used following the same procedures. MTT method was used to test the effect of rTα1-BP5 effect on thymic and splenic lymphocytes proliferation. Relative ratio of cell proliferation (%) = (experimental group OD_{570}/control group OD_{570}) × 100% [31, 32].

2.5. Immunization of chickens

All animal experiments were approved by the Henan University of Science and Technology Animal Care and Use Committee. Twenty-one-day-old SPF Roman chickens were randomly divided into six experimental groups of 25 chickens each and intramuscularly immunized two times on days 0 and 14 with (i) 100 μL PBS as a negative control, (ii) 100 μL H9N2 WIV (A/Chicken/Jiangsu/NJ08/05, 10^7 $TCID_{50}$/0.1 mL), (iii) a mixture of 100 μL H9N2 WIV and Tα1 (50 μg), (iv) a mixture of 100 μL H9N2 WIV and BP5 (50 μg), (v) a mixture of 100 μL H9N2 WIV and rTα1-BP5 (50 μg), and (vi) 100 μL oil-formulated inactivated H9N2 AIV vaccine (A/Chicken/Jiangsu/NJ08/05, 10^7 $TCID_{50}$/0.1 mL) as a positive control (**Table 2**).

Group	Vaccination on days 0 and 14[a]
1	100 μL PBS
2	10^7 $TCID_{50}$ H9N2 WIV
3	10^7 $TCID_{50}$ H9N2 WIV + 50 μg Tα1
4	10^7 $TCID_{50}$ H9N2 WIV + 50 μg BP5
5	10^7 $TCID_{50}$ H9N2 WIV + 50 μg rTα1-BP5
6	10^7 $TCID_{50}$ H9N2 AIV vaccine

[a] H9N2 WIV, inactivated H9N2 avian influenza whole-inactivated virus; H9N2 AIV vaccine, H9N2 avian influenza virus vaccine prepared with oil/water as an adjuvant.

Table 2. Animal groups and the experimental design.

The details of the animal experiment time points are shown in **Figure 1**.

2.6. Detection of antibodies in serum

Chicken (n = 5 per group) sera were collected on 7 and 21 days after the first immunization. Serum antibody (HI and antigen-specific antibodies) titers were determined using standard HI microliter and enzyme-linked immunosorbent assay (ELISA) as described [25, 33]. Briefly, to detect the HI titers in chicken serum, sera were inactivated by incubation for 30 min at 56°C and serially diluted twofold in PBS, then transferred in duplicate to 96-well round-bottomed

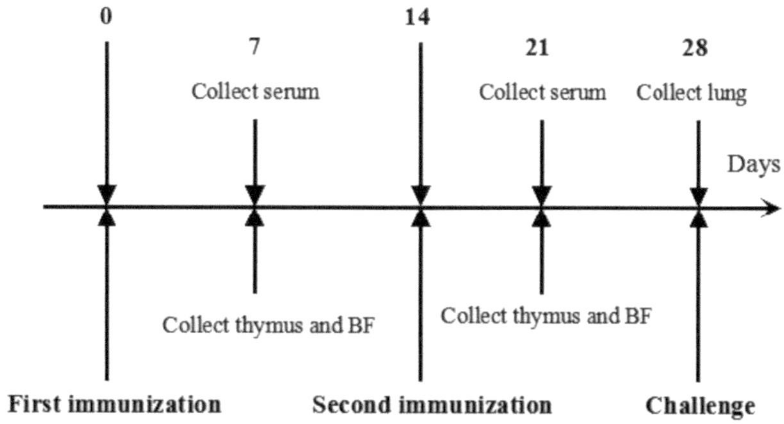

Figure 1. Experimental scheme of immunization, sample collection, and challenge.

plates. Standard avian influenza virus (A/Chicken/Shandong/6/96(H9N2)) antigen with four units was then added to each diluted serum samples in a volume of 50 μL, and followed by an equal volume of 0.5% chicken erythrocyte suspensions. The mixture was incubated for 1 h at room temperature before the results were read. The HI titers were defined as the highest serum dilution capable of preventing hemagglutination.

To evaluate the antigen-specific antibodies titers, ELISA plates were coated with 10-μg/mL recombinant influenza HA protein (expressed in *E. coli* BL21) and blocked with 1% bovine serum albumin (BSA) for 2 h at 37°C. Aliquots of diluted chicken sera were added to the plates, which were then incubated overnight, washed, and incubated with HRP-conjugated goat anti-chicken IgG. Finally, TMB was added and the reaction was stopped by the addition of 2N H_2SO_4 and the absorbance was read at OD_{450}. Each serum sample was repeated in quintuplicate. The results were plotted as OD versus dilution (log scale). Titers at half maximal OD were determined by linear interpolation [34].

2.7. Determination of AIV-neutralizing antibodies

Inactivated sera were incubated with 100 plaque-forming unit (pfu) of avian influenza virus (A/Chicken/Jiangsu/JS-1/2002(H9N2), and the titers of AIV-neutralizing antibodies determined as described [35].

2.8. Cytokine assays

On 7 and 21 days after the first immunization, the serum levels of Th1-type cytokine (IFN-γ) in chickens were determined using commercial Chicken cytokines gamma interferon ELISA kits (Cusabio Biotech, MD, USA), whereas Th2-type cytokine (IL-4) was determined with another commercial Chicken cytokines interleukin 4 ELISA kits (Cusabio Biotech, USA). The procedure followed the manufacturer's instructions.

2.9. Lymphocyte proliferation response

To detect changes in cellular immunity, lymphocyte proliferation response was performed. Thymus and bursa of Fabricius were collected from immunized chickens at 7 and 21 days after the first immunization. The thymus and BF lymphocytes were isolated and maintained in 1640 medium supplemented with 10% FBS at 37°C with 5% CO_2. The thymus lymphocytes (5×10^6 cells/mL) were seeded in a 96-well plate and incubated with 50 μL of ConA (40 μg/mL) at 40°C/5% CO_2 for 48 h, whereas the BF lymphocytes (5×10^6 cells/mL) were treated with 50 μL of PMA (1 μg/mL) in a 96-well plate at 40°C/5% CO_2 for 24 h. Then, the lymphocyte proliferation assay was performed using a standard MTT method as described previously [36, 37]. Then, the plate was incubated with 10 μL of 5 mg/mL MTT for 3 h. Finally, 100 μL of 10% (w/v) SDS in 0.01 M HCl was added into the plate and allowed to incubate for 2 h. A spectrophotometric measurement was taken at A_{570}.

2.10. Virus challenge experiment

Two weeks after the second vaccination, chickens (n = 15 per group) were intranasally challenged with 2.5×10^6 $TCID_{50}$ avian influenza virus A/chicken/Jiangsu/JS-1/2002(H9N2) in 100 μL PBS. Five chickens per group were humanely sacrificed at 3, 5, and 7 days after virus challenge and the viral titers in their lungs assessed by plaque formation assays using MDCK cells as described [35].

2.11. Statistical analysis

Statistical analyses were performed using unpaired *t*-tests or one-way analysis of variance (ANOVA) *F*-statistics followed by GraphPad Prism 6 software. Data are presented as the mean ± standard deviation (SD). Turkey multiple comparison tests were used to assess differences among the five experimental groups, with differences being considered significant at $P < 0.05$ or $P < 0.01$.

3. Results

3.1. Expression of the recombinant fusion peptide Tα1-BP5

The gene of Tα1-BP5 was amplified by SOE-PCR with the primers F1, F2, and F3. The PCR products were identified by electrophoresis, and then about 114bp strip was observed. The recombinant plasmid was extracted and identified with *Hind* III enzyme. The results showed that the recombinant plasmid was not digested by *Hind* III, indicating that the recombinant plasmid had deleted the *Hind* III restriction site (**Figure 2A**). Sequencing result showed that the gene of the recombinant fusion peptide Tα1-BP5 was inserted into pET32a vector, and it was consistent to the expected size (**Table 3**), which was suggested that the recombinant expression vector was constructed successfully, and it was named pET32a-Tα1-BP5. Then, pET32a-Tα1-BP5 was transferred into *E. coli* BL21 (DE3) for its expression, and the expressed products were detected by using SDS-PAGE. The result showed that Tα1-BP5 was expressed and purified with the molecular weight of 31.4 kDa (**Figure 2B**), which is consistent with its predicted molecular weight.

Name	Amino acid sequence
Tα1-BP5	Ser Asp Ala Ala Val Asp Thr Ser Ser Glu Ile Thr Thr Lys Asp Leu Lys Glu Lys Lys Glu Val Val Glu Glu Ala Glu Asn Gly Gly Gly Gly Ser Cys Lys Asp Val Tyr

Table 3. Amino acid sequence of recombinant fusion peptide Tα1-BP5.

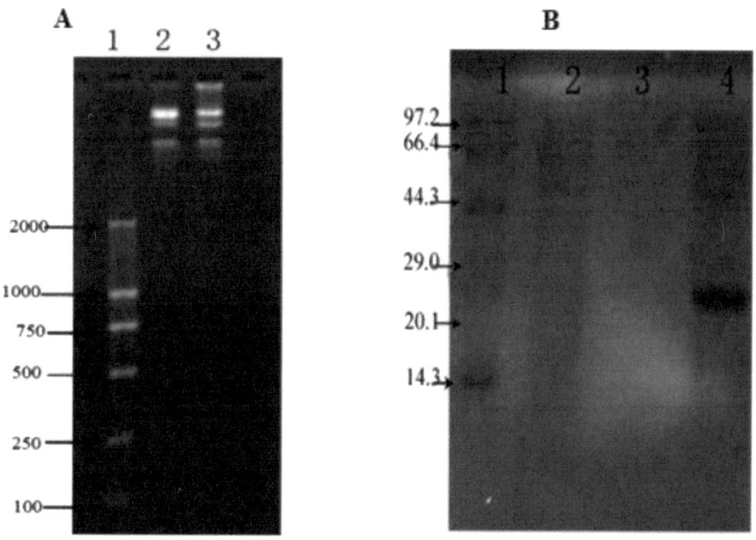

Figure 2. Identification of the recombinant plasmid pET32a-Tα1-BP5 and the expression of fusion peptide Tα1-BP5 in *E. coli*. (A) 1: DL2000 marker; 2: the recombinant plasmid pET32a-Tα1-BP5 after *Hind* III enzyme digestion; and 3: the recombinant plasmid pET32a-Tα1-BP5. (B) 1: low molecular weight protein marker; 2: not induced *E. coli* BL21 (DE3); 3: Not induced recombinant *E. coli* BL21 (DE3)/pET32a-Tα1-BP5; 4: induced recombinant *E. coli* BL21 (DE3)/pET32a-Tα1-BP5.

3.2. Activity of rTα1-BP5 in vitro

The expressed product of TBP5 recombinant bacteria was affinity chromatography purified through protein Ni column and quantified through spectrophotometer. MTT method was used to test the effect of rTα1-BP5 on the proliferation of mouse thymic and splenic lymphocytes. The results showed that all rTα1-BP5 with different concentrations (1.25, 2.5, 5.0, 10.0, and 20.0 μg/mL) could promote the proliferation of thymic and splenic lymphocytes compared to PBS group. rTα1-BP5 could stimulate thymic and splenic lymphocytes proliferation stronger than TP5 and BP5. The differences were significant ($P < 0.05$) on the concentrations of 5.0 and 20.0 μg/mL, and the differences were more significant ($P < 0.01$) on the concentrations of 10.0 μg/mL (**Figure 3A** and **B**). All these data demonstrated that rTα1-BP5 could promote the proliferation of mouse thymic T lymphocytes and splenic B lymphocytes.

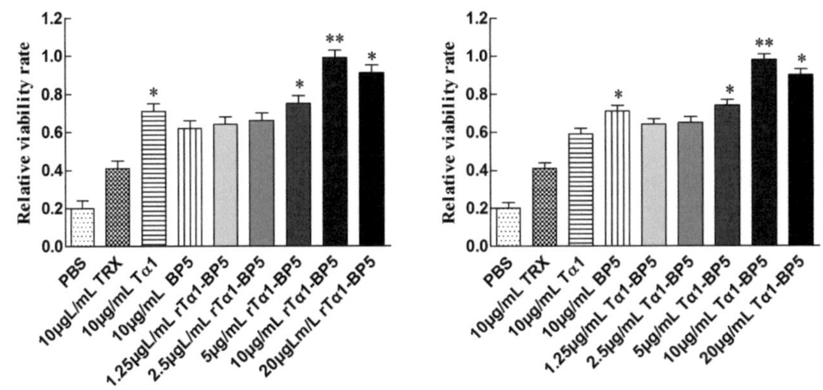

Figure 3. The effects of rTα1-BP5 on the proliferation of thymic lymphocytes (A) or splenic lymphocytes (B) from immunized mice. The data presented are of five replicates. *, $P < 0.05$, compared with mice immunized with PBS, and **, $P < 0.01$, compared with mice immunized with BP5 or Tα1.

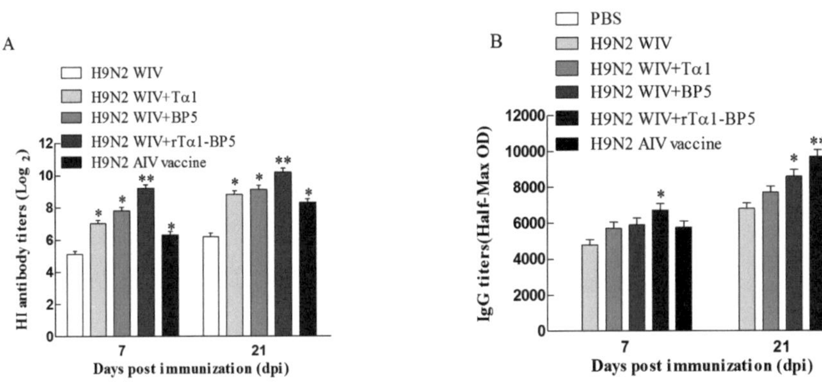

Figure 4. Effect of rTα1-BP5 to H9N2 AIV vaccination on antigen-specific HI titers and anti-HA IgG antibodies. Chickens were immunized two times, and chicken sera were collected on days 7 and 21 after the first immunization, and the serum HI titers (A) and IgG titers (B) were analyzed by HI assay and ELISA, respectively. The data presented are means ± SD of results from five replicates. *, $P < 0.05$, and **, $P < 0.01$, compared with chickens immunized with H9N2 WIV alone.

3.3. rTα1-BP5 stimulates significant antigen-specific immune responses

To determine antigen-specific immune responses to immunization, chickens were immunized two times, then sera were taken on days 7 and 21 after the first immunization and detected for HI and anti-HA antibody titers. HI antibody titers of chickens immunized with inactivated vaccine, Tα1 combined with H9N2 WIV and BP5 combined with H9N2 WIV increased significantly compared with chickens immunized with the H9N2 WIV alone at days 7 and 21 ($P < 0.05$). However, HI antibody titers in chickens immunized with rTα1-BP5 combined with H9N2 WIV were significantly higher than in chicken immunized with BP5 combined with

H9N2 WIV at days 7 and 21 ($P < 0.05$) (**Figure 4A**). Anti-HA IgG antibody was observed in immunized chickens on days 7 and 21 after the first immunization. rTα1-BP5 enhanced the secretion of IgG antibody on day 7 after the first immunization, and the effect was greater than that induced by H9N2 AIV vaccine, Tα1 combined with H9N2 WIV and BP5 combined with H9N2 WIV. On day 21 after the first immunization, BP5 significantly enhanced IgG antibody secretion levels compared with that induced by H9N2 vaccine, Tα1 combined with H9N2 WIV ($P < 0.05$), while the effect of rTα1-BP5 was the greatest than the other groups ($P < 0.01$) (**Figure 4B**). These results suggested that rTα1-BP5 stimulates significant antigen-specific immune responses.

3.4. rTα1-BP5 promoted the production of AIV-neutralizing antibody

To assess whether rTα1-BP5 can effectively enhance virus-neutralizing antibodies, chicken sera were collected on days 7 and 21 after the first immunization and the titers of AIV-neutralizing antibody were assessed. The result showed that the titers of neutralizing antibody of chickens immunized with Tα1 plus H9N2 WIV, BP5 plus H9N2 WIV, and H9N2 AIV vaccine were higher than that in chickens immunized with H9N2 WIV alone on day 7, while it was higher in chickens immunized with Tα1-BP5 plus H9N2 WIV than that of other groups. Consistent with this, AIV-neutralizing antibody titers of chicken injected with rTα1-BP5 plus H9N2 WIV were the highest on day 21 (**Table 4**). These results indicated that rTα1-BP5 significantly stimulates the production of AIV-neutralizing antibodies.

Treatment	**PRNT50**[a]	
	First boost	**Second boost**
PBS	–	–
H9N2 WIV	10 ± 0.38	19 ± 0.21
H9N2 WIV + Tα1	15 ± 0.30*	22 ± 0.25*
H9N2 WIV + BP5	18 ± 0.32*	28 ± 0.43*
H9N2 WIV + rTα1-BP5	22 ± 0.24**	32 ± 0.19**
Inactivated H9N2 AIV vaccine	16 ± 0.15*	25 ± 0.54**

a Chickens were vaccinated on days 0 (first boost) and 14 (second boost). Chicken sera ($n = 5$) were collected on days 7 and 21, and plaque-reducing neutralizing antibody titers were determined. The 50% plaque-reducing neutralizing titer ($PRNT_{50}$) was reported as the geometrical reciprocal of the serum dilution resulting in a 50% reduction in plaques. The data presented are means ± SD of results from five replicates.
*, $P < 0.05$, and
**, $P < 0.01$, compared with chickens immunized with H9N2 WIV alone.

Table 4. Titers of plaque-reducing neutralizing antibody in groups of chicken.

3.5. rTα1-BP5 increases the production of both Th1- and Th2-type cytokines

We then examined the levels of Th1 (IFN-γ) and Th2 (IL-4) cytokines from immunized chickens. Compared with stimulation with H9N2 WIV alone, both IFN-γ and IL-4 secretion were remarkably increased after immunization with inactivated H9N2 AIV vaccine, Tα1 plus

H9N2 WIV and BP5 plus H9N2 WIV at days 7 and 21, and the highest level of IFN-γ secretion was observed in the vaccination group with rTα1-BP5 plus H9N2 WIV ($P < 0.01$) (**Figure 5A** and **B**). Taken together, the results suggested that rTα1-BP5 promoted the secretion of both Th1 and Th2 cytokines.

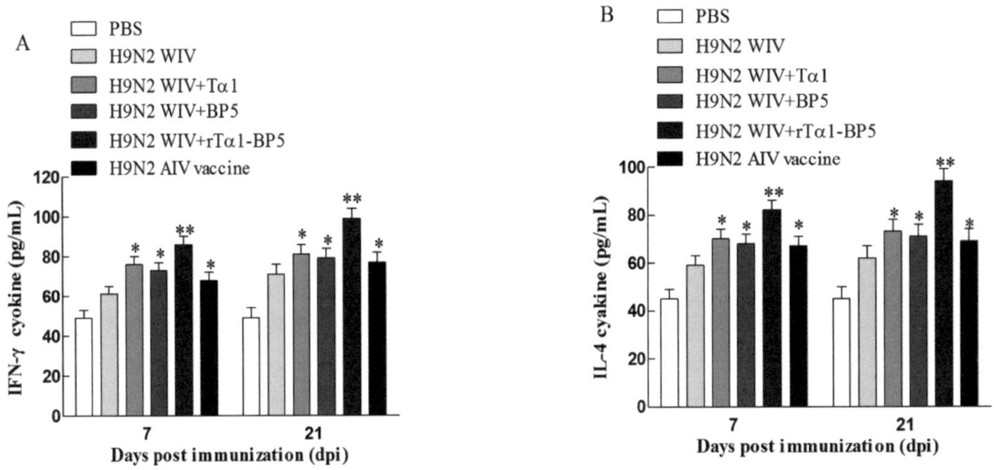

Figure 5. Effect of rTα1-BP5 to H9N2 AIV vaccination on cytokine production in chicken sera. Chickens were immunized two times, and chicken sera were collected on days 7 and 21 after the first immunization. Cytokine release was measured by using commercial chicken cytokines gamma interferon (IFN-γ) and interleukin 4 (IL-4) ELISA kits. The data presented are means ± SD of results from five replicates. *, $P < 0.05$, and **, $P < 0.01$, compared with chickens immunized with H9N2 WIV alone.

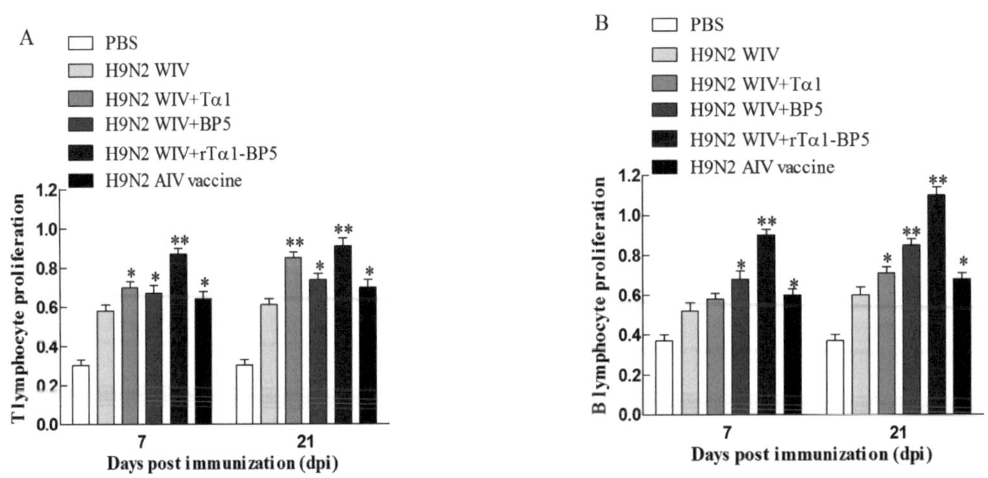

Figure 6. rTα1-BP5 significantly stimulates chicken T- and B-lymphocyte proliferation. Chickens were immunized two times, and chicken thymus and bursa of Fabricius were collected on days 7 and 21 after the first immunization. T- (A) and B (B)-lymphocyte proliferation assays were evaluated by MTT method. The data presented are means ± SD of results from five replicates. *, $P < 0.05$, and **, $P < 0.01$, compared with chickens immunized with H9N2 WIV alone.

3.6. rTα1-BP5 significantly enhances T- and B-lymphocyte proliferation

To investigate the effects of rTα1-BP5 on T- and B-lymphocyte proliferation, thymus and BF were collected from chickens immunized with rTα1-BP5 plus H9N2 WIV. T-lymphocyte proliferation responses of chickens immunized with Tα1 plus H9N2 WIV, BP5 plus H9N2 WIV, and H9N2 AIV vaccine were enhanced at 7 days compared with chickens immunized with H9N2 WIV alone ($P < 0.05$), whereas it was higher for that immunized with rTα1-BP5 plus H9N2 WIV ($P < 0.01$). On day 21, T-lymphocyte proliferation responses of chickens immunized with Tα1 plus H9N2 WIV and H9N2 AIV vaccine were higher than chickens immunized with H9N2 WIV alone ($P < 0.05$), while it was highest for that immunized with rTα1-BP5 plus H9N2 WIV ($P < 0.01$) (**Figure 6A**). Similarly, B-lymphocyte proliferation responses of chickens immunized with BP5 plus H9N2 WIV and H9N2 AIV vaccine were enhanced at 7 and 21 days compared with chickens immunized with H9N2 WIV alone ($P < 0.05$), whereas, it was highest for that immunized with rTα1-BP5 plus H9N2 WIV ($P < 0.01$) (**Figure 6B**). The data indicated that rTα1-BP5 promoted T- and B-lymphocyte proliferative responses.

3.7. rTα1-BP5 significantly promotes immune protection against H9N2 AIV challenge

To evaluate whether rTα1-BP5 promotes immune protection against H9N2 AIV infection, viral titers in chicken lungs were evaluated at 3, 5, and 7 days after viral challenge by plaque formation assays. Chickens immunized with Tα1 plus H9N2 WIV, BP5 plus H9N2 WIV, and H9N2 AIV vaccine showed significant virus removal from the lungs at 3, 5, and 7 days after challenge compared with H9N2 WIV groups ($P < 0.05$), while the viral titers of lungs from chicken immunized with rTα1-BP5 plus H9N2 WIV were significantly lower than that in the H9N2 AIV vaccine group ($P < 0.01$). Moreover, chickens immunized with rTα1-BP5 plus H9N2 WIV had almost no detectable virus particles in the lungs 7 days after challenge (**Figure 7A–C**). The data indicated that rTα1-BP5 significantly promoted immune protection against H9N2 AIV challenge.

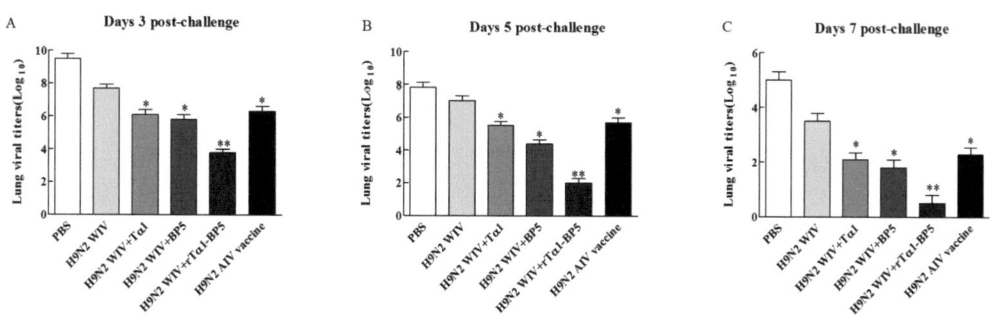

Figure 7. AIV-viral titers of lung in chickens. Lung samples from individual chicken in each group ($n = 5$) were collected on days 3, 5, and 7 post challenge with 2.5 × 106 $TCID_{50}$ avian influenza virus (A/chicken/Jiangsu/JS-1/2002(H9N2)). Each lung sample was diluted to 1 mL with 1640 media. The titers are presented as pfu per mL. The data presented are means ± SD of results from five replicates. *, $P < 0.05$, and **, $P < 0.01$, compared with chickens immunized with H9N2 WIV alone.

4. Discussion

In the event of an influenza pandemic, vaccination is one of the most effective ways of intervention in terms of reducing cost, disease, and even death. Appropriate adjuvant can enhance the immunogenicity of the vaccine and improve the immune responses [38, 39]. However, most of the adjuvants used in conjugation with antigen have unacceptable levels of side effects, only a few of them are used clinically [40]. Thus, we need to find new and optimal adjuvant candidates for vaccine. In recent years, some small peptide immunostimulants were reported in use for vaccine adjuvants [41–43]. Both Tα1 and BP5 are associated with immune regulation. Previous studies showed that both Tα1 and BP5 had high potential as an adjuvant for vaccines [26, 44].

In this study, the fusion peptide of rTα1-BP5 was designed and synthesized, and to investigate it as an adjuvant for inducing immune responses in chickens upon vaccination with inactivated H9N2 avian influenza virus (WIV). An effective adjuvant should be able to enhance the levels of both humoral and cell-mediated immunity. To investigate the effect of rTα1-BP5 on humoral responses, chickens were immunized with H9N2 WIV combined with Tα1-BP5, and then titers of HI antibody, antigen-specific antibodies, and AIV-neutralizing antibodies were assessed. Then, we found that rTα1-BP5 significantly enhanced HI antibody and antigen-specific IgG antibodies titers, promoted the secretion of AIV-neutralizing antibodies, which suggested that rTα1-BP5 enhanced the levels of humoral immune responses in chickens when it was co-immunized with H9N2 WIV.

In addition to humoral immune responses, cellular immunity also plays an important role in fighting influenza virus infections [45]. The levels of Th1- and Th2-type cytokines are important references to measure cellular immunity. And lymphocyte homeostasis is required for the maintenance of normal immune function [46]. Th1-type cytokines mainly include IL-2, TNF-α, and IFN-γ, whereas Th2-type cytokines include IL-4, IL-5, and IL-10 [47]. Our study though analyzed the production of Th1 (IFN-γ)- and Th2 (IL-4)-type cytokines, and T- and B-lymphocytes proliferation in vaccinated chickens post immunization to evaluate the cell-mediated immunity. The results suggested that rTα1-BP5 promoted the secretion of both Th1 and Th2 cytokines and T- and B-lymphocyte proliferative responses. Overall, this study found that rTα1-BP5 not only enhanced the humoral immune responses but also promoted the cell-mediated immune responses, and it had the potential to use as an adjuvant.

To further evaluate the influence of rTα1-BP5 as an adjuvant on the immunity protection provided by H9N2 AIV vaccine against AIV infection, chickens were intramuscularly challenged with H9N2 AIV (A/chicken/Jiangsu/JS-1/2002) on day 28 post immunization. After 3 days post challenge, the PBS group chickens that received the challenge virus were mildly depressed. No other clinical signs were observed in that group or any of the other groups, which is typical of low-pathogenicity AIV in chickens [48, 49]. At 7 days post challenge, only the PBS-challenged group had mild, grossly detectable lesions in both the respiratory and gastrointestinal tract. And we found that the viral titers of lungs from chicken immunized with rTα1-BP5 plus H9N2 WIV were significantly lower than all the other groups at 3 days. Chickens immunized with rTα1-BP5 plus H9N2 WIV had almost no detectable virus particles in the lungs at 7 days after challenge. Our data indicated that rTα1-BP5 could effectively inhibit the replication of H9N2 AIV in chickens and promote virus clearance in the lungs of chickens. Thus, rTα1-BP5 had the potential to be used in vaccine formulations to provide improved protection against H9N2 AIV infection in poultry.

In summary, this study demonstrated that inactivated H9N2 AIV vaccine with Tα1-BP5 as an adjuvant enhanced strong immune responses at both humoral and cellular levels against AIV infection in chickens. These data may provide a novel insight to find new adjuvant in vaccines.

Acknowledgements

This work was supported by Grant no. 31101792 from the National Natural Science Foundation of China and no. 2012GGJS-077 from the Foundation for University Key Teacher by Higher Education of Henan Province.

Author details

Chen Wang[1*], Chengshui Liao[1], Wufan Zhang[1], Deyuan Li[2] and Puyan Chen[2]

*Address all correspondence to: wangchen2001@126.com

1 Key Laboratory of Veterinary Oncological Immunology, Henan University of Science and Technology, Luoyang, China

2 Key Laboratory of Animal Bacteriology of China's Department of Agriculture, Nanjing Agricultural University, Nanjing, China

#C.WANG and C.S.LIAO equally contributed to this work.

References

[1] Fouchier RA, Munster V, Wallensten A, Bestebroer TM, Herfst S, Smith D, Rimmelzwaan GF, Olsen B, Osterhaus AD. Characterization of a novel influenza A virus hemagglutinin subtype (H16) obtained from black-headed gulls. Journal of Virology. 2005; 79: 2814–2822. DOI: 10.1128/JVI.79.5.2814-2822.2005

[2] Banet-Noach C, Perk S, Simanov L, Grebenyuk N, Rozenblut E, Pokamunski S, Pirak M, Tendler Y, Panshin A. H9N2 influenza viruses from Israeli poultry: a five-year outbreak. Avian Diseases. 2007; 51: 290–296. DOI: 10.1637/7590-040206R1.1

[3] Homme PJ, Easterday BC. Avian influenza virus infections. IV. Response of pheasants, ducks, and geese to influenza A-turkey-Wisconsin-1966 virus. Avian Diseases. 1970; 14: 285–290. DOI: 10.2307/1588473

[4] Shortridge KF. Pandemic influenza: a zoonosis? Seminars in Respiratory Infections. 1992; 7: 11–25.

[5] Sun Y. Proceedings of the Fourth International Symposium on Avian Influenza: avian influenza, a global problem: Georgia Center for Continuing Education, the University of Georgia, Athens, Georgia, USA, May 28–31, 1997. pp. 47–49.

[6] Alexander DJ. Proceedings of the Fourth International Symposium on Avian Influenza: Avian Influenza, A Global Problem: Georgia Center for Continuing Education, the University of Georgia, Athens, Georgia, USA, May 28–31, 1997. pp. 9–13

[7] Li C, Yu K, Tian G, Yu D, Liu L, Jing B, Ping J, Chen H. Evolution of H9N2 influenza viruses from domestic poultry in Mainland China. Virology. 2005; 340: 70–83. DOI: 10.1016/j.virol.2005.06.025

[8] Nicholson KG, Wood JM, Zambon M. Influenza. Lancet. 2003; 362: 1733–1745. DOI: 10.1016/S0140-6736(03)14854-4

[9] Nichol KL, Treanor JJ. Vaccines for seasonal and pandemic influenza. The Journal of Infectious Diseases. 2006; 194:S111–S118. DOI: 10.1086/507544

[10] Wareing MD, Tannock GA. Live attenuated vaccines against influenza; an historical review. Vaccine. 2001; 19: 3320–3330. DOI: 10.1016/S0264-410X(01)00045-7

[11] Singh M, O'Hagan D. Advances in vaccine adjuvants. Nature Biotechnology. 1999; 17(11): 1075–1781. DOI: 10.1038/15058

[12] Bungener L, Geeraedts F, Ter Veer W, Medema J, Wilschut J, Huckriede A. Alum boosts TH2-type antibody responses to whole-inactivated virus influenza vaccine in mice but does not confer superior protection. Vaccine. 2008; 26: 2350–2359. DOI: 10.1016/j.vaccine.2008.02.063

[13] Riedl K, Riedl R, von Gabain A, Nagy E, Lingnau K. The novel adjuvant IC31 strongly improves influenza vaccine-specific cellular and humoral immune responses in young adult and aged mice. Vaccine. 2008; 26: 3461–3468. DOI: 10.1016/j.vaccine.2008.04.029

[14] O'Hagan DT. MF59 is a safe and potent vaccine adjuvant that enhances protection against influenza virus infection. Expert Review of Vaccines. 2007; 6: 699–710. DOI: 10.1586/14760584.6.5.699

[15] Li J, Zheng L, Li P, Wang F. Intein-mediated expression, purification, and characterization of thymosin alpha 1-thymopentin fusion peptide in *Escherichia coli*. Protein Expression and Purification. 2012; 84: 1–8. DOI: 10.1016/j.pep.2012.04.013

[16] Lunin SM, Glushkova OV, Khrenov MO, Novoselova TV, Parfenyuk SB, Fesenko EE, Novoselova EG. Thymic peptides restrain the inflammatory response in mice with

experimental autoimmune encephalomyelitis. Immunobiology. 2013; 218: 402–407. DOI: 10.1016/j.imbio.2012.05.023

[17] Goldstein AL, Low TL, McAdoo M, McClure J, Thurman GB, Rossio J, Lai CY, Chang D, Wang SS, Harvey C, Ramel AH, Meienhofer J. Thymosin alpha1: isolation and sequence analysis of an immunologically active thymic polypeptide. Proceedings of the National Academy of Sciences of the United States of America.1977; 74: 725–729. DOI: 10.1073/pnas.74.2.725

[18] Ahmed A, Wong DM, Thurman GB, Low TL, Goldstein AL, Sharkis SJ, Goldschneider I. T-lymphocyte maturation: cell surface markers and immune function induced by T-lymphocyte cell-free products and thymosin polypeptides. Annals of the New York Academy of Sciences. 1979; 332: 81–94. DOI: 10.1111/j.1749-6632.1979.tb47100.x

[19] Hadden JW, Verastegui E, Hadden E. IRX-2 and thymosin alpha 1 (zadaxin) increase T lymphocytes in T lymphocytopenic mice and humans. Thymosins in Health and Disease: First International Symposium. Annals of the New York Academy of Sciences. 2007; 1112: 245–255. DOI: 10.1196/annals.1415.032

[20] Lao X, Liu M, Chen J, Zheng H. A tumor-penetrating peptide modification enhances the antitumor activity of thymosin alpha 1. PLoS One. 2013; 8: e72242. DOI: 10.1371/journal.pone.0072242

[21] Li YM, Chen H, Li X, Zhou WC, He MY, Chiriva-Internati M, Wachtel MS, Frezza EE. A new immunomodulatory therapy for severe sepsis: Ulinastatin Plus Thymosin {alpha} 1. Journal of Intensive Care Medicine. 2009; 24: 47–53. DOI: 10.1177/0885066608326970

[22] Audhya T, Kroon D, Heavner G, Viamontes G, Goldstein G. Tripeptide structure of bursin, a selective B-cell-differentiating hormone of the bursa of fabricius. Science. 1986; 231: 997–999. DOI: 10.1126/science.3484838

[23] Wang C, Wen WY, Su CX, Ge FF, Dang ZG, Duan XG, Cao RB, Zhou B, Chen PY. Bursin as an adjuvant is a potent enhancer of immune response in mice immunized with the JEV subunit vaccine. Veterinary Immunology and Immunopathology. 2008; 122: 265–274. DOI: 10.1016/j.vetimm.2007.11.010

[24] Wang C, Li XK, Wu TC, Li DY, Niu MF, Wang Y, Zhang CJ, Cheng XC, Chen PY. Bursin-like peptide (BLP) enhances H9N2 influenza vaccine induced humoral and cell mediated immune responses. Cellular Immunology. 2014; 292: 57–64. DOI: 10.1016/j.cellimm.2014.09.003

[25] Li DY, Xue MY, Wang C, Wang JB, Chen PY. Bursopentine as a novel immunoadjuvant enhances both humoral and cell-mediated immune responses to inactivated H9N2 avian influenza virus in chickens. Clinical and Vaccine Immunology. 2011; 18(9): 1497–1502. DOI: 10.1128/CVI.05133-11

[26] Li DY, Geng ZR, Zhu HF, Wang C, Miao DN, Chen PY. Immunomodulatory activities of a new pentapeptide (Bursopentin) from the chicken bursa of Fabricius. Amino Acids. 2011; 40(2): 505–515. DOI: 10.1007/s00726-010-0663-7

[27] Novak M, Moldoveanu Z, Schafer DP, Mestecky J, Compans RW. Murine model for evaluation of protective immunity to influenza virus. Vaccine. 1993; 11: 55–60. DOI: 10.1016/0264-410X(93)90339-Y

[28] Sha Z, Compans RW. Induction of CD4 (+) T-cell-independent immunoglobulin responses by inactivated influenza virus. Journal of Virology. 2000; 74: 4999–5005. DOI: 10.1128/JVI.74.11.4999-5005.2000

[29] OIE 2012. Manual of diagnostic tests and vaccines for terrestrial animals. Paris: Office International des Epizooties. [Internet]. Available from: http://www.oie.int/manual-of-diagnostic-tests-and-vaccines-for-terrestrial-animals/

[30] Horton RM, Hunt HD, Ho SN, Pullen JK, Pease LR. Engineering hybrid genes without the use of restriction enzymes: gene splicing by overlap extension. Gene. 1989; 77: 61–68. DOI: 10.1016/0378-1119(89)90359-4

[31] Mosmann T. Rapid colorimetric assay for cellular growth and survival: application to proliferation and cytotoxicity assays. Journal of Immunological Methods.1983; 65: 55–63. DOI: 10.1016/0022-1759(83)90303-4

[32] Yu L, Li JR, Huang YW, Liang XY, Meng SS. Enhanced immunogenicity of plasmid encoding polyprotein gene of infectious bursal disease virus by co-administration of chicken interleukin 2 (IL-2). Sheng Wu Gong Cheng Xue Bao. 2001; 17: 652–657. DOI: 10.3321/j.issn:1000-3061.2001.06.013

[33] Haan L, Verweij WR, Holtrop M, Brands R, van Scharrenburg GJ, Palache AM, Agsteribbe E, Wilschut J. Nasal or intramuscular immunization of mice with influenza subunit antigen and the B subunit of Escherichia coli heat-labile toxin induces IgA- or IgG-mediated protective mucosal immunity. Vaccine. 2001; 19: 2898–2907. DOI: 10.1016/S0264-410X(00)00556-9

[34] Fritz JH, Brunner S, Birnstiel ML, Buschle M, Gabain AV, Mattner F, Zauner W. The artificial antimicrobial peptide KLKLLLLLKLK induces predominantly a TH2-type immune response to co-injected antigens. Vaccine. 2004; 22: 3274–3284.DOI: 10.1016/j.vaccine.2004.03.007

[35] Rimmelzwaan GF, Baars M, van Beek R, van Amerongen G, Lovgren-Bengtsson K, Claas EC, Osterhaus AD. Induction of protective immunity against influenza virus in a macaque model: comparison of conventional and iscom vaccines. The Journal of General Virology. 1997; 78: 757–765. DOI: 10.1099/0022-1317-78-4-757

[36] Du L, Lyle CS, Obey TB, Gaarde WA, Muir JA, Bennett BL, Chambers TC. Inhibition of cell proliferation and cell cycle progression by specific inhibition of basal JNK activity:

evidence that mitotic Bcl-2 phosphorylation is JNK-independent. The Journal of Biological Chemistry. 2004; 279: 11957-11966. DOI: 10.1074/jbc.M304935200

[37] Wang C, Li XK, Zhang CJ, Wu TC, Li YJ, Cheng XC. A eukaryotic expression plasmid carrying chicken interleukin-18 enhances the response to Newcastle disease virus vaccine. Clinical and Vaccine Immunology. 2015; 22: 56–64. DOI: 10.1128/CVI.00636-14

[38] Bhardwaj N. Processing and presentation of antigens by dendritic cells: implications for vaccines. Trends in Molecular Medicine. 2001; 7: 388–394. DOI: 10.1016/S1471-4914(01)02101-3

[39] Schijns VE. Immunological concepts of vaccine adjuvant activity. Current Opinion in Immunology. 2000; 12: 456–463. DOI: 10.1016/S0952-7915(00)00120-5

[40] Petrovsky N, Aguilar JC. Vaccine adjuvants: current state and future trends. Immunology and Cell Biology. 2004; 82: 488–496. DOI: 10.1111/j.0818-9641.2004.01272.x

[41] Cai MH, Zhu F, Wu HC, Shen PP. A new recombinant hybrid polypeptide and its immunologic adjuvant activity for inactivated infectious bursal disease vaccine. Biotechnology Letters. 2014; 36: 1431–1437. DOI: 10.1007/s10529-014-1499-0

[42] Charoenvit Y, Goel N, Whelan M, Rosenthal KS, Zimmerman DH. CEL-1000—a peptide with adjuvant activity for Th1 immune responses. Vaccine. 2004; 22: 2368–2373. DOI: 10.1016/j.vaccine.2003.11.062

[43] Gagnon L, DiMarco M, Kirby R, Zacharie B, Penney CL. D-LysAsnProTyr tetrapeptide: a novel B-cell stimulant and stabilized bursin mimetic. Vaccine. 2000; 18: 1886–1892. DOI: 10.1016/S0264-410X(99)00374-6

[44] Li WY, Lu HM, Guo Q, Hu WM, Zhang ZD. Effects of thymosin alpha1 on immune effector molecules of mouse. Sichuan da xue xue bao Yi xue ban = Journal of Sichuan University Medical science edition. 2014; 45: 400–404.

[45] Kreijtz JH, Bodewes R, van Amerongen G, Kuiken T, Fouchier RA, Osterhaus AD, Rimmelzwaan GF. Primary influenza A virus infection induces cross-protective immunity against a lethal infection with a heterosubtypic virus strain in mice. Vaccine. 2007; 25: 612–620. DOI: 10.1016/j.vaccine.2006.08.036

[46] Wen L, Chen SJ, Zhang W, Ma HW, Zhang SQ, Chen L. hsBAFF regulates proliferation and response in cultured CD4(+) T lymphocytes by upregulation of intracellular free Ca(2+) homeostasis. Cytokine. 2011; 53: 215–222. DOI: 10.1016/j.cyto.2010.11.006

[47] Kumar DA, Manikandan P, Sumitra M, Raju KV, Gayathri C, Arutselvan N, Puvanakrishnan R. A novel peptide derivative exhibits anti inflammatory and antioxidant activity in adjuvant induced arthritis in rats. Molecular and Cellular Biochemistry. 2002; 229: 9–17. DOI: 10.1023/A:1017980024029

[48] Lee CW, Song CS, Lee YJ, Mo IP, Garcia M, Suarez DL, Kim SJ. Sequence analysis of the hemagglutinin gene of H9N2 Korean avian influenza viruses and assessment of the

pathogenic potential of isolate MS96. Avian diseases. 2000; 44: 527–535. DOI: 10.2307/1593091

[49] Soda K, Asakura S, Okamatsu M, Sakoda Y, Kida H. H9N2 influenza virus acquires intravenous pathogenicity on the introduction of a pair of di-basic amino acid residues at the cleavage site of the hemagglutinin and consecutive passages in chickens. Virology Journal. 2011; 8: 64. DOI: 10.1186/1743-422X-8-64

Chapter 7

Cholesteryl Pullulan Nanoparticles-Encapsulated TNF-α: An Effective Mucosal Vaccine Adjuvant Against Influenza

Tsunetaka Ohta

Additional information is available at the end of the chapter

http://dx.doi.org/10.5772/64366

Abstract

We encapsulated tumor necrosis factor-α (TNF-α), a major proinflammatory cytokine, into cholesteryl pullulan (CHP) to prepare TNF/CHP nanoparticles. In this chapter, the immune response-enhancing capability of the nanoparticles to act as a vaccine adjuvant against influenza is described. TNF/CHP nanoparticles showed excellent storage stability, and they enhanced host immune responses to external immunogens. We applied the nanoparticles in a mouse model of influenza virus infection to investigate their adjuvant ability. Nasal administration of TNF/CHP nanoparticles combined with a conventional split vaccine was effective at inducing systemic IgG_1 as well as mucosal IgA, and it protected mice against a lethal challenge of A/PR/8/34 (H1N1) influenza virus. Mechanistic studies showed that the nanoparticles enhanced antigen uptake by dendritic cells (DCs) and moderately induced the expression of inflammation-related genes in nasal-associated lymphoid tissue (NALT), leading to the activation of both B and T cells. A preliminary safety study revealed no severe toxicity to TNF/CHP nanoparticles. Slight-to-moderate influences in nasal mucosa were observed only after repeated administration and they were reversible. Our data show that TNF/CHP nanoparticles effectively enhance both humoral and cellular immunity via nasal administration and could be a potential adjuvant for vaccines against infectious diseases like influenza.

Keywords: adjuvant, mucosal, nanoparticle, CHP, TNF-α

1. Introduction

Vaccines are the most effective interventions against infectious diseases such as influenza. Many vaccines, however, are only effective at preventing onset and aggravation of symptoms, and less effective at preventing infection, particularly with respiratory infections. One reason for this is that the major administration routes of conventional vaccines, including subcutaneous (*s.c.*) and intramuscular (*i.m.*), induce neutralizing IgG antibody in blood but not mucosal IgA antibody, which is more effective at preventing infection. The efficacy of IgG antibody against variant or mutated viruses is very limited because it has highly restricted cross-protective capabilities. Conversely, IgA antibody on mucosa shows wide cross-protection and can block infection [1, 2]. When immunizations are delivered at the mucosa, IgA antibody is induced on mucosal surfaces throughout the body and IgG antibody is produced in the blood. Since mucosal vaccination induces immunity in both the systemic and mucosal compartments [3, 4], enhanced antigen-specific mucosal immunity is a clear goal for next-generation vaccines. Mucosal, especially nasal, vaccines are ideal because of their effectiveness in preventing infection via the respiratory tract. Nasal vaccines have the additional benefit of improved patient compliance and greater clinical convenience as well.

One significant drawback of mucosal vaccines is that they generally do not induce strong enough immune responses. The recent component-split vaccines, while avoiding many negative patient reactions, tend to be less immunogenic by themselves even in the case of intravenous (*i.v.*) or *i.m.* administration. Generally, children and the elderly tend to respond less to vaccinations, which may lower the preventive power of the population [5]. Therefore, adjuvants must be administered simultaneously with the vaccine in order to enhance vaccine-specific immune responses. Alum salts are the most commonly used adjuvant, but they are neither suitable for all vaccines nor always capable of eliciting the desired immune responses. Other types of adjuvants are being tested, such as liposomes, emulsions, and their combinations [6, 7]. The development of safe, effective, and suitable adjuvants is an important component in the future of mucosal vaccines.

Several groups have examined the use of cytokines (proteinaceous bioactive substances) as a new type of vaccine adjuvant due to their potent effects on the immune system [8–10]. Although some encouraging results have been reported, cytokines are not yet in the practical use as adjuvants. One of the important points to consider is the type of drug delivery system (DDS). Recently, our group tried to generate a new type of vaccine adjuvant by combining cytokines and biocompatible saccharide materials. This chapter describes the creation of human tumor necrosis factor-α (TNF-α) encapsulated by cholesteryl pullulan (CHP) resulting in TNF/CHP nanoparticles. We investigated the potential of the nanoparticles as a nasal vaccine adjuvant by examining its ability to protect against lethal influenza infection in a mouse model and conducting further mechanistic analyses on innate and acquired immunity.

http://dx.doi.org/10.5772/64366

2. Tumor necrosis factor-α (TNF-α)

TNF-α is a major proinflammatory cytokine primarily produced by T cells and macrophages, and it is bioactive in a homotrimeric form [11]. It was first described as a potent anti-tumor factor, but it is now known to play an integral role in host defense. It activates innate and adaptive immunity by stimulating dendritic cell (DC) maturation and subsequent T cell activation as well as contributing to inflammatory responses [12, 13] (**Figure 1**).

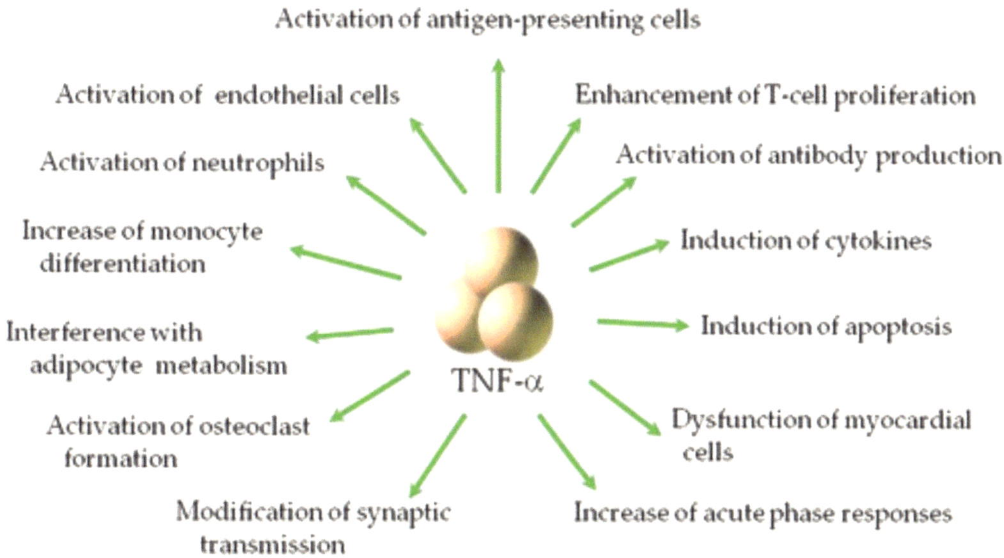

Figure 1. Various actions of TNF-α.

Interestingly, it was recently shown that TNF-α exerted adjuvant activities against pathogenic infections [14, 15]. Although there were some attempts to develop TNF-α (as well as other cytokines) as a vaccine adjuvant, successful practical results have not been reported. This is probably because TNF-α causes unfavorable biological reactions when administered systemically, and it is rapidly degraded when delivered at the mucosal surface. To overcome these obstacles, some investigators have attempted to generate protease-resistant mutant TNF-α molecules and have reported some potential as a vaccine adjuvant at the experimental level [16, 17].

3. Pullulan and cholesteryl pullulan (CHP)

One method of establishing a safer and more effective way to administer bioactive substances that is gaining popularity is a nanoparticle DDS. For nanoparticle materials, polysaccharides have been shown to possess several favorable characteristics in comparison with synthetic polymers currently used. Unlike synthetic polymers that could accumulate in the body to levels beyond the renal clearance, saccharides are biocompatible, meaning they are degraded by intrinsic enzymes inside the body [18, 19]. In this study, we used pullulan to create DDS nanoparticles.

Pullulan is a natural and chemically neutral homopolysaccharide consisting of α-1, 6-linked maltotriose units (maltotriose is three glucose molecules linked with α-1, 4 glycosidic bonds). It is produced primarily by fermentation of starch by strains of the fungus *Aureobasidium pullulans* [20]. By introducing hydrophobic moieties onto the hydrophilic pullulan molecule, amphiphilic coploymers can be generated. A representative is cholesteryl pullulan (CHP) [21, 22] (**Figure 2**).

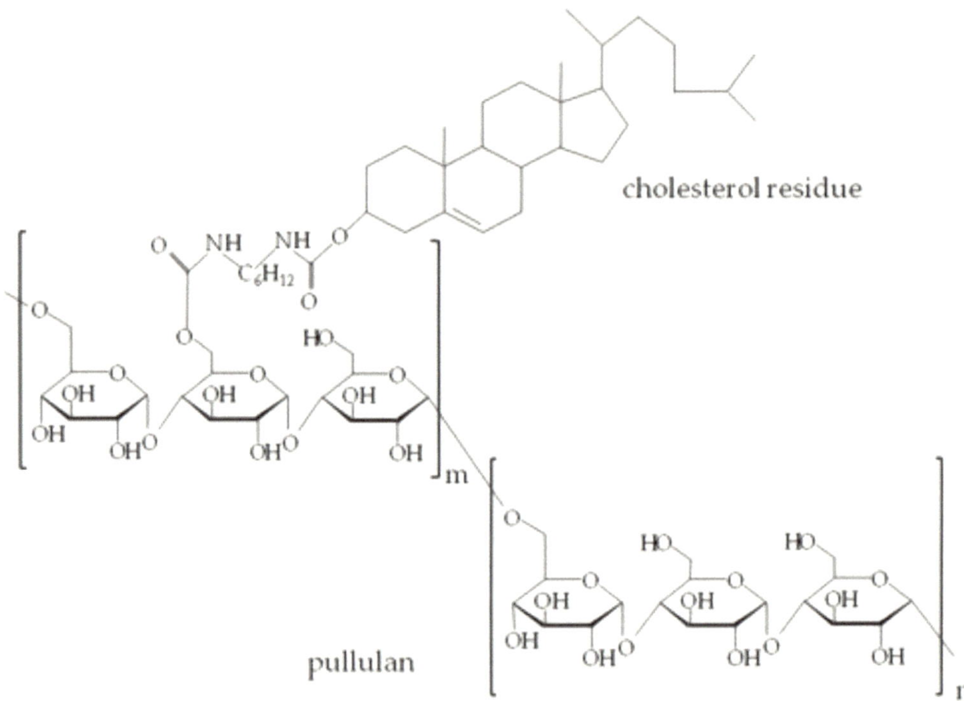

Figure 2. Chemical structure of CHP. m, n; integer values. In PUREBRIGHT CP-100T (NOF Co., Tokyo, Japan), 1–3% of glucose units are modified with cholesterol residues.

CHP self-assembles into nanoparticles in aqueous solution and entraps various molecules in its internal space through hydrophobic interactions. The hydrophilic shell serves as a stabilizing interface between the hydrophobic core and the external aqueous environment. It also protects the entrapped molecule from mechanical, chemical, or enzymatic attacks from outside the particle, and it acts as a superior carrier for delivery. It also allows slow release of the encapsulated materials [23–25]. Furthermore, the CHP nanoparticles showed prolonged circulation and thermodynamic stability in animal models [26].

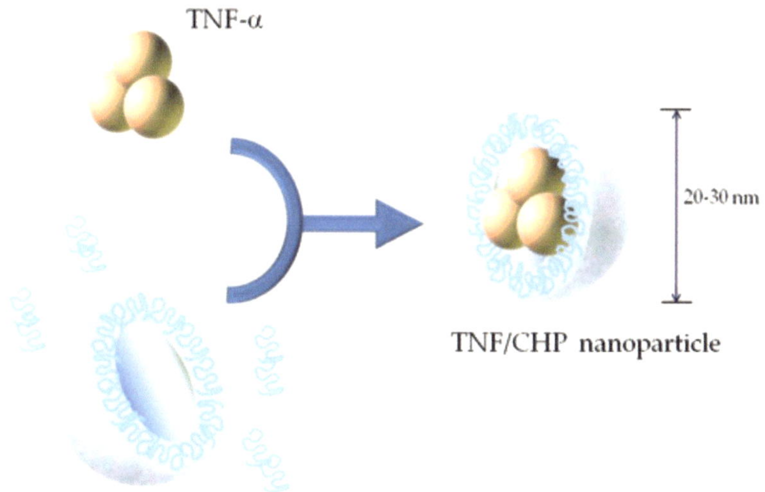

Figure 3. Schematic model of self-assembling of TNF/CHP nanoparticles. TNF-α is shown in the trimeric, bioactive form. The diameter of the particle is approximately 20–30 nm.

Pullulan-based nanoparticles have been used for the delivery of proteins, anticancer drugs, imaging agents, and nucleotides. CHP nanoparticles are efficiently transferred to antigen-presenting cells such as macrophages and/or DCs, and they elicit strong immune responses [27, 28]. CHP is under vigorous investigation for establishing novel vaccine therapies against several types of cancers [29–31]. We created CHP nanoparticles containing TNF-α, which are described in the following sections (**Figure 3**).

4. TNF/CHP nanoparticles

4.1. Preparation of TNF/CHP nanoparticles

In this study, we used TNF-α derived from a human lymphoblastoid cell line, BALL-1 [32], and CHP (PUREBRIGHT CP-100T) from NOF Corporation. CHP encapsulated active trimeric TNF-α to form stable nanoparticles as schematically shown in **Figure 3**. The encapsulating process was time- and temperature-dependent; at 37°C, more than 95% of the TNF-α was encapsulated into CHP complexes after 5 days of incubation; at 4°C, very few, if any, TNF/CHP nanoparticles were formed.

The resulting nanoparticles were relatively uniform. The mode and average sizes of the particles were 27.2 and 42.4 nm based on dynamic light scattering (DLS) results. This was not very different from the size of the blank CHP particles with a mode of 27.6 nm and an average of 42.8 nm (**Figure 4**). Stoichiometric analyses showed that a TNF/CHP nanoparticle consisted of a TNF-α active trimer (ca. 50 kDa) in a CHP tetrameric complex (ca. 400 kDa).

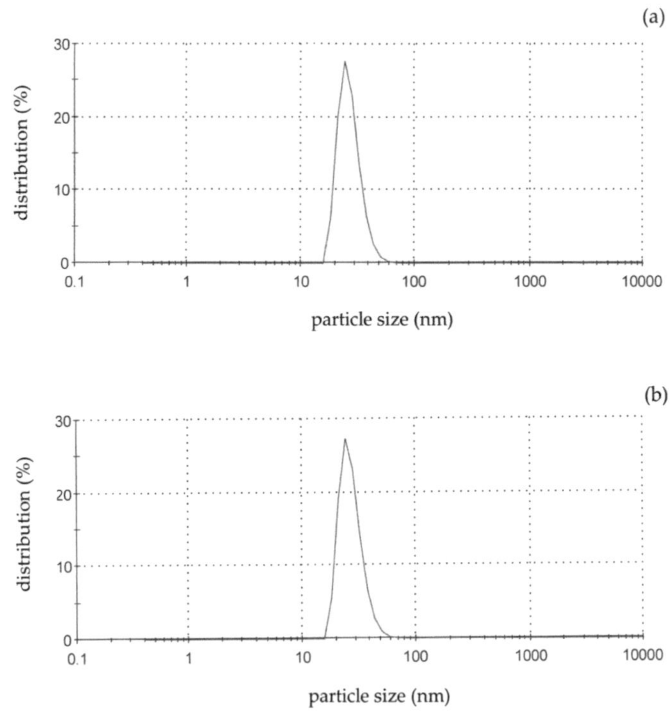

Figure 4. Size distribution of TNF/CHP nanoparticles. Two hundred fifty μg/mL TNF-α and 12 mg/mL CHP were mixed, sterilized by filtration, and incubated at 37°C for 5 days. CHP self-assembled with TNF-α molecules to form nanoparticles. The particle size was determined by DLS with a Zetasizer Nano ZS (Malvern Instruments Ltd., Malvern, UK). (a) TNF/CHP nanoparticles, (b) blank CHP particles. Reproduced with permission from Nagatomo D. et al., [33].

4.2. Storage stability of TNF/CHP nanoparticles

Stability of the nanoparticles was evaluated after various treatments by measuring the level of TNF-α. To estimate the amount of encapsulated TNF-α, methyl-β-cyclodextrin (Me-β-CD) was used to disrupt the CHP complex and release the TNF-α as previously described [26]. The results showed that the nanoparticle retained its integrity and kept TNF-α molecules active inside the complex in aqueous solution at room temperature for at least 21 days (**Figure 5a**). Furthermore, even after five cycles of freezing and thawing, 80% of the particles remained intact (**Figure 5b**). These results show that the TNF/CHP nanoparticles have excellent storage stability. However, upon contact with high concentrations of dissolved proteins, such as serum albumin, the nanoparticles rapidly released the encapsulated TNF-α (data not shown), probably replaced by proteins from the external environment as reported [34]. This calls an attention to the usage of the nanoparticles, such as *i.v.* injection.

Me-β-CD is known to interact with cholesteryl groups and disrupt CHP complexes to release the substance inside the particles [26]. The amount of Me-β-CD required to disrupt the TNF/CHP nanoparticles was approximately 100 mg/mL, much higher than the 0.3 mg/mL reported for Interleukin-12 (IL-12)/CHP nanoparticles [35], suggesting that the affinity between TNF-α and CHP was much stronger than that of IL-12 and CHP. The molecular interaction of TNF-α and CHP that creates this strength is an interesting area for further study.

Many medical formulations, especially biologicals, require storage at low temperatures or freezing. On the contrary, the TNF/CHP nanoparticles could be stored in solution and without refrigeration. Our formulation offers improved convenience of handling and transportation.

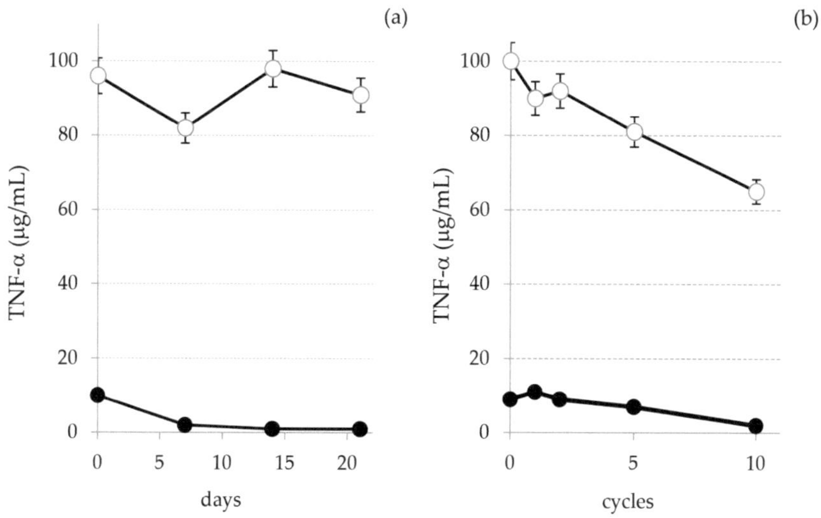

Figure 5. Stability of TNF/CHP nanoparticles *in vitro*. TNF/CHP nanoparticles were incubated in Dulbecco's phosphate buffer at 25°C or repeatedly freeze-thawed (–80°C/25°C). An aliquot was examined for the amount of active TNF-α. Samples were treated with 100 mg/mL Me-β-CD at 37°C for 2 h to release TNF-α from the particles. The amount of TNF-α was determined by an enzyme-linked immunosorbent assay (ELISA) system. (a) storage stability at 25°C; (b) stability through freeze-thaw cycles. Open circle, treated with Me-β-CD; closed circle, without Me-β-CD. (mean ± SD, *n* = 3).

5. Immune responses induced by TNF/CHP nanoparticles administered nasally

Although TNF-α is known to have immune-enhancing activity [14], severe and unfavorable effects have hampered its practical use. Based on the stability described in the previous section, we hypothesized that delayed release of TNF-α from TNF/CHP nanoparticles would promote the beneficial effects of TNF-α while avoiding harmful events. We examined the adjuvant activity of the TNF/CHP nanoparticles, for example, enhanced induction of antigen-specific antibodies in mice, particularly in the case of nasal administration. We used a commercial influenza virus hemagglutinin vaccine (IVV), which is a component-split and trivalent vaccine for seasonal influenza. It consists of the inactivated hemagglutinin (HA) antigens from A/Brisbane/59/2007 (H1N1), A/Uruguay/716/2007 (H3N2), and B/Brisbane/60/2008. The nasally administered TNF/CHP nanoparticles combined with the IVV induced significant levels of

IgA in the nasal wash, as well as IgG_1 in blood plasma (**Figure 6a, b**). These are comparable to those of the positive control cholera toxin B subunit (CTB), the most powerful adjuvant in experimental settings [35]. Furthermore, IVV with CHP alone (without TNF-α) or with free TNF-α failed to induce significant levels of antibodies when compared to IVV with no adjuvant. The TNF/CHP nanoparticles alone did not induce a measurable antibody response against IVV. To further examine antigen specificity, we performed hemagglutinin (HA)-specific hemagglutination inhibition (HI) assay for the different types of influenza virus included in the vaccine. The TNF/CHP nanoparticles with IVV induced significant HI activity against all types of HA used (A/H1N1, A/H3N2, and B) (**Figure 6c**).

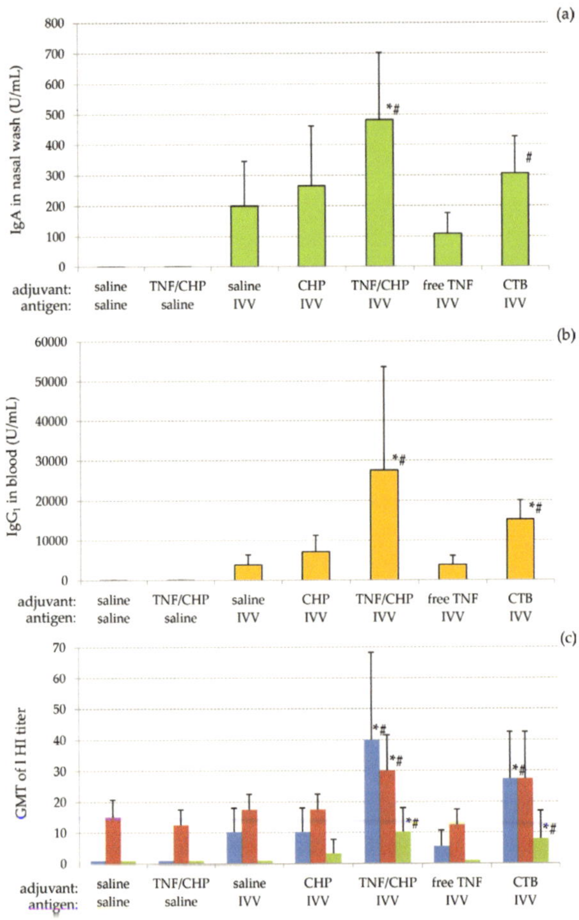

Figure 6. Adjuvant effects of TNF/CHP nanoparticles administered nasally. BALB/c mice were nasally given IVV (SEIKEN, Denka Seiken Co., Ltd., Japan) (0.3 μg/mouse) and TNF/CHP nanoparticles (5 μg/mouse of TNF-α) or CTB (0.8 μg/mouse) once a week for 4 weeks. The nasal wash and blood plasma were prepared from the mice, and the levels of IVV-specific IgA and IgG_1 were determined by ELISA. (a) IgA levels in nasal wash, (b) IgG_1 levels in blood plasma, (c) HI titer in blood plasma against different HA types of influenza virus expressed in GMT (geometric mean titer). Blue column, type A/H1N1; red column, type A/H3N2; green column, type B. (mean ± SEM, n = 8). *, $P < 0.05$ vs. saline/IVV; #, $P < 0.05$ vs. free TNF/IVV. Adapted with permission from Nagatomo D. et al., [33].

http://dx.doi.org/10.5772/64366

These data indicate that TNF/CHP nanoparticles administered nasally can induce not only mucosal but also systemic immunity significantly and efficiently, comparable to the effects of CTB. In addition, the nasal vaccination covers a broad range of antigenicity as previous reports suggested [1, 2]. Also, just for reference, the induction of specific antibodies was seen for other antigens, such as Hepatitis virus type A vaccine, diphtheria toxoid, and cedar pollen allergen (data not shown). Those suggest that TNF/CHP nanoparticles have the potential as a vaccine adjuvant with a broad range of applications, as well as influenza.

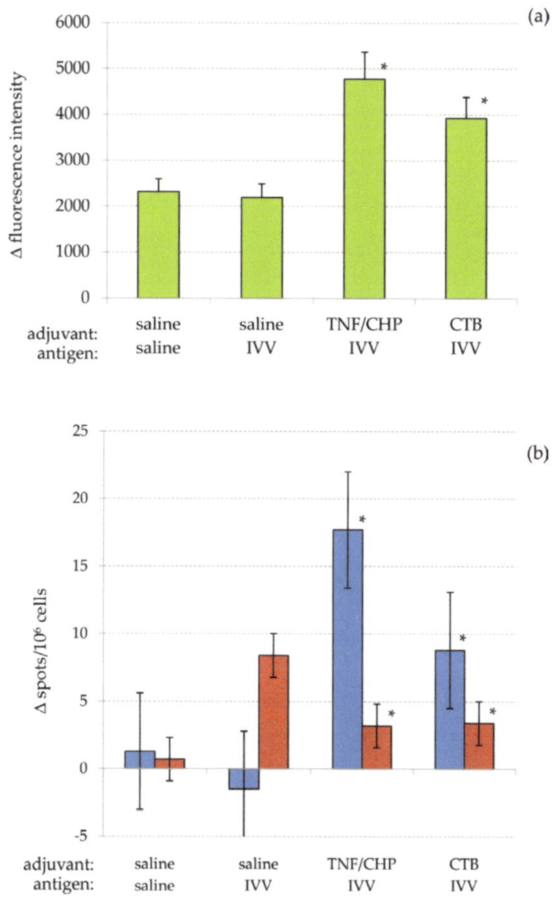

Figure 7. Proliferation and cytokine production by splenocytes from mice nasally administered TNF/CHP nanoparticles and IVV. BALB/c mice were given IVV (0.3 μg/mouse) and TNF/CHP nanoparticles (5 μg/mouse as TNF-α) or CTB (0.8 μg/mouse) by the nasal route as previously described. Splenocytes were prepared from the mice. Then, IVV-specific proliferation and IL-4/IFN-γ-producing cells were examined with alamarBlue and ELISpot, respectively. The results represent the difference (Δ) between data from experiments with and without IVV antigen stimulation. (a) proliferation response. (b) cytokine production. Blue column, IL-4 production; red column, IFN-γ production (mean ± SEM, n = 8). *, $P < 0.05$ vs. saline/IVV. Adapted with permission from Nagatomo D. et al. [33].

The antigen-specific T cell responses of the vaccinated animals were examined by challenging their isolated splenocytes with IVV. IVV-specific proliferation in the TNF/CHP nanoparticle group was comparable to that of CTB (**Figure 7a**). We also measured cytokine production to understand what kind of T cell response occurred. IVV alone increased IFN-γ production, while the addition of either adjuvant (TNF/CHP nanoparticle or CTB) suppressed IVV-induced Interferon-γ(IFN-γ) production. The TNF/CHP nanoparticles combined with IVV also produced IL-4 cytokine to a higher level than IVV with CTB (**Figure 7b**). These experiments suggest that the nasally administered adjuvant shifted the Th1/Th2 balance to a Th2-dominant state, which confirms previous results obtained with a mutant TNF-α [17].

6. Protective effect of TNF/CHP nanoparticles in lethal challenge of influenza virus on mice

To directly address the stimulatory effect of the TNF/CHP nanoparticle adjuvant on protective immunity, we challenged immunized mice with a lethal dose of influenza virus. Mice were nasally immunized with IVV with or without TNF/CHP nanoparticles once a week for 3 weeks. Then, they were challenged with the antigenically distinct influenza virus A/Puerto Rico/8/34 strain at a lethal dose (**Figure 8**). The mice that received only IVV died by 8 days post challenge, which was comparable to mice without IVV immunization. The TNF/CHP nanoparticles without the IVV slightly delayed the time to death, but all of the animals eventually died. On the contrary, combined administration of IVV and TNF/CHP nanoparticles showed a highly protective effect with 90% of the mice surviving lethal challenge. The effect was comparable to that of the CTB adjuvant. Free TNF also showed a somewhat protective effect. Interestingly,

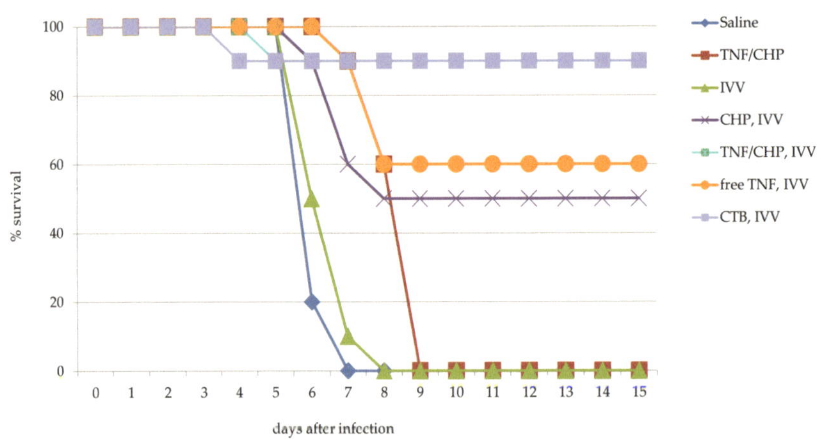

Figure 8. Protective effect of TNF/CHP nanoparticles adjuvant against lethal influenza virus challenge in mice. BALB/c mice were nasally administered with IVV with or without an adjuvant once a week for 3 weeks. Seven days after the final immunization, mice were challenged nasally with influenza virus (Puerto Rico/8/34, 10 LD_{50}) and then monitored daily. Mice that were moribund or that had lost more than 20% of their body weight were considered to have reached an experimental endpoint and were humanely euthanized by anesthetization. Blue diamond, saline only; red square, TNF/CHP nanoparticles only (5 μg/mouse of TNF-α); green triangle, IVV only (0.3 μg/mouse); purple cross, IVV with blank CHP nanoparticles (240 μg/mouse); blue square, IVV with TNF/CHP nanoparticles (5 μg/mouse of TNF-α); orange circle, IVV with free TNF (5 μg/mouse); purple dot, IVV with CTB (0.8 μg/mouse) (n = 10). Reproduced with permission from Nagatomo D. et al. [33].

CHP only (without TNF-α) provided a certain level of protection as an adjuvant, as we observed 50% survival. Importantly, the nasally administered TNF/CHP nanoparticles induced significant protective immunity in spite of the distinct antigenicities [36], suggesting that they have a potential for inducing broad cross-protection.

Antibodies became detectable after the second or third vaccination and reached plateau levels thereafter in mice vaccinated with TNF/CHP nanoparticles. The surviving animals immunized with IVV and TNF/CHP nanoparticles had immunological memory, including IgG_1 in plasma, and IgA in nasal/vaginal wash and feces. This memory was maintained at high levels for more than 90 days, and these mice responded to a boosting challenge of the IVV to further elevate the antibody levels (**Table 1**). These data indicate that the nanoparticles induced systemic immunity and long-lived memory, a critical feature for successful vaccine adjuvants. Overall, our data demonstrate that TNF/CHP nanoparticles are effective as a vaccine adjuvant for nasally delivered IVV.

TNF/CHP nanoparticles enhanced an IgA response not only at the site of application (e.g., in the nasal wash) but also at distant mucosal sites, such as the intestine (feces), vaginal, and salivary glands (data not shown). IgA antibody elicited at the mucosa is of vital importance as the natural route of infection for influenza is via the respiratory mucosa. Hence, local mucosal protection against pharyngeal carriage is likely to be decisive for preventing disease [37]. Conventional parenteral vaccines are not able to stimulate mucosal immune responses, thus restricting their efficacy in infections of mucosal surfaces such as the respiratory tract [1]. Our nasal vaccine/adjuvant formulation consisting of the IVV and TNF/CHP nanoparticles effectively induced both systemic and mucosal protective immunity.

			IgG_1 titer in plasma (U/mL)				**IgA titer in feces extract (U/mL)**	
Adjuvant	**Unimmunized**	**None**	**TNF/CHP nanoparticles**	**CTB**	**Unimmunized**	**None**	**TNF/CHP nanoparticles**	**CTB**
1 day before boost								
Day 90	n.d.	21,338 ± 2,438.9	16,917 ± 9,392.0	8,700 ± 5,510.3	n.d.	4.2 ± 3.5	14.4 ± 16.7	13.1 ± 10.8
12 days after boost								
Day 112	36.6 ± 43.2	19,764 ± 13,601.2	53,769 ± 29,893.7	37,729 ± 29,281.3	34.6 ± 33.3	19.8 ± 8.3	64.4 ± 63.4	58.2 ± 37.1

BALB/c mice were nasally administered with IVV (0.3 μg/mouse), with or without TNF/CHP nanoparticles (5 μg/mouse of TNF-α) or CTB (0.8 μg/mouse) once a week for 4 weeks. Ninety-one days after the immunization, the mice were boosted with IVV (0.9 μg/mouse). Twenty-one days after the boosting challenge, the blood plasma was prepared and the feces were extracted with 10 volumes of water. The IgG_1 in blood plasma and IgA in feces extract were examined (mean ± SEM, $n = 8$).
n.d., not detected.

Table 1. Induction of immunological memory by TNF/CHP nanoparticles.

Muraoka et al. proposed that CHP-based nanoparticles preferentially deliver antigen to antigen-presenting cells in the lymph nodes, which potentiates effective immune responses [38]. This might be the reason why the TNF/CHP nanoparticles induced excellent protective immunity. They, however, reported that CHP itself did not show an adjuvant effect in the context of a tumor vaccine [31]. Interestingly, CHP only (without TNF-α) showed a certain level of protective efficacy in our study. The reason for the discrepancy between their results and ours is not clear. It is unlikely, given the short time frame, that TNF-α was replaced *in vivo* by IVV antigens to form IVV/CHP nanoparticles that were then delivered to the lymph node. Another factor that is critical for adjuvant activity is particle size [39]; however, size is not an issue in our case since the DLS analyses showed no difference in particle size between the TNF/CHP nanoparticles and empty CHP particles (**Figure 4**). Most probably, the difference has to do with varying mechanisms to elicit protection against external pathogens, such as influenza virus, and internal antigens, such as tumor antigen.

7. Mechanistic analyses of effects of TNF/CHP nanoparticles

7.1. Activation of immune cells in NALT

Being focused on the nasal route of vaccination, we examined immune cells in nasal tissues after immunization. The mucosal surfaces contain abundant B cells, T cells, and plasma (or DC) cells. After repeated immunization of animals for 3 weeks, cells from the nasal-associated lymphoid tissues (NALT) were prepared from mice, and expression of a surface marker for DCs (CD11c) and activation markers for B cells (CD80 and CD86) were examined by flow cytometry. The ratios of $CD80^+/CD11c^+$ cells; $CD86^+/CD11c^+$ cells were 0.20; 0.33, 0.30; 0.44, and 0.33; 0.50% for saline, IVV, and IVV with TNF/CHP nanoparticles, respectively (data not shown). Even though the degree was small, IVV vaccination with or without TNF/CHP nanoparticles activated DCs and B cells. Also, TNF/CHP nanoparticles did not have a prominent effect on DC or B cell activation.

7.2. Antigen uptake and activation of NALT and nasal passage cells

We next focused on the early immune response of nasal mucosal tissues. Uptake of antigen by the mucosal tissues is essential for the induction of immune responses [40]. Therefore, we examined antigen uptake by NALT-resident and nasal passage DCs, the inductive sites of the common mucosal immune system [41]. In these experiments, we used ovalbumin (OVA) as a model antigen and assessed antigen uptake by DCs in the NALT and nasal passage cells by flow cytometry at 6 h after immunization. Immunization of mice with OVA combined with TNF/CHP nanoparticle activated antigen uptake by both NALT and nasal passage DCs. TNF/CHP nanoparticles stimulated DCs most in the nasal passage mucosal immune tissue (**Figure 9**). We also found that TNF/CHP nanoparticles enhanced expression of DC and B cell activation markers (CD40, 80, and 86) in a bone marrow-derived immature DC preparation *in vitro* (data not shown).

http://dx.doi.org/10.5772/64366

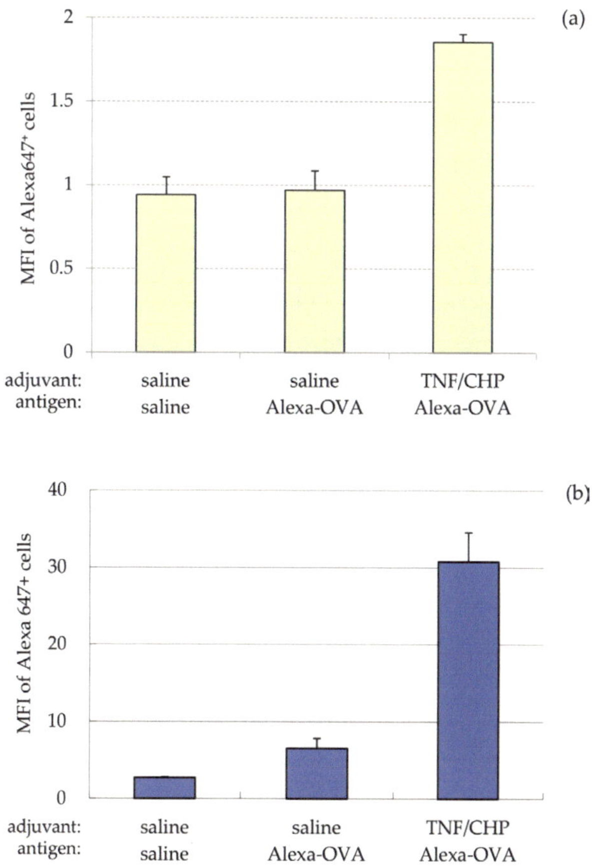

Figure 9. Antigen uptake of NALT and nasal passage DCs after TNF/CHP nanoparticles administration. BALB/c mice were nasally immunized with 10 μg of Alexa 647-labeled OVA antigen with or without TNF/CHP nanoparticles as an adjuvant. Six hours after the immunization the NALT and the nasal passage cells were prepared [42] and subjected to flow cytometric analysis. Antigen uptake was determined by detecting the Alexa 647 florescence intensity and the DC marker ($CD11c^+$ cells) in parallel, for example, ratio of Alexa $647^+/CD11c^+$. (a) NALT DCs, (b) nasal passage DCs. MFI, mean fluorescence intensity (mean ± SD, n = 4). Adapted with permission from Nagatomo D. et al. [33].

7.3. Expression of inflammatory signals in NALT

Vaccine adjuvants trigger the innate immune system allowing enhanced humoral and cellular responses against the co-administered vaccine antigens. To understand innate immune system activation caused by the TNF/CHP nanoparticles after immunization, we conducted gene expression profiling in NALT cells 2, 6, and 26 h after nasal administration of IVV antigen with or without the nanoparticles. By scattering analyses, the gene expression of inflammation- and immunity-related molecules was found to be significantly upregulated (data not shown). These included the triggering receptor expressed on myeloid cells 1, fibronectin 1, CD14, Toll-like receptor (TLR) 2, TLR3, IL-1β, IL-1 family 9, and IL-6. We confirmed the level of inflammation-related molecules in activated NALT cells by quantitative polymerase chain reaction (PCR) analysis. Expression of the inflammatory markers was enhanced when an adjuvant was included (TNF/CHP nanoparticles, free TNF, or CTB), while CHP itself did not show significant enhancing activity. Among the molecules tested, significant increases in expression occurred for IFN-γ, IL-1α, IL-1β, IL-6, CXCL2, IL-12β, CD14, and lipopolysaccharide (LPS)-binding protein (**Figure 10**). The degree of enhancement varied from gene to gene, but the greatest increase of expression was observed for IL-6 and IL-12β.

Overall, free exogenous TNF-α elicited the strongest increase in expression of inflammatory markers, and the enhancement tended to be highest at 2 h post-immunization. TNF/CHP nanoparticles elicited a moderate increase in gene expression by comparison, but the pattern over time was similar to that of free TNF-α. One reason for the discrepancy in gene expression between free TNF and the nanoparticles could be that the nanoparticles cause a slow release of TNF-α, prolonging the immune-stimulatory effect. The pattern of expression over time was very different for most genes when stimulated with CTB adjuvant. For example, although the expression of IL-12β was prominent at 6 h post-immunization when CTB was used as an adjuvant, the IL-12β response was much lower with TNF/CHP nanoparticles at the same time point.

Taken together, TNF/CHP nanoparticles delayed activation of innate immunity. By prolonging and dampening the stimulatory effect of TNF-α CHP seemed to minimize the unfavorable effects of TNF-α while promoting its beneficial activities. One important safety issue related to the development of nasal vaccines is the potential dissemination of vaccine antigens to the central nervous system (CNS). Past reports suggested that nasal administration of CTB allowed it to reach the CNS and accumulate in olfactory tissues. It caused Bell's Palsy in clinical studies, probably due to IL-12β production, and the use of CTB in humans was prohibited [43, 44]. In this context, the lower expression level of IL-12β seen in our experiments with TNF/CHP nanoparticles could be a beneficial safety feature.

Regarding CHP itself, a shell of the nanoparticles did not show immune-enhancing activity, such as increasing IgG_1 and IgA or the expression of inflammation-related genes (**Figure 10**). However, CHP did confer a certain level of protection in a lethal influenza virus challenge (**Figure 8**). We cannot easily account for these conflicting observations; there are other pathways and mechanisms likely involved and waiting to be clarified.

8. Safety study of TNF/CHP nanoparticles

General safety was preliminarily examined according to the OECD guidelines for testing chemicals [45]. Mice nasally administered with a combination of TNF/CHP nanoparticles and IVV either once or four times were subjected to an acute or a repeated toxicity study, respectively.

8.1. General symptoms, ophthalmic examination, body weight, and body temperature

No general symptoms or behavioral anomalies in either male or female animals were correlated with the IVV with TNF/CHP nanoparticles treatment during the study period. In ophthalmic examinations, there were no test material-related ocular findings observed. Body

http://dx.doi.org/10.5772/64366

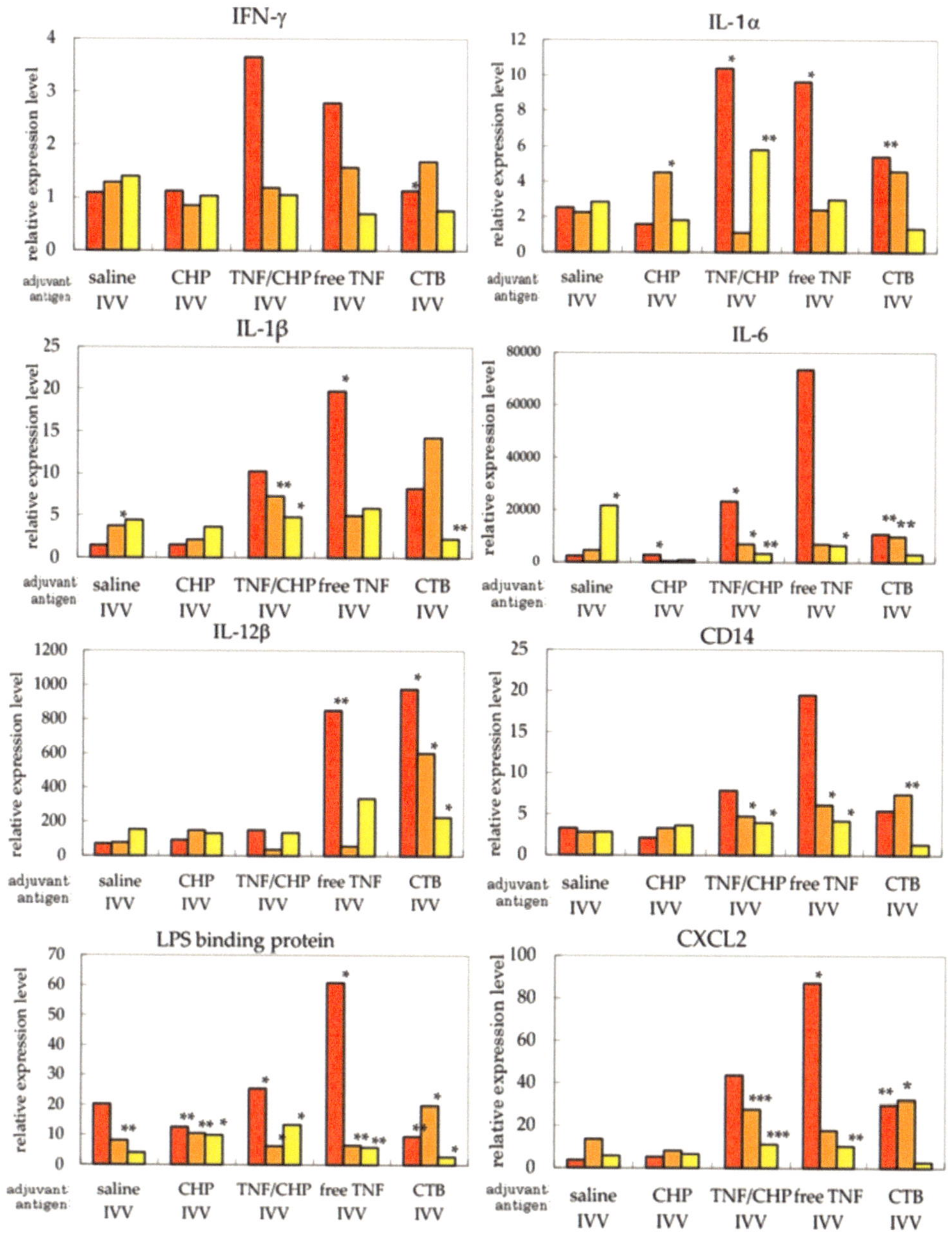

Figure 10. Gene expression in NALT after TNF/CHP nanoparticles administration. mRNA was prepared from NALT cells of BALB/c mice 2, 6, and 26 h after administration of TNF/CHP nanoparticles and IVV. Gene expression related to innate and adaptive immune responses was analyzed by quantitative PCR and normalized to glyceraldehyde 3-phosphate dehydrogenase (GAPDH) expression. Data are shown as relative level vs. control (means of quadruple experiments). Red column, 2 h; orange column, 6 h; yellow column, 26 h post treatment. *, $P < 0.05$; **, $P < 0.01$; ***, $P < 0.001$ vs. saline control. Adapted with permission from Nagatomo D. et al. [33].

weight and body temperature were not statistically different among the treatment groups (data not shown).

8.2. Hematology, blood biochemistry, and urinalysis

Hematology evaluations were performed during and at the end of study. There were no differences in any of the tested parameters (white blood cell, red blood cell, hematocrit, lymphocyte, neutrophil, eosinophil, basophil, and monocyte) between controls and TNF/CHP nanoparticles with the IVV treatment. For blood biochemistry, we examined total protein, albumin, urea nitrogen, creatinine, Na^+, K^+, Cl^-, Ca^{2+}, inorganic phosphate, aspartate aminotransferase (AST), alanine aminotransferase (ALT), lactate dehydrogenase (LDH), amylase (AMY), γ-glutamyl transpeptidase (γ-GT), total cholesterol, triglyceride, high density lipoprotein (HDL)-cholesterol, total bilirubin, and glucose. Urobilinogen, bilirubin, ketone body, glucose, protein, pH, specific gravity, nitrite salt, and leucocytes were examined during the study period. All differences found during the study fell within historical control value ranges and were not considered test material-related (data not shown).

8.3. Pathology and major organ weights

Gross pathology of all the animals was examined at the end of the study. The major organs (brain, heart, lung, kidney, liver, ovary, testis, spleen, adrenal, and thymus) were weighed at the end of the study in all of the animals. No change was noted as test material-related (data not shown).

8.4. Histopathology

The histopathology of tissues from animals in each group was examined. As discussed in Section 7.3, there were some concerns of possible harmful effects on the CNS. However, no abnormalities in the brain, especially olfactory bulb, were noted in any animals after histological examination. There were some effects observed at the administration site (nasal mucosal tissue). While single administration showed no effect, repeated administration with IVV alone showed a slight infusion and TNF/CHP nanoparticles combined with IVV induced slight-to-moderate infusion and infiltration of inflammatory cells (lymphocytes, neutrophils, eosinophils, and mast cells). However, the response was reversed with time since the infusion diminished to trace proportions after the 2-week cessation period. No excessive inflammatory symptoms, such as formation of edema or fibrosis, were noted (data not shown).

Overall, no obvious immunotoxicity was detected. Although further evaluation is required, our results demonstrate that the toxicity of TNF/CHP nanoparticles is relatively low and safe as a nasal vaccine adjuvant against influenza.

Very recently, Onishi et al. reported that hydroxypropyl-β-cyclodextrin (HP-β-CD), another type of saccharide-based material that can form nanoparticles, exhibited adjuvant activity and elicited a strong protective effect against influenza virus in mice and cynomolgus macaques [46]. They suggested the involvement of follicular helper T cells via myeloid differentiation primary gene 88 (MyD88)- and TANK-binding kinase (TBK)-dependent pathways. Their findings may shed some light on additional mechanisms at play with nanoparticles as vaccine adjuvants. However, they mentioned the cytotoxicity of HP-β-CD at more than 0.5% *in vitro*, probably because of β-CD's ability to extract cholesterol out of cell membranes [47]. TNF/CHP nanoparticles might represent a preferable alternative.

A probable precaution for the practical use of TNF/CHP nanoparticles is avoiding contact with high concentrations of dissolved proteins as mentioned in Section 4.2. Unless, encapsulated TNF-α would be released from the nanoparticles and the adjuvant activity would be diminished. This means that the nanoparticles is not suitable for *i.v.* administration and premixed formulation with vaccine antigen. For the best performance, we recommend to administer the TNF/CHP nanoparticles on mucosa, such as nasal surface, after mixing with the vaccine antigen just before use.

9. Conclusions

The results of this study demonstrate that TNF/CHP nanoparticles are effective as a vaccine adjuvant against influenza when administered via the nasal mucosal route. Moreover, the ability of TNF/CHP nanoparticles to stimulate comparatively balanced systemic and mucosal immune responses makes them a potentially promising vaccine adjuvant for inducing immunity against infectious pathogens. In the short term, TNF/CHP nanoparticles may aid the development of new nasal influenza vaccines. Looking further ahead, we propose that combining TNF/CHP nanoparticles with next-generation vaccine platforms that do not rely on the cold chain will offer valuable alternatives for vaccination in a variety of settings.

Acknowledgements

The author is very grateful to Dr. Ayato Takada of Research Center for Zoonosis Control, Hokkaido University for his expertise with influenza challenge of mice. The author is also thankful to the staff of R&D Center, Hayashibara Co., Ltd. for their excellent technical assistance, especially Mr. Daiki Nagatomo and Ms. Madoka Taniai for the mechanistic analyses of action, and Dr. Shigeyuki Arai for the histopathological examination.

Author details

Tsunetaka Ohta

Address all correspondence to: tsunetaka.ota@hb.nagase.co.jp

R&D Center, Hayashibara Co. Ltd., Okayama, Japan

References

[1] Kikuta K, Hirabayashi Y, Nagamine T, Aizawa C, Ueno Y, Oya A, Kurata T, and Tamura S. Cross-protection against influenza B type virus infection by intranasal inoculation of the HA vaccines combined with cholera toxin B subunit. Vaccine. 1990;8:595–599.

[2] Ichinohe T, Kawaguchi A, Tamura S, Takahashi H, Sawa H, Ninomiya A, Imai M, Itamura S, Odagiri T, Tashiro M, Chiba J, Sata T, Kurata T, and Hasegawa H. Intranasal immunization with H5N1 vaccine plus Poly I:Poly C12U, a Toll-like receptor agonist, protects mice against homologous and heterologous virus challenge. Microbes Infect. 2007;9:1333–1400.

[3] Holmgren J and Czerkinsky C. Mucosal immunity and vaccines. Nat. Med. 2005;11:S45–S53.

[4] Kiyono H and Fukuyama S. NALT-versus Peyer's-patch-mediated mucosal immunity. Nat. Rev. Immunol. 2004;4:699–710.

[5] Goodwin K, Viboud C, and Simonsen L. Antibody response to influenza vaccination in the elderly: a quantitative review. Vaccine. 2006;24:1159–1169.

[6] Garcon N, Leroux-Roels G, and Cheng WF. Chapter 4, Vaccine adjuvants. In: Garçon N, Stern PL, Anthony L. Cunningham AL, edited. Understanding Modern Vaccines: Perspectives in Vaccinology. Amsterdam: Elsevier; 2011;1: pp. 89–113. ISSN 2210–7630.

[7] De Gregorio E, Caproni E, and Ulmer JB. Vaccine adjuvants: mode of action. Front. Immunol. 2013;4:214. doi:10.3389/fimmu.2013.00214.

[8] Boyaka PN, Lillard JW, and McGhee J. Interleukin 12 and innate molecules for enhanced mucosal immunity. Immunol. Res. 1999;20:207–217.

[9] Tovey MG and Lallemand C. Adjuvant acitivity of cytokines. Methods Mol. Biol. 2010;626:287–309.

[10] Boyaka PN and McGhee JR. Cytokines as adjuvants for the induction of mucosal immunity. Adv. Drug Deliv. Rev. 2001;51:71–79.

[11] Aggarwal BB, Kohr WJ, Hass PE, Moffat B, Spencer SA, Henzel WJ, Bringman TS, Nedwin GE, Goeddel DV, and Harkins RN. Human tumor necrosis factor, production, purification, and characterization. J. Biol. Chem. 1985;260:2345–2354.

[12] Wajant H, Pfizenmaier K, and Scheurich P. Tumor necrosis factor signaling. Cell Death Differ. 2003;10:45–65.

[13] Calzascia T, Pellegrini M, Hall H, Sabbagh L, Ono N, Elford AR, Mak TW, and Ohashi PS. TNF-alpha is critical for antitumor but not antiviral T cell immunity in mice. J. Clin. Invest. 2007;117:3833–3845.

[14] Brunner C, Seiderer J, Schlamp A, Bidlingmaier M, Eigler A, Haimerl W, Lehr HA, Krieg AM, Hartmann G, and Endres S. Enhanced dendritic cell maturation by TNF-alpha or

cytidine-phosphate-guanosine DNA drives T cell activation *in vitro* and therapeutic anti-tumor immune responses *in vivo*. J. Immunol. 2000;165:6278–6286.

[15] Chen Z, Huang H, Chang T, Carlsen S, Saxena A, Marr R, Xing Z, and Xiang J. Enhanced HER-2/neu-specific antitumor immunity by cotransduction of mouse dendritic cells with two genes encoding HER-2/neu and alpha tumor necrosis factor. Cancer Gene Ther. 2002;9:778–786.

[16] Kayamuro H, Abe Y, Yoshioka Y, Katayama K, Nomura T, Yoshida T, Yamashita K, Yoshikawa T, Kawai Y, Mayumi T, Hiroi T, Itoh N, Nagano K, Kamada H, Tsunoda S, and Tsutsumi Y. The use of a mutant TNF-α as a vaccine adjuvant for the induction of mucosal immune responses. Biomaterials. 2009;30:5869–5876. doi:10.1016/j.biomaterials.2009.07.009.

[17] Kayamuro H, Abe Y, Yoshioka Y, Katayama K, Yoshida T, Yamashita K, Yoshikawa T, Kawai Y, Mayumi T, Hiroi T, Itoh N, Nagano K, Kamada H, Tsunoda S, and Tsutsumi Y. Mutant TNF-alpha, mTNF-K90R, is a novel candidate adjuvant for a mucosal vaccine against HIV. Pharmazie. 2010;65:254–256.

[18] Kean T and Thanou M. Biodegradation, biodistribution and toxicity of chitosan. Adv. Drug Deliv. Rev. 2010;62:3–11. doi:10.1016/j.addr.2009.09.004.

[19] Toole TB. Hyaluronan: from extracellular glue to pericellular cue. Nat. Rev. Cancer. 2004;4:528–539.

[20] Lethers TD. Biotechnological production and applications of pullulan. Appl. Microbiol. Biotechnol. 2003;62:468–473.

[21] Prajapati VD, Jani GK, and Khanda SM. Pullulan: an exopolysaccharide and its various applications. Carbohydr. Polym. 2013;95:540–549. doi:10.1016/j.carbpol.2013.02.082.

[22] Akiyama E, Morimoto N, Kujawa P, Ozawa Y, Winnik FM, and Akiyoshi K. Self-assembled nanogels of cholesteryl-modified polysaccharides: effect of the polysaccharide structure on their association characteristics in the dilute and semidilute regimes. Biomacromolecules. 2007;8:2366–2373.

[23] Akiyoshi K, Kobayashi S, Shichibe S, Mix D, Baudys M, Kim SW, and Sunamoto J. Self-assembled hydrogel nanoparticle of cholesterol-bearing pullulan as a carrier of protein drugs: complexation and stabilization of insulin. J. Control. Release. 1998;54:313–320.

[24] Akiyoshi K, Sasaki Y, and Sunamoto J. Molecular chaperone-like activity of hydrogel nanoparticles of hydrophobized pullulan: thermal stabilization with refolding of carbonic anhydrase B. Bioconj. Chem. 1999;10:321–324.

[25] Shimizu T, Kishida T, Hasegawa U, Ueda Y, Imanishi J, Yamagishi H, Akiyoshi K, Otsuji E, and Mazda O. Nanogel DDS enables sustained release of IL-12 for tumor immunotherapy. Biochem. Biophys. Res. Commun. 2008;367:330–335.

[26] Letchford K and Burt H. A review of the formation and classification of amphiphilic block copolymer nanoparticulate structures: micelles, nanospheres, nanocapsules and polymersomes. Eur. J. Pharm. Biopharm. 2007;65:259–269.

[27] Kobiyama K, Aoshi T, Narita H, Kuroda E, Hayashi M, Tetsutani K, Koyama S, Mochizuki S, Sakurai K, Katakai Y, Yasutomi Y, Saijo S, Iwakura Y, Akira S, Coban C, and Ishii KJ. Nonagonistic Dectin-1 ligand transforms CpG into a multitask nanoparticlate TLR9 agonist. Proc. Natl. Acad. Sci. U.S.A. 2014;111:3086–3092. doi:10.1073/pnas.1319268111.

[28] Mody KT, Popat A, Mahony D, Cavallaro AS, Yu C, and Mitter N. Mesoporous silica nanoparticles as antigen carriers and adjuvants for vaccine delivery. Nanoscale. 2013;5:5167–5179. doi:10.1039/c3nr00357d.

[29] Shiku H, Wang L, Ikuta Y, Okugawa T, Schmitt M, Gu X, Akiyoshi K, Sunamoto J, and Nakamura H. Development of a cancer vaccine: peptides, proteins, and DNA. Cancer Chemother. Pharmacol. 2000;46:S77–S82.

[30] Kageyama S, Wada H, Muro K, Niwa Y, Ueda S, Miyata H, Taniguchi S, Sugino SH, Miyahara Y, Ikeda H, Imai N, Sato E, Yamada T, Osakao M, Ohnishi M, Harada N, Hishida T, Doki Y, and Shiku H. Dose-dependent effects of NY-ESO-1 protein vaccine complexed with cholesteryl pullulan (CHP-NY-ESO-1) on immune responses and survival benefits of esophageal cancer patients. J. Transl. Med. 2013;11:246. doi: 10.1186/1479-5876-11-246.

[31] Kageyama S, Kitano S, Hirayama M, Nagata M, Imai H, Shiraishi T, Akiyoshi K, Scott AM, Murphy R, Hoffman EW, Old LJ, Katayama N, and Shiku H. Humoral immune responses in patients vaccinated with 1-146 HER2 protein complexed with cholesteryl pullulan nanogel. Cancer Sci. 2008;99:601–607.

[32] Fukuda S, Ando S, Sanou O, Taniai M, Fujii M, Masaki N, Nakamura K, Ando O, Torigoe K, Sugimoto T, and Kurimoto M. Simultaneous production of natural human tumor necrosis factor-α, -β and interferon-α from BALL-1 cells stimulated by HVJ. Lymphokine Res. 1988;7:175–185.

[33] Nagatomo D, Taniai M, Ariyasu H, Taniguchi M, Aga M, Ariyasu T, Ohta T, and Fukuda S. Cholesteryl pullulan encapsulated TNF-α nanoparticles are an effective mucosal vaccine adjuvant against influenza virus. BioMed Res. Int. 2015;2015:471468. doi: 10.1155/2015/471468.

[34] Ayame H, Morimoto N, and Akiyoshi K. Self-assembled cationic nanogels for intracellular protein delivery. Bioconjug. Chem. 2008;19:882–890. doi:10.1021/bc700422s.

[35] Wu HY, and Russell M. Induction of mucosal and systemic immune responses by intranasal immunization using recombinant cholera toxin B subunit as an adjuvant. Vaccine. 1998;16:286–292.

[36] Ichinohe T, Watanabe I. Ito S, Fujii H, Moriyama M, Tamura S, Takahashi H, Sawada H, Chiba J, Kurata T, Sata T, and Hasegawa H. Synthetic double-stranded RNA

poly(I:C) combined with mucosal vaccine protects against influenza virus infection. J. Virol. 2005;79:2910–2919.

[37] Patel H, Yewale C, Rathi MN, and Misra A. Mucosal immunization: a review of strategies and challenges. Crit. Rev. Ther. Drug Carrier Syst. 2014;31:273–303.

[38] Muraoka D, Harada N, Hayashi T, Tahara Y, Momose F, Sawada SI, Mukai SA, Akiyoshi K, and Shiku H. Nanogel-based immunologically stealth vaccine targets macrophages in the medulla of lymph node and induces potent antitumor immunity. ACS Nano. 2014;8:9209–9218. doi:10.1021/nn502975r.

[39] Oyewumi MO, Kumar A, and Cui Z. Nano-microparticles as immune adjuvants: correlating particle sizes and the resultant immune responses. Expert Rev. Vaccines. 2010;9:1095–1107. doi:10.1586/erv.10.89.

[40] Yuki K and Kiyono H. New generation of mucosa adjuvants for the induction of protective immunity. Rev. Med. Virol. 2003;13:293–310.

[41] Mestecky J and McGhee JR. Immunoglobulin A (IgA): molecular and cellular interactions involved in IgA biosynthesis and immune response. Adv. Immunol. 1987;40:153–245.

[42] Rodriguez-Monroy MA, Rojas-Hernandez S, and Morefno-Fierros L. Phenotypic and functional differences between lymphocytes from NALT and nasal passages of mice. Scand. J. Immunol. 2007;65:276–288.

[43] Mutsch M, Zhou W, Rhodes P, Bopp M, Chen RT, Linder T, Spyr C, and Steffen R. Use of the inactivated intranasal influenza vaccine and the risk of Bell's palsy in Switzerland. N. Engl. J. Med. 2004;350:896–903.

[44] van Ginkel FW, Jackson RJ, Yuki Y, and McGhee JR. Cutting edge: The mucosal adjuvant cholera toxin redirects vaccine proteins into olfactory tissues. J. Immunol. 2000;165:4778–4782.

[45] OECD. OECD Guidelines for the testing of chemicals and related documents [Internet]. Available from: http://www.oecd.org/chemicalsafety/testing/oecdguidelinesforthetestingofchemicals.htm. [Accessed: 2016-03-18].

[46] Onishi M, Ozasa K, Kobiyama K, Ohata K, Kitano M, Taniguchi K, Homma T, Kobayashi M, Sato A, Katakai Y, Yasutomi Y, Wijaya E, Igarashi Y, Nakatsu N, Ise W, Inoue T, Yamada H, Vandenbon A, Standley DM, Kurosaki T, Coban C, Aoshi T, Kuroda E, and Ishii KJ. Hydroxypropyl-β-cyclodextrin spikes local inflammation that induces Th2 cell and T follicular helper cell responses to the coadministered antigen. J. Immunol. 2015;194:2673–2682. doi:10.4049/jimmunol.1402027.

[47] Atger VM, de la Llera Moya M, Stoudt GW, Rodrigueza WV, Phillips MC, and Rothblat GH. Cyclodextrins as catalysts for the removal of cholesterol from macrophage foam cells. J. Clin. Invest. 1997;99:773–780.

Chapter 8

Development of Vaccines for Poultry Against H5 Avian Influenza Based on Turkey Herpesvirus Vector

Atsushi Yasuda, Motoyuki Esaki,
Kristi Moore Dorsey, Zoltan Penzes, Vilmos Palya,
Darrell R. Kapczynski and Yannick Gardin

Additional information is available at the end of the chapter

http://dx.doi.org/10.5772/64348

Abstract

Avian influenza (AI) remains a major threat to public health as well as to the poultry industry. AI vaccines are considered a suitable tool to support AI control programs in combination with other control measures such as good biosecurity and monitoring programs. We constructed recombinant turkey herpesvirus (HVT) vector vaccines expressing the hemagglutinin gene of AI virus H5 subtype (rHVT-H5) and evaluated their characteristics and efficacy against AI. We found that the cytomegalovirus (CMV) promoter is the most suitable for expression of the hemagglutinin gene among three promoters we evaluated. The rHVT-H5 vaccine did not cause any adverse reactions and did not revert to virulence after passages in chicken. Finally, efficacy of the rHVT-H5 vaccine was evaluated. We demonstrated that it provided protection against diverse AI H5 viruses belonging to different clades and reduced virus shedding from the challenged chicken. We also proved that efficacy provided by the rHVT-H5 vaccine was not significantly affected by presence of maternally derived antibodies (MDA) against AI virus. Furthermore, the rHVT-H5 vaccine could be applicable to the differentiating infected from vaccinated animals (DIVA) strategy. In summary, we successfully developed a HVT vector AI vaccine that possesses features that could be beneficial to AI control.

Keywords: avian influenza, turkey herpesvirus, vector vaccines, DIVA, hemagglutinin gene

1. Introduction

Avian influenza (AI) is an important zoonotic disease and it remains a major threat to public health and to the poultry industry. The highly pathogenic (HP) H5N1 outbreaks were first reported in China in 1996 and then spread to other parts of the world. These HP avian influenza viruses (AIV) have become endemic in several countries including China, Indonesia, Vietnam, and Egypt [1]. Between 2003 and 2015, 846 confirmed human cases of AI (H5N1) have been reported and 449 of those human patients have died (WHO, 2016). Most recently, HP H5N2 and H5N8 viruses caused outbreaks in the United States from December 2014 to June 2015, which resulted in depopulation of more than 48 million chickens and turkeys. These outbreaks cost farmers, the government, and consumers in the United States billions of dollars. France has also been hit by HP H5 viruses since November 2015 and the outbreaks have caused significant damages to its poultry industry. These recent HP H5 AIV continued to evolve into various clades as defined by the World Health Organization (WHO)/World Organisation for Animal Health (OIE)/Food and Agriculture Organization (FAO) H5N1 Evolution Working Group according to phylogenetic topology based on *hemagglutinin* (HA) gene sequences [2]. Another significant event of AI is the series of human infections in China caused by H7N9 AIV since March 2013. Although these viruses are low pathogenic (LP) for poultry, 277 human deaths have been reported out of 693 confirmed cases (WHO, 2016). These cases emphasize importance of controlling AIV in poultry for the industry as well as for public health.

Control of HP AI in poultry has been achieved traditionally through (1) education, (2) biosecurity, (3) diagnostics and surveillance, and (4) elimination of infected poultry (stamping-out) [3]. Viruses were successfully eradicated through a combination of those measures in many countries affected by HP AIV. However, in endemically infected countries, viruses had spread widely before executing effective measures, and therefore, it was impossible to identify and eliminate all of infected birds. In such endemic situations, vaccines are considered suitable and powerful tools to support AI eradication or control programs in combination with other control measures such as good biosecurity and monitoring programs [4–6]. When used properly, vaccines for AI have been demonstrated to protect poultry against clinical signs and mortality, increase resistance to infection, and reduce virus shedding markedly, thus decreasing the possibility of virus spreading among birds [7]. Most frequently used AI vaccines have been oil-adjuvanted, inactivated whole-virus vaccines and fowlpox virus or Newcastle disease virus (NDV)-vectored vaccines are also available. However, efficacy of these vaccines is limited especially against antigenically distant viruses [8–10]. Also, efficacy of these vaccines is known to be severely impaired by maternally derived antibodies (MDA) [11, 12]. Furthermore, oil-adjuvanted, inactivated whole-virus vaccines impede virus surveillance programs based on serology because serological responses elicited by the inactivated whole-virus vaccines are indistinguishable to those elicited by live field viruses. Therefore, development of novel vaccines which are efficacious in the face of MDA and are compatible with so-called differentiate infected from vaccinated animals (DIVA) strategy is necessary.

Turkey herpesvirus (HVT), or the meleagrid herpesvirus 1, belongs to the family of *Herpesviridae*, the subfamily of *Alphaherpesvirinae*, and the genus *Mardivirus*. It is classified as part of the Marek's disease virus (MDV) group and designated as serotype 3 MDV. HVT is non-oncogenic and antigenically related to oncogenic serotype 1 MDV. The virus has been utilized extensively as a vaccine against Marek's disease for over 30 years and considered extremely safe [13, 14]. It is administered at hatcheries either to day-of-age chicks by subcutaneous (SQ) route or in ovo to chicken embryos at 18–19 days of incubation and is known to elicit strong cell-mediated immunity as well as humoral immunity [15–17]. Furthermore, since HVT becomes latent and persists in inoculated chickens [18], a longer period of protection is expected. Indeed, HVT-vectored Newcastle disease vaccine has been shown to be efficacious for 72 weeks after inoculation into day-of-age chicks [19]. For aforementioned reasons and also because of its large genome that can be potentially used for insertion of heterologous genes [20], HVT has been evaluated as vectors expressing protective antigen gene(s) of various poultry pathogens including NDV, infectious bursal disease virus (IBDV), and infectious laryngotracheitis virus (ILTV) [21–26]. These HVT vector vaccines have shown to be very safe and induce effective humoral and cellular immunity that is long lasting. Also, the efficacy of HVT vector vaccines does not appear to be excessively affected by the presence of MDA, probably because HVT replicates in a cell-associated manner [22]. Here, we intended to apply the HVT vector technology to develop an effective poultry vaccine against AI. Several HVT vector vaccines expressing *HA* gene of H5 AIV (rHVT-H5) were constructed and evaluated for their characteristics and efficacy against AI.

2. Construction of rHVT-H5 vaccines

2.1. Construction of recombinant viruses

A number of HVT vector vaccines have been constructed and evaluated for their characteristics and efficacy against avian pathogens [21–26]. There are three important elements in HVT vector vaccines that can impact efficacy of these vaccines in chicken: insertion sites, antigen genes, and promoters. Several insertion sites including US2, US10, UL39 [21], and an intergenic region between UL45 and UL46 (UL45/46) [24–26] have been evaluated. Out of these potential insertion sites, we demonstrated that insertion of extraneous genes at the UL45/46 site did not alter their capacity to replicate [26]. Furthermore, using the UL45/46 as the insertion site, we were successful in constructing HVT vector vaccines having antigen genes of NDV, IBDV, or ILTV that are highly efficacious against these pathogens [24–26]. Therefore, we decided to use the UL45/46 site for insertion of antigen genes of AIV.

Eight segments of genomic RNA of influenza A virus encode three membrane-associated proteins, HA, neuraminidase (NA), and Matrix (M) 2, five internal proteins, nucleoprotein (NP), PB1, PB2, PA, and M1, and two nonstructural (NS) proteins, NS1 and NS2. Out of these viral proteins, the HA surface glycoprotein is known to be the major antigen and elicits neutralizing antibodies that provide protection against the disease [27]. We used the *HA* gene cloned from LP A/turkey/Wisconsin/68 (H5N9) strain or HP A/Swan/Hungary/4999/2006

(H5N1) clade 2.2 strain. The cleavage site of the *HA* gene from A/Swan/Hungary/4999/2006 (H5N1) strain was altered to a typical cleavage site sequence of LP AIV strains.

Selection of promoters that control the expression of antigen genes is also an important factor. Tsukamoto et al. compared the cytomegalovirus (CMV) promoter and CMV/chicken β-actin chimera (Pec) promoter for expression of IBDV *VP2* gene in HVT vectors and found that the Pec promoter expressed more VP2 protein and provided superior protection against challenge with IBDV [24]. In MDV serotype 1 (MDV1) vectors expressing NDV *fusion* gene, less potent MDV glycoprotein B promoter gave better protection than the simian virus 40 (SV40) late promoter when tested in chickens with MDA [28]. Another group compared five different promoters for expression of the *HA* gene of AIV H9N2 subtype in MDV vectors and found that two MDV endogenous promoters (pp38 and gB) with relatively low expression activities provided better protection than the other three promoters (CMV, SV40, and p1.8 kb) [29]. In this experiment, to find the most appropriate promoter to express the *HA* gene of AIV H5 subtype in HVT vectors, we compared three different promoters: the CMV promoter, the chicken β-actin (Bac) promoter, and the Pec promoter.

To prepare for construction of recombinant HVT, HVT insertion site sequences (*UL45* and *UL46* genes) were isolated by polymerase chain reaction (PCR) and cloned into pUC18. Homology plasmids were then constructed by inserting the *HA* gene with the promoter into the insertion site (between *UL45* gene and *UL46* gene) of the HVT sequences. The homology plasmid along with HVT infectious genomic DNA was transfected into chicken embryo fibroblasts (CEF), where homologous recombination took place. Recombinant HVT with the inserted gene was identified by an in situ immunostaining assay called black plaque assay (BPA) using anti-HA (H5) antibodies. Recombinant HVT was purified from HVT parent through several rounds of screening process by the BPA.

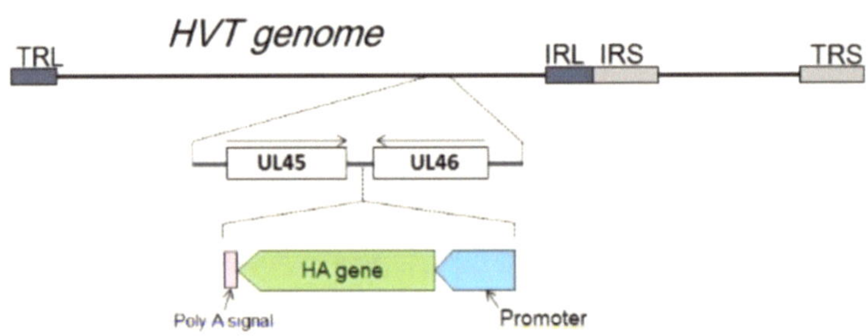

Figure 1. Genomic structure of rHVT-H5 vaccines.

2.2. In vitro characterization of rHVT-H5

Figure 1 shows genomic structures of the constructed rHVT-H5 vaccines. The genomic structures of the rHVT-H5 vaccines were confirmed by PCR assays with one primer binding to the insert sequence and the other primer binding to the HVT insertion site sequences (data not shown). The genomic structures were further confirmed by Southern blot analysis using

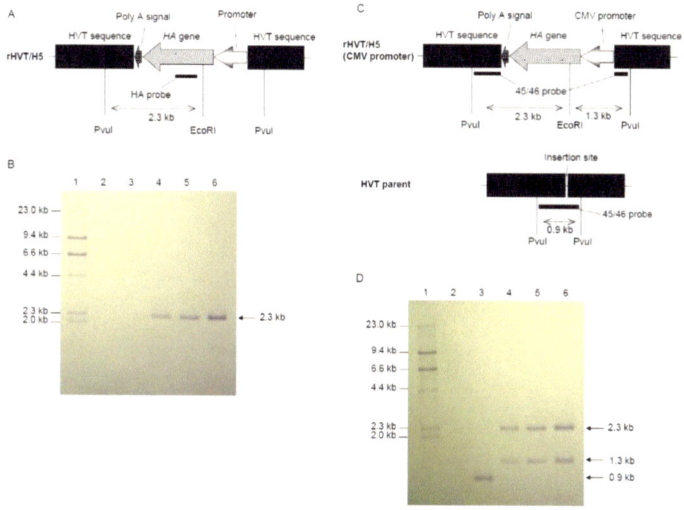

Figure 2. (A) Gene structure of rHVT/H5 and expected annealing site of the HA probe. (B) Result of Southern blot using the HA probe. Lane 1 = DNA molecular weight marker II, DIG-labeled (Roche); Lane 2 = uninoculated CEF control; Lane 3 = HVT parent; Lane 4 = rHVT/H5; Lane 5 = rHVT/H5 passage 5; Lane 6 = homology plasmid. (C) Gene structure of rHVT/H5 with CMV promoter and HVT parent and expected annealing site of the 45/46 probe. (D) Result of Southern blot using the 45/46 probe. Lane 1 = DNA molecular weight marker II, DIG-labeled (Roche); Lane 2 = uninoculated CEF control; Lane 3 = HVT parent; Lane 4 = rHVT/H5 with CMV promoter; Lane 5 = rHVT/H5 with CMV promoter passage 5; Lane 6 = homology plasmid.

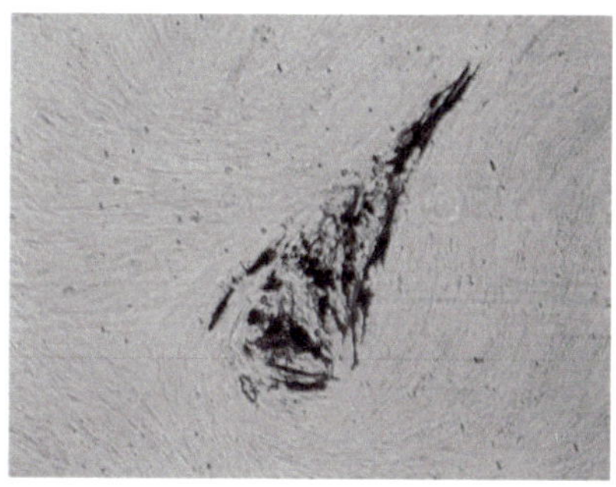

Figure 3. Black plaque assay on a rHVT/H5 plaque detecting expression of the HA protein of AIV H5 subtype. CEF monolayer infected with rHVT/H5 was incubated for 5 days and fixed with methanol:acetone. The monolayer with rHVT/H5 plaques was reacted with chicken anti-AIV HA serum, then with biotinylated anti-chicken IgG antibody and finally with streptavidin-alkaline phosphatase conjugates. Plaques expressing HA protein were stained by addition of BCIP/NBT solution.

digoxigenin-labeled probes specific to the *HA* gene or HVT insertion site sequences (**Figure 2**). Expression of the HA protein by the rHVT-H5 vaccines was confirmed by BPA using the chicken anti-HA serum (**Figure 3**). Western blot analysis using the chicken anti-HA serum detected a 75-kDa band with CEF infected with the rHVT-H5 (**Figure 4**). This band corresponds to non-cleaved HA protein that is produced by the rHVT-H5. Since the cleavage sites of the expressed HA proteins are those of LP AIV strains, the HA protein was not cleaved to HA1 and HA2 subunits in CEF.

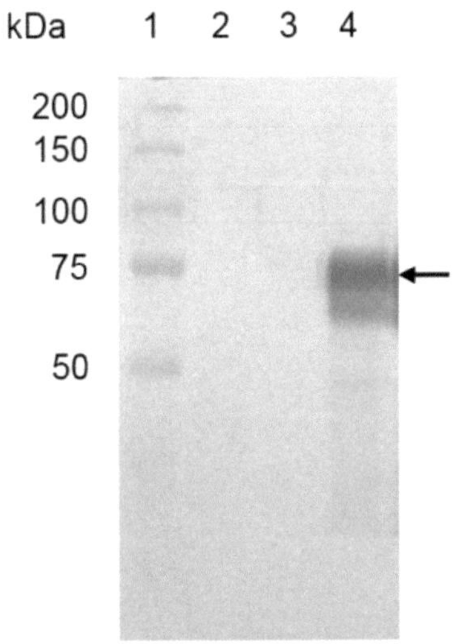

Figure 4. Western blot assay detecting expression of the HA protein by rHVT/H5. Lane 1 = Precision Plus Protein All Blue Standards (Bio-Rad Laboratories); Lane 2 = CEF control; Lane 3 = HVT FC126 parent strain; Lane 4 = rHVT/H5. An arrow indicates the HA protein with a molecular weight of 75 kDa.

In order to assess genetic and phenotypic stability of the rHVT-H5 vaccines, the viruses were passed in CEF 20 times. Viruses after the passages were characterized by PCR, Southern blot, BPA, and western blot. Results obtained with the passed viruses were identical to those obtained with the viruses before the passage (data not shown), and therefore, it was concluded that these viruses were genetically and phenotypically stable.

2.3. Evaluation of promoters for expression of HA gene

In order to identify the most suitable promoter among the CMV promoter, the Bac promoter, and the Pec promoter for expression of the *HA* gene, we compared three rHVT-H5 vaccines harboring the *HA* gene from A/turkey/Wisconsin/68 (H5N9) strain with one of these promoters. The rHVT-H5 vaccines with the CMV promoter, the Bac promoter, and the Pec promoter were designated as HVT-CMV-H5Wis68, HVT-Bac-H5Wis68, and HVT-Pec-H5Wis68, respectively.

One-day-old specific pathogen free (SPF) White Leghorn chicks were vaccinated subcutaneously with one of the rHVT-H5 vaccines. A group of chickens was held as a non-inoculated negative control group and another group of chickens was vaccinated subcutaneously with inactivated A/turkey/Wisconsin/68 (H5N9) vaccine at 3 weeks of age as an inactivated vaccine control group. Chickens in each group were bled each week between 3 and 7 weeks of age (6 and 7 weeks of age for the inactivated vaccine control group) and obtained sera were evaluated by the AIV hemagglutination inhibition (HI) test and AIV enzyme-linked immunosorbent assay (ELISA). The AIV HI tests were conducted using four hemagglutination units of an inactivated AIV homologous antigen of the A/turkey/Wisconsin/68 (H5N9) strain according to the standard procedure [30].

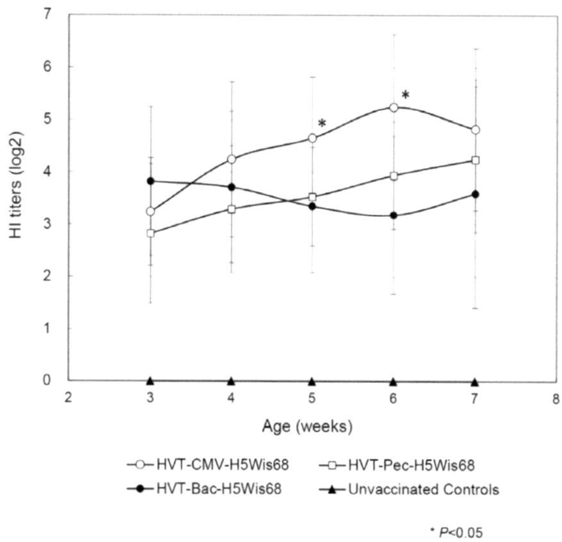

Figure 5. HI titers in chickens vaccinated with rHVT-H5 vaccines with different promoters.

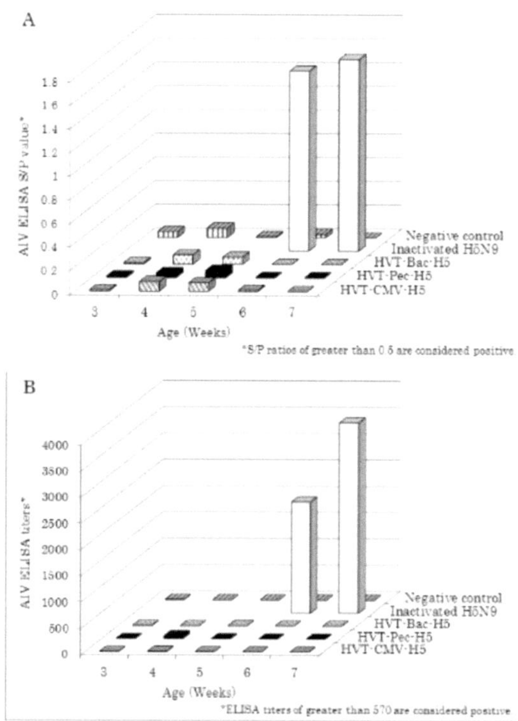

Figure 6. ELISA titers in chickens vaccinated with three rHVT-H5 vaccines using (A) FlockChek™ AIV Ab kit (Idexx Laboratories) and (B) ProFLOK® AIV Ab test kit (Zoetis).

As shown in **Figure 5**, the rHVT-H5 vaccines induced increased HI titers as early as 3 weeks of age and the increased titers were maintained through 7 weeks of age. Chickens vaccinated with HVT-CMV-H5Wis68 had higher mean HI titers than HVT-Pec-H5Wis68 and HVT-Bac-H5Wis68 vaccinated groups had between 4 and 7 weeks of age, with the differences statistically significant at 5 and 6 weeks of age. As expected, the inactivated A/turkey/Wisconsin/68 (H5N9) vaccine induced high HI titers at 6 and 7 weeks of age (3 and 4 weeks post-vaccination), confirming validity of the assay. When tested with the commercial AIV ELISA kits, Flock-Chek™ AIV Ab kit (Idexx Laboratories) and ProFLOK® AIV Ab test kit (Zoetis), sera collected from the rHVT-H5 vaccinated chickens were negative between 3 and 7 weeks of age, whereas sera collected from the inactivated vaccine control chickens showed highly positive ELISA titers with both kits (**Figure 6**).

This result demonstrated that the CMV promoter was the most suitable for expression of the *HA* gene in HVT vector vaccines. Furthermore, sera from the rHVT-H5 vaccinated chickens were found to be negative by the commercially available ELISA kits, although they were highly positive by the AIV HI test. This is most likely because these ELISA kits are designed to detect antibodies to more conserved internal protein, NP, of AIV, in order to detect antibodies to many different subtypes of AIV. This feature of the rHVT-H5 vaccines will be useful in differentiating chicken infected with field AIV viruses from vaccinated chicken (DIVA).

3. Safety of rHVT-H5 vaccine

Based on the results described above, the CMV promoter was selected for the expression of the *HA* gene. The rHVT-H5 vaccine with the CMV promoter attached to the *HA* gene from A/Swan/Hungary/4999/2006 (H5N1) strain (rHVT-H5h) was evaluated further for its safety and efficacy.

Safety of the rHVT-H5h vaccine was evaluated by an overdose study and a backpassage study. For the overdose study, SPF embryos at 18 days of incubation or day-of-age SPF chicks received rHVT-H5h at 10 times the typical field dose. In ovo application of rHVT-H5h at overdose did not affect hatchability and the vaccinated chickens remained free from any clinical signs or adverse reactions until 18 weeks of age. Chickens were necropsied at 18 weeks of age and no gross lesions were observed in any of the vaccinated chickens. Similarly, rHVT-H5h did not cause any clinical signs, adverse reactions, or gross lesions in other avian species such as turkeys, quail, pheasants, and pigeons.

For the backpassage study, to confirm that the rHVT-H5h vaccine will not revert to virulence, rHVT-H5h was passed five times in SPF chickens by using heparinized blood from chickens in the previous passage to inoculate a new set of SPF chicks. Chickens inoculated with the virus at the fifth passage, that is, inoculated with the heparinized blood from the fourth passage, were observed closely for any clinical signs for 45 days. Chickens were then necropsied and observed for grossly observable lesions. No chickens had any clinical signs, adverse reactions, or gross lesions. Therefore, it was concluded that rHVT-H5h did not revert to virulence after backpassages in chickens.

We conducted another study to evaluate the ability of the rHVT-H5h vaccine to transmit from vaccinated chickens to non-vaccinated chickens in contact. Day-of-age SPF chickens vaccinated in ovo with rHVT-H5h or parental HVT were commingled in isolators with non-vaccinated contact chickens. Virus isolation was attempted from the peripheral mononuclear blood lymphocytes collected from chickens at 10, 14, and 21 days of age. No virus was isolated from any of the contact chickens at any time points while the viruses were isolated from the vaccinated chickens, indicating that neither rHVT-H5h nor parental HVT spread from vaccinated chickens to non-vaccinated contact chickens. It appears that transmissibility of HVT parent and the rHVT-H5h vaccine between chickens is negligible.

In summary, similar to parent HVT vaccines and other HVT vector vaccines, the rHVT-H5h vaccine is extremely safe causing no adverse effects and does not revert to virulence after passages in chickens. The lack of transmission of the rHVT-H5h vaccine further strengthens the safety profile of this vaccine in terms of containment of the genetically modified organism.

4. Efficacy of rHVT-H5 vaccine

4.1. Efficacy against homologous challenge

Finally, efficacy of the rHVT-H5h vaccine was evaluated. After vaccination, humoral immune response was evaluated by the AIV HI tests. After challenge with HP AIV, vaccine efficacy was evaluated for (1) protection against mortality and clinical signs and (2) reduction of challenge virus shedding from challenged birds. Both the criteria are important for AI vaccines because these features will ensure that the vaccine will be beneficial as a measure to contain spread of field AI viruses as well as to reduce economical burdens in both endemic and emergent situations [4, 31].

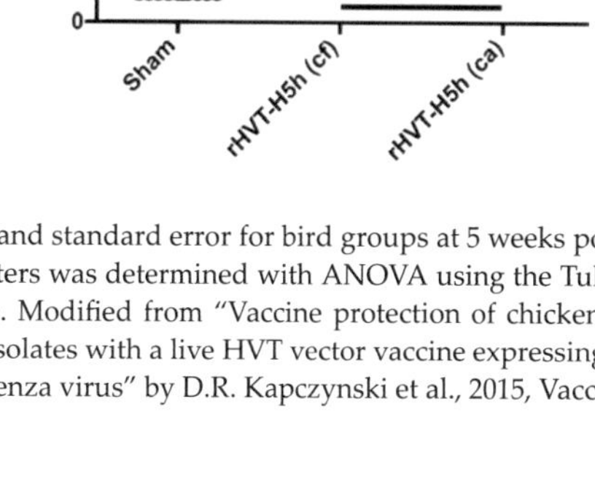

Figure 7. Individual HI titers (log_2) and standard error for bird groups at 5 weeks post-vaccination (prechallenge). Statistical significance between mean titers was determined with ANOVA using the Tukey's multiple comparison test ($p < 0.05$). NS = no significant difference. Modified from "Vaccine protection of chickens against antigenically diverse H5 highly pathogenic avian influenza isolates with a live HVT vector vaccine expressing the influenza hemagglutinin gene derived from a clade 2.2 avian influenza virus" by D.R. Kapczynski et al., 2015, Vaccine, 33, p1200.

Initial evaluation of the rHVT-H5h vaccine efficacy was conducted using homologous AIV as a challenge virus [32]. Day-of-age SPF chicks were vaccinated subcutaneously with either a frozen, cell-associated (ca) form or a lyophilized, cell-free (cf) form of the rHVT-H5h vaccine. At 5 weeks of age before challenge, increased HI titers were observed in all the rHVT-H5h vaccinated chicken with mean titers of $2^{6.3}$ for the ca group and $2^{5.1}$ for the cf group (**Figure 7**) when using homologous antigen.

Chickens were challenged with 10^6 mean embryo infectious dose (EID_{50}) HP H5N1 AIV A/Whooper Swan/Mongolia/3/2005 clade 2.2 strain at 6 weeks of age. The *HA* gene from the A/Whooper Swan/Mongolia/3/2005 strain has 100% gene homology with the A/Swan/Hungary/4999/2006 (H5N1) *HA* gene sequence. All chickens in the diluent-vaccinated, challenge control group died within 3 days. However, none of the rHVT-H5h vaccinated chickens succumbed to challenge and all the chickens were free from clinical signs of AI.

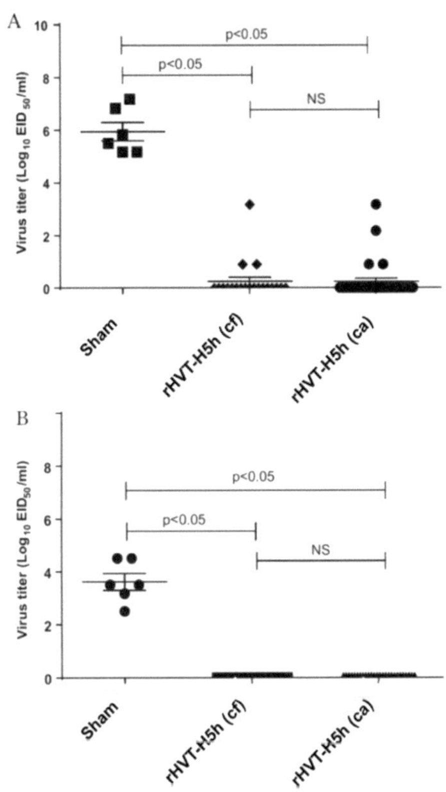

Figure 8. Viral titers from oral (A) and cloacal swabs (B) on day 2 post-challenge. Birds were vaccinated with a single dose rHVT-H5h in cell-associated (ca) or cell-free (cf) form at 1 day-of-age and challenge at 6 weeks with homologous HPAI H5N1. Viral titers are expressed as $\log_{10}EID_{50}$ per milliliter. The lower limit of detection is 0.9 $\log_{10}EID_{50}$ per milliliter. Statistical significance between mean titers was determined with ANOVA using Tukey's multiple comparison test ($p < 0.05$). NS = no significant difference. Modified from "Vaccine protection of chickens against antigenically diverse H5 highly pathogenic avian influenza isolates with a live HVT vector vaccine expressing the influenza hemagglutinin gene derived from a clade 2.2 avian influenza virus" by D.R. Kapczynski et al., 2015, Vaccine, 33, p1200.

We observed 3–6 $\log_{10}$ reduction of challenge virus shedding in the rHVT-H5h vaccinated chickens. From oropharyngeal swabs at 2 days post-challenge (dpc), only 4/30 (13%) chickens in the ca rHVT-H5h group and 3/20 (15%) chickens in the cf rHVT-H5h group shed virus with minimal virus titers (10^1–10^3 EID_{50}/ml), while all the challenge controls shed significant amounts (10^5–$10^7 EID_{50}$/ml) of virus (**Figure 8A**). From cloacal swabs, no virus was isolated from any of the rHVT-H5h vaccinated chickens at 2 dpc, while all the challenge controls shed virus at 10^2–$10^5 EID_{50}$/ml (**Figure 8B**).

These results demonstrated high potential of the rHVT-H5h vaccine as an excellent tool to support control of AI. Therefore, we proceeded to further evaluation of the rHVT-H5h, especially for protection against heterologous virus challenge and effects of MDA. Since the ca form appeared to provide slightly better immunogenicity than the cf form, the following evaluation was conducted using the ca form of the vaccine.

4.2. Efficacy against heterologous challenge

Since HP H5 viruses have become diverse and have evolved into various different clades, it is highly important that AI vaccines exert broad "cross-clade" efficacy against diverse AIV strains. Indeed, one of the limitations of conventional oil-adjuvanted, inactivated vaccines is that they are not as effective against heterologous viruses as homologous viruses [8–10]. Therefore, we tested efficacy of the rHVT-H5h vaccine against various AIV HP H5 strains.

Day-of-age SPF broiler chicks were vaccinated with the rHVT-H5h vaccine. A commercially available inactivated vaccine based on H5N2 Mexican strain (iH5N2) was used as a control and injected into birds at 10 days of age. Challenge was conducted at 4 weeks of age using the Indonesian A/chicken/WestJava Sbg/29/2007 H5N1 strain (CW07). The CW07 virus belongs to clade 2.1.3 and sequence similarity of the HA gene between the rHVT-H5h insert and the CW07 virus was 93%. After challenge, all chickens in the sham-vaccinated, challenge control group died within 2 days. In the group vaccinated with rHVT-H5h, 80% (16/20) of the chickens survived the challenge, while only one bird (5%) vaccinated with iH5N2 survived the challenge. When rHVT-H5h vaccinated chickens received boost with iH5N2 vaccine at 10 days of age, protection increased to 90% (18/20). Reduction in virus shedding up to 3 $\log_{10}$ was observed in rHVT-H5h vaccinated chickens compared to the challenge control. When the homologous antigen was used, rHVT-H5h, either with or without boost with iH5N2 vaccine, it induced average HI titers of 2^5–2^6 prior to challenge. HI titers were much lower with the heterologous CW07 antigen with average between 2^1 and 2^2. These results indicate that cell-mediated immunity as well as mucosal immunity provided by HVT vector vaccines might be involved in protective efficacy against heterologous CW07 strain.

In the next trial, another AIV HP H5 strain, A/Viet Nam/1203/04 (H5N1) (VN04), was used for challenge. The VN04 virus belongs to clade 1 and shares 96.5% HA gene similarity with the rHVT-H5h insert. Vaccination was conducted at the day of age to SPF layer chicks and challenge was conducted at 4 weeks of age. Protection was 85% (17/20) while all challenge control chickens died and reduction of virus shedding of 3 $\log_{10}$ was observed in the rHVT-H5h group.

Since these two trials using heterologous HP H5 strains demonstrated that the rHVT-H5h provided "cross-clade" efficacy, we went further and conducted another efficacy trial using Mexican H5N2 HP strain which shares only 82% HA gene similarity with the rHVT-H5h insert. Day-of-age chicks vaccinated with rHVT-H5h were challenged with A/chicken/Queretaro/14588-19/95 (H5N2) strain at 4 weeks of age. Nineteen out of 20 (95%) chickens survived the challenge, while all the challenge control died. This result demonstrated very broad cross-protective efficacy provided by rHVT-H5h.

We further evaluated efficacy of the rHVT-H5h vaccine against various HP AIV H5 isolates including several Egyptian isolates and a recent 2014 H5N8 isolate from Germany, as summarized in **Figure 9**. Protection in rHVT-H5h vaccinated chickens ranged between 60 and 100% with significant reduction in virus shedding, further strengthening evidence of very broad "cross-clade" efficacy provided by the rHVT-H5h vaccine. In one study where layer chickens were vaccinated and raised under field conditions in Egypt, a single rHVT-H5h vaccination at day of age conferred a high level of protection (60–73%) for a relatively extended period (up to 19 weeks of age) against an Egyptian isolate [33].

Type of bird	with MDA against:		HPAIV used for challenge			Challenge	% Protection		Reference
	HVT	AIV	Strain	S.type	Clade	at:	Vaccinated	Not vaccinated	
SPF CK	No	No	A/CK/Viet Nam/1203/2004	H5N1	1	4 woa	85%	0%	Perez D. 2012
COM BR	Yes	No	A/Duck/Hungary/11804/2006	H5N1	2.2	2 woa	90%	0%	De Vriese J. et al. 2009
COM BR	Yes	Yes (H5N2)	A/Duck/Hungary/11804/2006	H5N1	2.2	2 woa	100%	20%	De Vriese J. et al. 2009
COM BR	Yes	Yes (H5N2)	A/Duck/Hungary/11804/2006	H5N1	2.2	3 woa	90%	0%	De Vriese J. et al. 2009
SPF CK	No	No	A/CK/Egypt/1709-1 VIR08/2007	H5N1	2.2.1	3 woa	100%	0%	Rauw F. et al. 2011
SPF CK	No	No	A/CK/Egypt/1709-6/2008	H5N1	2.2.1.1	3 woa	100%	0%	Rauw F. et al. 2011
COM BR	Yes	No	A/CK/Egypt/1709-6/2008	H5N1	2.2.1.1	4 woa	90%	0%	Rauw F. et al. 2012
COM BR	Yes	Yes (H5N1)	A/CK/Egypt/1709-6/2008	H5N1	2.2.1.1	4 woa	100%	0%	Rauw F. et al. 2012
COM BR	Yes	Yes (H5N1)	A/CK/Egypt/1709-1 VIR08/2007	H5N1	2.2.1	4 woa	90%	0%	Rauw F. et al. 2012
COM BR	Yes	Yes (H5N1)	A/CK/Egypt/1709-6/2008	H5N1	2.2.1.1	4 woa	70%	0%	Rauw F. et al. 2012
COM BR	Yes	Yes (H5N1)	A/CK/West Java Subang/29/2007	H5N1	2.1.3	4 woa	80%	0%	Soejoedono R. D. et al. 2012
COM BR	Yes	Yes (H5N1)	A/CK/Puwakarta-Cilingga/142/2010	H5N1	2.1.3	4 woa	95%	0%	Soejoedono R. D. et al. 2012
SPF CK	No	No	A/Whooper Swan/Mongolia/3/2005	H5N1	2.2	6 woa	100%	0%	Kapczynski D.R. et al. 2015
SPF CK	No	No	A/CK/West Java Subang/29/2007	H5N1	2.1.3	4 woa	80%	0%	Kapczynski D.R. et al. 2015
SPF CK	No	No	A/CK/Queretaro/14588/1995	**H5N2**	-	4 woa	95%	0%	Kapczynski D.R. et al. 2015
SPF CK	No	No	A/CK/Egypt/1709-6/2008	H5N1	2.2.1.1	4 woa	100%	0%	Rauw F. et al. 2012
SPF CK	No	No	A/CK/Egypt/1709-6/2008	H5N1	2.2.1.1	8 woa	100%	0%	Rauw F. et al. 2012
COM BR	Yes	Yes (H5N1)	A/CK/Egypt/1709-6/2008	H5N1	2.2.1.1	4 woa	93%	0%	Kilany W. H. et al. 2012
COM BR	Yes	Yes (H5N1)	A/CK/Egypt-63/2010 "variant"	H5N1	2.2.1.1	5 woa	80%	0%	Kilany W. H. et al. 2012
SPF CK	No	No	A/CK/Germany/2014	**H5N8**	2.3.4.4	4 woa	100%	0%	Steensels M. et al. 2015
SPF CK	No	No	A/CK/Bangladesh/11RS1 984-33/2011	H5N1	2.3.2.1	4 woa	100%	0%	Bonfante F. et al. 2013
COM LY	Yes	Yes (H5N1)	A/CK/Egypt/128s/2012	H5N1	2.2.1	19 woa	73%	0%	Kilany W. H. et al. 2014
COM LY	Yes	Yes (H5N1)	A/CK/Egypt/128s/2012	H5N1	2.2.1	19 woa	60%	0%	Kilany W. H. et al. 2014
SPF TK	No	No	A/WS/Mongolia/2005	H5N1	2.2	4 woa	96%	0%	Kapczynski et al. 2012

SPF CK = SPF Chickens
SPF TK = SPF Turkeys
COM BR = Commercial broilers
COM LY = Commercial Layers
S.type = serotype
woa = weeks of age

Figure 9. Summary of challenge experiments conducted with the rHVT-H5 vaccine. Modified from "Experimental and field results regarding immunity induced by a recombinant HVT-H5 vector vaccine against H5N1 and other H5 Highly Pathogenic Avian Influenza Virus challenge." by Y. Gardin et al., 2016, Avian Dis, in press.

To see if cellular immunity indeed is involved in this broad protective efficacy, we conducted in vitro cytotoxicity assay. Splenic lymphocytes collected from chickens vaccinated with the rHVT-H5h vaccine were incubated with chicken lung cells infected with either H5N9, H6N2, H7N2, or H9N2 low pathogenic AIV. The highest level of lysis by splenic cytotoxic T cells was observed with H5-infected target cells. Lysis was also observed with other heterologous AIV (H6, H7, or H9), although to a lower degree. Negligible lysis was observed with naïve uninfected lung cells. These results indicated that the rHVT-H5h vaccine induced AIV-specific cytotoxic T-cell activity and it may contribute in part to broad protective immunity induced by the rHVT-H5h.

4.3. Efficacy of rHVT-H5 in chicken with maternally derived antibodies

In endemic countries, most breeders are vaccinated with AI vaccines and/or exposed to field AIV challenge and therefore, their progeny possess MDA against AIV. Efficacy of oil-adjuvanted, inactivated AIV vaccines and fowlpox-vectored AI vaccines has been shown to be significantly impaired in the presence of MDA. On the other hands, HVT vector vaccines have been shown not to be excessively affected by the presence of MDA against inserted antigens. Indeed, with the rHVT-H5h vaccine, several studies demonstrated lack of significant interference on its protective efficacy by the presence of MDA when administered to day-of-age chicks [10, 34].

4.4. DIVA

AI surveillance is conducted through serological assays including ELISA and HI. Except in endemic countries, positive serological response in those assays will lead to immediate and extreme actions including "stamping-out." Also, there are trade implications because many countries ban importation of poultry from AI-positive countries. Therefore, when AI vaccination is introduced, it is critical that AI vaccines do not interfere with the AI surveillance. It is highly favorable that serological responses elicited by AI vaccines may be distinguished from those elicited by infection of field AIV. Since conventional inactivated vaccines elicit humoral immune responses that lead to positive titers in both ELISA and HI tests, these vaccines do interfere with the surveillance [7].

The rHVT-H5h vaccine elicits antibodies against the HA protein and the antibody responses can be detected by the HI tests. However, those sera from vaccinated chickens were negative in commercial ELISA kits because the ELISA kits are designed to detect antibodies against more conserved internal protein (NP) in order to offer coverage over different subtypes of AIV. When we examined serological responses in chickens that were vaccinated with the rHVT-H5h and then challenged with HP AIV, we found positive ELISA titers in chickens that excreted challenge viruses. These results demonstrated that the rHVT-H5h vaccines may be applied to the DIVA strategy and do not interfere with AI surveillance.

5. Conclusions

Our studies demonstrated that the rHVT-H5h vaccine possesses characteristics that could be beneficial to control of AI in endemic countries and in emergency situations. Those characteristics are (1) broad "cross-clade" protective efficacy against diverse AIV H5 isolates, (2) lack of interference by MDA, (3) applicability to hatchery vaccination, and (4) applicability to DIVA. The rHVT-H5h vaccine has been approved by authorities in Egypt, Mexico, and Bangladesh and is in use in the field. An independent survey conducted by FAO, General Organization for Veterinary Services in Egypt, and Centre International de Recherche en Agriculture pour le Développement in France concluded that day-of-age vaccination utilizing the rHVT-H5h vaccine at hatcheries is more efficient than the program using the inactivated vaccines at farms and it would have a positive impact for disease control in Egypt [35].

It is clear that vaccines alone cannot solve all the problems associated with AI. However, we believe that in conjunction with active and efficient surveillance and strict biosecurity measures, the rHVT-H5h vaccine can contribute to disease control by increasing resistance against infection and decreasing the amount of virus shed to the environment. It would also remove economical burdens from farmers and consumers and improve animal welfare by protecting chickens from mortality and clinical signs. In conclusion, we successfully developed a HVT vector AI vaccine that possesses many features that could be beneficial to AI control. It remains to be seen whether this vaccine is truly useful in the field.

Author details

Atsushi Yasuda[1*], Motoyuki Esaki[1], Kristi Moore Dorsey[2], Zoltan Penzes[3], Vilmos Palya[3], Darrell R. Kapczynski[4] and Yannick Gardin[5]

*Address all correspondence to: atsushi.yasuda@ceva.com

1 Ceva Animal Health, Yokohama, Japan

2 Ceva Animal Health, Lenexa, Kansas, USA

3 Ceva Animal Health, Budapest, Hungary

4 Exotic and Emerging Avian Viral Disease Research Unit, Southeast Poultry Research Laboratory, U.S. National Poultry Research Center, Athens, Georgia, USA

5 Ceva Animal Health, Libourne, France

References

[1] Food and Agriculture Organization (FAO). Approaches to controlling, preventing and eliminating H5N1 highly pathogenic avian influenza in endemic countries. Rome; 2011.

[2] WHO/OIE/FAO H5N1 Evolution Working Group. Continued evolution of highly pathogenic avian influenza A (H5N1): updated nomenclature. Influenza and Other Respiratory Viruses. 2012;6:1–5.

[3] Swayne D.E., Suarez D.L., Sims L.D. Influenza. In: Swayne DE, Glisson JR, McDougald LR, Nair V, Nolan LK, Suarez DL, editors. Diseases of Poultry. 13th ed. Ames, IA: Wiley-Blackwell; 2013. pp. 181–218.

[4] Swayne D.E. The role of vaccines and vaccination in high pathogenicity avian influenza control and eradication. Expert Review of Vaccines. 2012;11:877–880.

[5] Capua I., Alexander D.J. Avian influenza vaccines and vaccination in birds. Vaccine. 2008;26:D70–D73.

[6] Sims L.D. Lessons learned from Asian H5N1 outbreak control. Avian Diseases. 2007;51:174–181.

[7] Swayne D.E. Vaccines for list A poultry diseases: Emphasis on avian influenza. Developmental Biology (Basel). 2003;114:201–212.

[8] Abdelwhab E.M., Grund.C, Aly M.M., Beer M., Harder T.C., Hafez H.M. Multiple dose vaccination with heterologous H5N2 vaccine: immune response and protection against variant clade 2.2.1 highly pathogenic avian influenza H5N1 in broiler breeder chickens. Vaccine. 2011;29:6219–6225.

[9] Swayne D.E., Kapczynski D. Strategies and challenges for eliciting immunity against avian influenza virus in birds. Immunolgical Reviews. 2008;225:314–331.

[10] Rauw F., Palya V., Gardin Y., Tatar-Kis T., Dorsey K.M., Lambrecht B. et al. Efficacy of rHVT-AI vector vaccine in broilers with passive immunity against challenge with two antigenically divergent Egyptian clade 2.2.1 HPAI H5N1 strains. Avian Diseases 2012;56:913–922.

[11] Abdelwhab E.M., Grund C., Aly M.M., Beer M., Harder T.C., Hafez H.M. Influence of maternal immunity on vaccine efficacy and susceptibility of one day old chicks against Egyptian highly pathogenic avian influenza H5N1. Veterinary Microbiology. 2012;155:13–20.

[12] De Vriese J., Steensels M., Palya V., Gardin Y., Dorsey K.M., Lambrecht B. et al. Passive protection afforded by maternally-derived antibodies in chickens and the antibodies' interference with the protection elicited by avian influenza-inactivated vaccines in progeny. Avian Diseases. 2010;54:246–252.

[13] Schat K.A., Nair V. Marek's disease. In: Swayne D.E., Glisson J.R., McDougald L.R., Nolan L.K., Suarez D.L., Nair V, editors. Diseases of Poultry. 13th ed. Hoboken, NJ: Wiley-Blackwell; 2013. pp. 515–552.

[14] Okazaki W., Purchase H.G., Burmester B.R. Protection against Marek's disease by vaccination with a herpesvirus of turkeys. Avian Diseases. 1970;14:413–429.

[15] Heller E. D., Schat K.A. Enhancement of natural killer cell activity by Marek's disease vaccines. Avian Pathology. 1987;16:51–60.

[16] Kitamoto N., Ikuta K., Kato S., Yamaguchi S. Cell-mediated cytotoxicity of lymphocytes from chickens inoculated with herpesvirus of turkey against a Marek's disease lymphoma cell line (MSB-1). Biken Journal. 1979;22:11–20.

[17] Rauw F., Gardin Y., Palya V., Anbari S., Lemaire S., Boschmans M. et al. Improved vaccination against Newcastle disease by an in ovo recombinant HVT-ND combined with an adjuvanted live vaccine at day-old. Vaccine. 2010;28:823–833.

[18] Witter R.L., Offenbecker L. Duration of vaccinal immunity against Marek's disease. Avian Diseases. 1978;22:396–407.

[19] Palya V., Tatár-Kis T., Mató T., Felföldi B., Kovács E., Gardin Y. Onset and long-term duration of immunity provided by asingle vaccination with a turkey herpesvirus vector ND vaccine in commercial layers. Veterinary Immunology and Immunopathology. 2014;158:105–115.

[20] Afonso C.L., Tulman E.R., Lu Z., Zsak L., Rock D.L., Kutish G.F. The genome of turkey herpesvirus. Journal of Virology. 2001;75:971–978.

[21] Darteil R., Bublot M., Laplace E., Bouquet J.F., Audonnet J.C., Rivière M. Herpesvirus of turkey recombinant viruses expressing infectious bursal disease virus (IBDV) VP2 immunogen induce protection against an IBDV virulent challenge in chickens. Virology. 1995;211:481–490.

[22] Morgan R.W., Gelb J. Jr, Schreurs C.S., Lütticken D., Rosenberger J.K., Sondermeijer P.J.. Protection of chickens from Newcastle and Marek's diseases with a recombinant herpesvirus of Turkeys vaccine expressing the Newcastle disease virus fusion protein. Avian Diseases. 1992;36:858–870.

[23] Ross L.J., Binns M.M., Tyers P., Pastorek J., Zelnik V., Scott S. Construction and properties of a turkey herpesvirus recombinant expressing the Marek's disease virus homologue of glycoprotein B of herpes simplex virus. Journal of General Virology. 1993;74:371–377.

[24] Tsukamoto K., Saito S., Saeki S., Sato T., Tanimura N., Isobe T. et al. Complete, long-lasting protection against lethal infectious bursal disease virus challenge by a single vaccination with an avian herpesvirus vector expressing VP2 antigens. Journal of Virology. 2002;76:5637–5645.

[25] Esaki M., Godoy A., Rosenberger J.K., Rosenberger S.C., Gardin Y., Yasuda A. et al. Protection and antibody response caused by turkey herpesvirus vector Newcastle disease vaccine. Avian Diseases. 2013;57:750–755.

[26] Esaki M., Noland L., Eddins T., Godoy A., Saeki S., Saitoh S. et al. Safety and efficacy of a turkey herpesvirus vector laryngotracheitis vaccine for chickens. Avian Diseases. 2013;57:192–198.

[27] Swayne D.E., Suarez D.L., Sims L.D. Influenza. In: Swayne D.E., Glisson J.R., McDougald L.R., Nolan L.K., Suarez D.L. and Nair V, editors. Diseases of Poultry. 13th ed. Hoboken, NJ: Wiley-Blackwell; 2013. pp. 181–218.

[28] Sonoda K., Sakaguchi M., Okamura H., Yokogawa K., Tokunaga E., Tokiyoshi S. et al. Development of an effective polyvalent vaccine against both Marek's and Newcastle diseases based on recombinant Marek's disease virus type 1 in commercial chickens with maternal antibodies. Journal of Virology. 2000;74:3217–3226.

[29] Ma C., Zhang Z., Zhao P., Duan L., Zhang Y., Zhang F. et al. Comparative transcriptional activity of five promoters in BAC-cloned MDV for the expression of the hemagglutinin gene of H9N2 avian influenza virus. Journal of Virological Methods. 2014;206:119–127.

[30] Pedersen J.C. Hemagglutination-Inhibition Test for Avian Influenza Virus Subtype Identification and the Detection and Quantitation of Serum Antibodies to the Avian Influenza Virus. Methods in Molecular Biology. 2008;436:53–66.

[31] Gardin Y., Palya V., Dorsey K.M., El-Attrache J., Bonfante F., de Wit S. et al. Experimental and field results regarding immunity induced by a rHVT-H5 vector vaccine against H5N1 and other H5 type highly pathogenic avian influenza viruses. Avian Diseases. Forthcoming. DOI: 10.1637/11144-050815-ResNote.1

[32] Kapczynski DR, Esaki M, Dorsey KM, Jiang H, Jackwood M, Moraes M, Gardin Y. Vaccine protection of chickens against antigenically diverse H5 highly pathogenic avian influenza isolates with a live HVT vector vaccine expressing the influenza hemagglutinin gene derived from a clade 2.2 avian influenza virus. Vaccine. 2015;33:1197–1205.

[33] Kilany W.H., Dauphin G., Selim A., Tripodi A., Samy M., Sobhy H. et al. Protection conferred by recombinant turkey herpesvirus avian influenza (rHVT-H5) vaccine in the rearing period in two commercial layer chicken breeds in Egypt. Avian Pathology. 2014;43:514–523.

[34] Kilany W.H., Hassan M.K., Safwat M., Mohammed S., Selim A., VonDobschuetz S. et al. Comparison of the effectiveness of rHVT-H5, inactivated H5 and rHVT-H5 with inactivated H5 prime/boost vaccination regimes in commercial broiler chickens carrying MDAs against HPAI H5N1 clade 2.2.1 virus. Avian Pathology. 2015;44:333–341.

[35] Peyre M., Choisy M., Sobhy H., Kilany W.H., Gély M., Tripodi A. et al. Added value of avian influenza (H5) day old chick vaccination for disease control in Egypt. Avian Diseases. Forthcoming. DOI: 10.1637/11131-050715-ResNote.1

Section 3

Response to Vaccines

Chapter 9

Maternal Influenza: Infection, Vaccination, and Compelling Questions

Jill M. Manske

Additional information is available at the end of the chapter

http://dx.doi.org/10.5772/64368

Abstract

Influenza presents a significant risk for increased morbidity and mortality to pregnant women and infants based on evidence from previous influenza pandemics, seasonal epidemics, and the recent H1N1 pandemic. Since 2004, influenza vaccine has been recommended for pregnant women during any trimester of pregnancy to reduce this risk. This chapter presents an overview of influenza risks associated with pregnancy as well as a review of our current understanding of vaccine effectiveness in pregnant women, neonates, and young infants. In addition, some of the current compelling questions related to influenza risk and prevention across all trimesters of pregnancy are explored.

Keywords: influenza vaccine, pregnancy, effectiveness, maternal immunization

1. Introduction

Influenza is a highly contagious, acute respiratory infection (ARI). Each year, it is estimated that 5–10% of adults and 20–30% of children worldwide will become infected with influenza [1]. Pregnant women and infants are at particular risk for influenza. Influenza infection during pregnancy or during the first 6 months of life is a substantial cause of morbidity. Prevention of influenza in these populations is of global health importance.

2. Maternal influenza

Pregnant women are considered a high-risk group for serious illness and complications from influenza. While annual influenza incidence rates in pregnant women are similar to those of nonpregnant women [2–4], influenza infection is associated with increased morbidity and mortality in this subpopulation, with pregnant women having an increased risk of influenza-attributed hospitalizations compared to nonpregnant women [4, 5]. Most likely this is associated with the interaction of the infection with the physiologic and immunologic changes that occur during pregnancy.

Pregnancy-associated changes such as decreased lung capacity, reduced tidal volume, and increased cardiac output likely reduce the capacity of the respiratory and cardiac system to respond to the stress of influenza infection [2, 6]. In addition, during pregnancy there is a progressive suppression of cellular (T-cell mediated) immunity. While this immune suppression serves to protect the developing fetus from maternal cytotoxic T-cell immunity, it can impair the maternal response to viral infections such as influenza [7–11].

The combination of these factors contributes to an increased risk of negative outcomes from influenza infection. If respiratory disease develops, especially during the later stages of pregnancy, it can lead to high morbidity among the pregnant women [6, 12–14]. In a study of hospital admissions records of women admitted between 1994 and 2000 with respiratory conditions during pregnancy, the hospitalization rate was 150/100,000, an admission rate considerably higher than that of nonpregnant women (17/100,000) and corresponding to the rate for people aged 65–69 [5]. Healthy pregnant women ages 20–34 were estimated to be 18 times more likely to be hospitalized for influenza than their nonpregnant peers [5].

While hospitalization rates are increased in all trimesters of pregnancy [4, 15, 16], they are the highest during the third trimester [5, 14, 16–18]. Likewise, there is a strong association of maternal morbidity with this trimester of pregnancy. In a 2003 study, Hartert et al. showed that cardiovascular hospitalization during influenza season increased with each trimester, nearly threefold higher by the third trimester compared to the first trimester [18]. In a study of 8323 healthy pregnant and postpartum women, Lindsay et al. found that the strength of association between influenza exposure and influenza-like illness (ILI) increased as the stage of pregnancy progressed, reporting an odds ratio (OR) of 1.12 (CI, 0.79–1.59) during the first trimester, 1.30 (CI, 0.97–1.73) during the second trimester, and 1.84 (CI, 1.31–2.59) for the third trimester [14]. Other studies have reported that by the third trimester, healthy pregnant women with no comorbidity have the same risk for ILI-associated hospitalization as nonpregnant women with chronic or comorbid conditions [4, 5].

Pregnant women with comorbid conditions such as asthma, diabetes, heart disease, or chronic obstructive pulmonary disease are even more likely to be hospitalized than are pregnant women without chronic conditions [5, 14, 16–18]. Neuzil et al. reported event rates for influenza for low-risk women of 3, 6, and 10 per 10,000 women months in the first, second, and third trimesters, respectively. The event rate in nonpregnant women was 2 per 10,000 women months. Among women with chronic comorbid conditions, rates of 31, 16, and 21 per 10,000 women months were observed during these trimesters, respectively [4].

http://dx.doi.org/10.5772/64368

While considerable data demonstrate increased morbidity and hospitalization from seasonal influenza in pregnant women, mortality appears to be rare in healthy pregnant women during non-pandemic seasons [7, 19, 20]. A study of seasonal influenza among pregnant women over an 8-year period reported an average of five deaths per year and a mean mortality ratio of 2.9 per million live births [21]. However, during pandemics, influenza infection presents a significant increased risk of both morbidity and mortality in pregnant women.

For example, during the pandemic of 1918, pneumonia was reported in 50% of previously healthy pregnant women, leading to case-fatality rates of over 50% [22–26]. In the 1957 pandemic, 50% of the women of childbearing age who died of influenza were pregnant. Furthermore, 10% of all influenza deaths during this pandemic occurred in pregnant women, with the majority occurring during the third trimester [23, 24].

Increased rates of morbidity and mortality in pregnant women also were observed more recently during the 2009 influenza A(H1N1)pdm09 pandemic. In fact, the first reported death of an adult in the United States during this pandemic was a pregnant woman [27]. Of the 45 deaths reported early in the pandemic, 6 (13.3%) were pregnant women, all of whom developed viral pneumonia and respiratory distress syndrome [27–29].

A study of pregnant US women with confirmed or probable influenza during the first month of the outbreak reported 11/34 cases (32.4%) resulted in hospitalization—admissions rates four times higher than those in the general population [30]. Deaths were reported in all three trimesters and were independent of preexisting risk factors. In a California study, pregnant women who were hospitalized with or died from pH1N1 were less likely than nonpregnant women to have a predisposing or comorbid medical condition [31].

A review of published studies following the 2009 pandemic documented that pregnant women were disproportionately represented among hospitalizations, ICU admissions, and deaths. The 120 papers that were included in the review reported 3110 pregnant women from 29 countries with A(H1N1)pdm09 influenza infection, including 1625 (52.3%) who were hospitalized with 2009 H1N1, of whom 378 (23.3%) were admitted to an ICU and 130 (8%) died [32]. Pooling the data from all of the studies included in the review, the authors reported that pregnant women, who represent approximately 1% of the population of United States and Australia, accounted for 6.3% of hospitalizations, 5.9% of ICU admissions, and 5.7% of deaths [32].

Using data from the Centers for Disease Control (CDC) and the Pregnancy Mortality Surveillance System, Callaghan et al. estimated the total burden of pregnancy-related mortality resulting from the 2009 to 2010 pandemic. Confirmed and possible deaths resulting from A(H1N1)pdm09 infection represented the leading cause of pregnancy-related mortality in the United States between the months of April 2009 and June 2010. Of 915 total pregnancy-related deaths during this period, 12% of pregnancy-related deaths were attributed to influenza, 75 (8.2%) classified as confirmed influenza A(H1N1)pdm09 deaths, and 34 (3.7%) classified as possible influenza infection deaths [33]. The authors calculated the pregnancy-related morality ratio for confirmed and possible influenza deaths at 2.2 per 100,000 live births. This represents a significant burden of mortality. The number of deaths (109) during the 2009–2010 influenza season was 20 times greater than the mean number (5) of annual possible influenza deaths reported in a 1998–2005 cohort of pregnancy-related deaths in non-pandemic years [33].

Infants born to influenza-infected women during the pandemic also experienced increased risks of poor clinical outcomes, mostly due to preterm birth. Reports of preterm birth rates ranged from 15 to 30% among infected women [32, 34–36]. Infection with A(H1N1)pdm09 was associated with increased risk of cesarean delivery [32]. In most cases, cesarean delivery was an attempt to improve worsening maternal status rather than out of concern for the infant [32]. Siston et al. reported a cesarean delivery rate of 58% in pregnant women with 2009 H1N1 compared to a baseline cesarean rate of 30.5% [32, 34, 37]. While cesarean deliveries were commonly described, it is likely that this rate was over-reported, since many of the studies reported only severely affected women. Many deliveries were emergencies and performed outside of controlled operating room settings, indicating the urgent nature of these deliveries and the critical status of the women [32].

3. Influenza infection and fetal development

While there is no clear consensus on transplacental transmission of influenza virus or direct viral effects on the fetus [2], the spread of virus beyond the respiratory tract during acute infection is unusual, and vertical transmission, although documented [38–40], appears to be rare [41, 42]. However, even in the absence of vertical transmission, adverse fetal effects can occur, most likely due to the systemic maternal immune response to the infection [43, 44]. Studies have documented inflammatory responses in fetal tissues in response to influenza infection. Such responses could impact the maternal-fetal interface, the placenta, or the fetus directly, leading to pregnancy loss [43]. In addition to direct damage from inflammatory responses, it is hypothesized that maternal hyperthermia can result in adverse fetal outcomes [28, 45]. Maternal hyperthermia during the first trimester of pregnancy, regardless of the cause, has been associated with an increased risk for neural tube defects [46], while fever during labor has been associated with adverse outcomes including neonatal seizures, cerebral palsy, encephalopathy, and death [2, 47–50].

In a large population-based study of influenza infection in over 100,000 women, Hansen et al. observed an increased risk for fetal abnormalities (e.g., central nervous system malfunctions in the fetus, chromosomal abnormalities, suspected damage to the fetus from viral disease) was present in both seasonal (OR 1.53, CI, 1.19–1.95) and pandemic infections (OR 1.48, CI, 1.27–1.73) [51].

A review and meta-analysis of 33 studies published from 1953 to 2013 of first-trimester influenza exposure found that influenza exposure during the first trimester of pregnancy was associated with an increase in congenital abnormalities [adjusted odds ratio (AOR) 2.00, CI, 1.62–4.28]. Anomalies included neural tube defects [odds ratio (OR) 3.33, CI, 2.05–5.40], hydrocephaly (OR 5.74, 1.10–30.00), congenital heart defects (OR 1.56, 1.13–2.14), cleft lip (OR 3.12, CI, 2.20–4.42), digestive system anomalies (OR 1.72, CI, 1.09–2.68), and limb reduction defects (OR 2.03, CI, 1.27–3.27) [52]. A major limitation of this study concerns the fact that it defined influenza exposure as any reported influenza, influenza-like illness, or fever with or without clinical confirmation. The inclusion of wide clinical symptoms without laboratory confirmation of influenza likely resulted in overestimation of the number of infants exposed to influenza during gestation. It therefore cannot be determined whether congenital abnormalities were associated with general, all cause hyperthermia or whether influenza infection poses a unique and specific risk for these outcomes. Nonetheless, these observations suggest that prevention of influenza during the first trimester of pregnancy may reduce risk for congenital abnormalities.

Fetal demise is associated with influenza infection as well. Women with influenza, especially those with pneumonia, had high rates of spontaneous abortion and preterm birth, with 52% of pregnancies ending in spontaneous abortion or preterm delivery during the 1918 pandemic [22, 23, 25].

Using a large nationwide registry, Haberg et al. examined the risk of fetal death after maternal exposure to pandemic influenza infection. The researchers found that pregnant women with a clinical diagnosis of influenza had a nearly twofold increase in the risk of fetal death (adjusted hazard ratio, 1.91; 95% CI, 1.07–3.41) as compared to women who were not exposed to influenza [53].

Pierce et al. assessed perinatal outcomes of maternal A(H1N1)pdm09 infection. The authors found that perinatal mortality was higher in infants born to infected women than in infants of uninfected women (39 per 1000 live births versus 7 per 1000 total births, respectively, $p = 0.001$). This was principally explained by an increase in the rate of stillbirth (27 per 1000 total births versus 6 per 1000 total births, $p = 0.001$) [54].

4. Influenza infection in neonates and young infants

Infants younger than 6 months of age are at a heightened risk for serious illness from influenza, exhibiting the highest rates of severe influenza compared to other pediatric populations [41]. This age group has higher rates of hospitalization, more prolonged ICU stays, and higher fatality rates (0.33 per 100,000 children) than almost any other age group [55–59]. In the United States, estimates of hospitalization rates for young infants (less than 6 months of age) range between 1.8 and 7.2 per 1000 infants, higher than reported rates of hospitalization for children up to 4 years of age (0.14 per 1000) [60] and people 65–80 years of age (0.56–2.13 per 1000) [60–63]. Childhood deaths associated with influenza are most frequent in infants during the first months of life, with mortality rates in infants 0–6 months old more than four times higher than those in older children [59].

Libster et al. [64] documented particularly high mortality rates for infants during the 2009 H1N1 pandemic in Argentina. Of 251 infants and children hospitalized with confirmed A(H1N1)pdm09 infection, 13 (5%) died, for an overall death rate of 1.1 per 100,000 children. Infants were at particularly high risk for fatality, representing the highest death rate at 7.6 per 100,000 children. By comparison, this death rate was 10 times the reported US infant death rate during the relatively serious seasonal influenza season of 2003–2004 [59, 64].

Taken together, these observations highlight the impact of influenza on infants, especially the youngest, and underscore the need for prevention in this vulnerable population.

5. Maternal influenza vaccination

A large body of evidence collected over several decades demonstrates that pregnant women and young infants are at increased risk for complications from influenza, making control of influenza infection in these populations an important public health challenge. Influenza vaccines have been used since 1945 and currently are the primary strategy for preventing influenza infection [65].

Due to the frequent changes of the influenza viral antigens, a vaccine is formatted during the end of the previous season to include the specific antigens of the influenza strains expected to circulate in the following season, with a goal of conferring protection against the upcoming season's strains. Each year, the trivalent inactivated influenza vaccines (IIV3) are formulated to contain three viral components: two influenza A subtypes and one influenza B virus. In 2012, the US Food and Drug Administration (FDA) approved the use of a quadrivalent influenza vaccine (IIV4). The quadrivalent vaccine contains two influenza A subtypes and two influenza B subtypes. In 2009, a monovalent H1N1 vaccine was prepared because the newly recognized strain was identified too late in the season to be included in the trivalent seasonal vaccines [66].

The current inactivated influenza vaccines (IIVs) are composed of inactivated (killed) virus that has been chemically disrupted and purified to form a split-inactivated virus preparation. Such split-virus vaccines contain purified HA and NA antigens and have fewer side effects and reactions than inactivated whole virus vaccines. The IIVs currently available in the United States are split virus or subunit virus similar to the split virus [66].

The other vaccine available in the United States is a live, attenuated influenza vaccine (LAIV). This vaccine is composed of live, attenuated, cold-adapted, temperature-sensitive virus administered directly into the nasal passage. The type A and B strains of influenza in this vaccine can replicate in the nasal passages, stimulating an immune response, but cannot replicate in the lower respiratory tract [67]. While LAIV has been licensed in the United States since 2003, it is not recommended for use in pregnant women [68].

A strategy to increase the effectiveness of IIVs is the addition of adjuvants. Adjuvants are compounds that stimulate the immune system to mount a more robust and protective response to the vaccine. The most commonly used adjuvants in influenza vaccines are the oil-based compounds AS03 and MF59. Adjuvants can allow for the use of lower doses of antigen, resulting in more available doses of vaccine, which may be useful in times of high demand such as during pandemics. While adjuvanted vaccines are not approved for use in pregnant women in the United States, in Canada, and in many European countries, the pandemic vaccine was formulated with adjuvant and administered to pregnant women [69].

Vaccination of pregnant women with IIV has taken place since the 1960s. Universal recommendation for vaccinating woman at all stages of pregnancy has been recommended by the

CDC's Advisory Committee on Immunization Practices (ACIP) since 2004 [65, 70, 71] and by the World Health Organization (WHO) since 2005 [1]. The Advisory Committee on Immunization Practices does not preferentially recommend a specific formulation—trivalent or quadrivalent—of the influenza vaccine [72]. In response to the 2009 H1N1 pandemic, the WHO placed pregnant women, along with caregivers of infants younger than 6 months old, health-care and emergency services personnel, individuals between 6 months and 24 years, and those aged 25 years or older with chronic medical conditions, in the highest priority group to receive vaccines [73].

The American College of Obstetrics and Gynecology (ACOG) considers prevention of influenza to be an "essential element of prenatal care" [74]. In full support of the ACIP recommendations, ACOG issued new guidelines in September of 2010 stating that all unvaccinated pregnant women at any gestational age be vaccinated against influenza [74].

It is well documented that the antibody (Ab) response to influenza vaccine in pregnant women is similar to that of age-matched, nonpregnant women [75–79]. These observations support a conclusion that influenza vaccination will lead to an effective immune response in pregnant women and thereby provide an important tool in prevention of influenza in this population.

5.1. Effectiveness of maternal influenza vaccines

Pregnant women and neonates are high-risk groups for complications from influenza infection. Control of influenza in this population is an important public health concern. However, due in part to ethical concerns related to enrolling pregnant women in clinical studies, experimental data on influenza vaccination during pregnancy has been scarce, and the quality of the evidence is not consistently high overall [80].

Prior to 2010, there were few well-designed studies specifically addressing vaccine effectiveness in pregnant women. From 1964 to 2008, four studies specifically addressed vaccine effectiveness in pregnant women (**Table 1**). These studies covered eight different influenza seasons and included 51,547 pregnant women.

During a 1962–1963 outbreak of Asian influenza, Hulka measured vaccine effectiveness in pregnant women by asking immunized and nonimmunized patients if they had experienced influenza symptoms during the influenza season. While fewer immunized than unimmunized patients reported respiratory illness with fever (11% versus 20%, respectively), there was no significant difference in reports of respiratory illness between these patients [76].

Black et al. assessed vaccine effectiveness in almost 50,000 pregnant women across five influenza seasons. Vaccine effectiveness was determined by the number of outpatient visits for ILI or hospitalization for influenza or pneumonia. Using these outcomes, the risk of medical visit for respiratory symptoms was no different between vaccinated and unvaccinated women, and hospitalization was rare in both groups [81]. Using the adjusted hazard ratios (AHR = 1.151; CI, 0.979–1.352) from this study, Skowronski and De Serres calculated a vaccine effectiveness of −15% (CI, −35 to 2%) for this study population [7].

In a retrospective case-control study of five influenza seasons (1995–2003), Munoz et al. estimated the potential protective effect of vaccination by recording the occurrence of acute respiratory infection (ARI) in vaccinated and unvaccinated women. The researchers reported a nonsignificant ($p = 0.24$) trend toward lower incidence of medically attended ARI in vaccinated women as compared to unvaccinated women (22.6% of the vaccinated cohort versus 18.9% of the unvaccinated cohort) [82]. Among the women who developed ARI, the number of episodes of ARI was the same, 1.4 illnesses/person in both groups. However, there was a difference in the timing of these episodes, with 9% of the vaccinated cohort reporting ARI episodes during the peak of the influenza season, while 19% of the ARI events in the unvaccinated cohort occurred during the peak ($p = 0.01$, CI, 0.1–0.8) [82]. In this study, only three women were diagnosed with ILI, one vaccinated and two unvaccinated women, all during the peak influenza seasons of 1999–2000 and 2000–2001. These low rates of ILI as well as the small number of vaccinated women in the study population (vaccination rate was 3.5%) are limitations of this study. Using the relative risks reported in the study, vaccine effectiveness was −20% for ARI any time during pregnancy (CI, −59 to 9%) and 39% (CI, −56 to 76%) during the peak of the influenza season [7].

Study	Study period	Participants	Outcomes measured	Influenza vaccine protection
Studies of seasonal IIV during pregnancy				
Hulka [76]	1962–1963	544 pregnant women -363 immunized -181 nonimmunized 176 nonpregnant women -138 immunized -38 nonimmunized	Incidence of influenza-like illness (ILI)	Nonsignificant reduction in incidence of ILI (20% versus 11%)
Black et al. [81]	1997–2002	49,585 pregnant women -3707 immunized -45,878 nonimmunized	Medical visit for respiratory symptoms	No difference in medical visits ($p = 0.088$) Adjusted hazard ratio = 1.151; (CI, 0.979–1.352) Clinical effectiveness: −15% Excluding medical visits for asthma, no difference ($p = 0.988$) Adjusted hazard ratio = 1.001 (CI, 0.838–1.196) Clinical effectiveness: 0%
Munoz et al. [117]	1998–2003	Pregnant women -252 immunized -826 nonimmunized	Medically attended acute respiratory illness (ARI)	Nonsignificant trend toward lower incidence of ARI (22.6% versus 18.9%; $p = 0.24$) Clinical effectiveness: −20% (CI, −59.5 to 9%) any time during pregnancy

http://dx.doi.org/10.5772/64368

Study	Study period	Participants	Outcomes measured	Influenza vaccine protection
				39% (CI, −56 to 76%) during peak of influenza season
Zaman et al. [79]	2004–2005	340 pregnant women -172 immunized with TIV -168 immunized with pneumococcal vaccine	Respiratory illness with fever	Significant reduction of respiratory illness with any fever: Risk difference: −14.2 (CI, −25.5 to 2.9) Clinical effectiveness: 35.8% (CI, 3.7–57.2%) Reduction in respiratory disease with fever over 38 °C: Risk difference: −7.3% (CI, −14.5 to 0.1%) Clinical effectiveness: 43.1% (CI, −9.0 to 70.3%)
Madhi et al. [83]	2011–2012	2116 pregnant women -1062 immunized with IIV3 -1054 received placebo	RT-PCR-confirmed influenza	Clinical effectiveness: 50.4% (CI, 14.5–71.2%)
Thompson et al. [84]	2010–2012	Pregnant women -100 with confirmed influenza -192 with ARI negative for influenza -200 control negative for influenza	RT-PCR-confirmed influenza	Clinical effectiveness: 44% (CI, 5–67%) compared to influenza-negative controls 53% (CI, 24–72%) compared to ARI-negative controls
Studies of PH1N1 vaccine during pregnancy				
Richards et al. [101]	2009–2010	1125 vaccinated 1581 non-vaccinated (unadjuvanted vaccine)	RT-PCR or medical visit during pregnancy with influenza-related ICD-9 diagnosis code	Clinical effectiveness: 61.5% (CI, 15.5–82.5%)
Haberg et al. [53]	2009–2010	117,347 pregnant women (adjuvanted vaccine)		Clinical effectiveness: 70% (AHR, 0.30; (CI), 0.25–0.34)

Table 1. Clinical effectiveness of IIV and A(H1N1)pdm09 influenza vaccine during pregnancy.

The authors of this study speculate that while the receipt of an influenza vaccine may not prevent infection, it is likely to reduce the severity of the disease. However, they provided no data on clinical severity or evidence of such an association with vaccination status. Since there was no confirmation of influenza infection in most patients with ARI, it is impossible to confirm whether clinical symptoms were associated with influenza infection or with other respiratory viruses.

In 2008, Zaman et al. published the first randomized, double-blind, controlled clinical trial (RCT) of influenza vaccine in pregnant women. In this study, 340 pregnant women were randomized to receive either trivalent influenza vaccine (IIV3) or pneumococcal polysaccharide vaccine during the third trimester of pregnancy. This study was part of The Mother's Gift project, a randomized trial with the primary goal of assessing the safety and immunogenicity of pneumococcal vaccines. Therefore, the control arm consisted of mothers who received the pneumococcal vaccine, providing a control for an active, non-influenza vaccine. The authors measured nonspecific respiratory illness with fever and found that vaccinated women were significantly less likely to have respiratory illness, reporting a clinical effectiveness of 35.8% (CI, 3.7–57.2%) for respiratory illness with any fever and 43.1% for fever over 38 °C (CI, −9.0 to 70.3%) [79].

All of these studies share the common weakness that they use clinical symptoms, and not laboratory-confirmed influenza, as the primary outcome. Influenza vaccines are specifically targeted to influenza viruses. Many other respiratory pathogens can cause symptoms similar to influenza, but influenza vaccines are not designed to prevent other causes of influenza-like illness. Hence, clinical symptoms without laboratory confirmation are nonspecific outcomes. Interpretation and quantification of true vaccine effectiveness using only clinical outcomes are problematic, potentially leading to inaccurate estimates of effectiveness. For this reason, laboratory confirmation, either by reverse transcription polymerase chain reaction (RT-PCR) or viral culture, remains the best diagnostic tool for confirming influenza and evaluating vaccine efficacy (VE) and effectiveness.

In 2014, two studies began to address this deficiency in the literature. The research teams estimated influenza vaccine effectiveness in preventing illness among pregnant women using laboratory-confirmed (RT-PCR) influenza as the primary outcome.

Madhi et al. examined maternal and fetal outcomes in 2116 HIV-negative South African women during the 2011–2012 influenza season. 1062 women who received IIV3 were compared to women who received a placebo. Overall vaccine effectiveness at preventing laboratory-confirmed (RT-PCR) influenza in this population was 50.4% (CI, 14.5–71.2) [83].

Using a large health plan database, the Pregnancy and Influenza Project evaluated seasonal vaccine efficacy during the 2010–2011 and 2011–2012 influenza seasons. The authors compared the proportion of vaccinated women among 100 RT-PCR-confirmed influenza cases with the proportion vaccinated among 192 women with ARI who tested negative for influenza, and 200 controls matched by season, site, and trimester [84]. The adjusted vaccine efficacy against influenza was of 44% (CI, 5–67%) using the influenza-negative controls and 53% (CI, 24–72%) for the ARI-negative controls [84].

The 2009 A(H1N1) pandemic provided an opportunity to improve understanding of influenza vaccination during pregnancy. The pandemic allowed an evaluation of the effectiveness of maternal vaccination during an influenza season in which there was a high rate of viral circulation, as well as a close match between the vaccine strain and the circulating viral strain.

Pregnant women were prioritized to receive the vaccine and were strongly advised to be vaccinated [85], resulting in higher than usual vaccination rates [86].

Since the 2009 pandemic, a number of studies have examined monovalent pandemic A(H1N1) vaccination of pregnant women. Synthesizing evidence from this new and expanding database should increase our understanding of maternal influenza vaccination. While most of these studies measured either seroconversion and hemagglutinin inhibition (HAI) titers [87–92] or safety and/or birth outcomes [93–100], two studies specifically examined clinical efficacy of pandemic A(H1N1) vaccine during pregnancy.

In a retrospective cohort study, Richards et al. evaluated influenza infection in 1125 vaccinated and 1581 non-vaccinated women. In this study, influenza infection was defined as testing positive for influenza by RT-PCR or having a medical visit during pregnancy with influenza-related *ICD-9* diagnosis code during the period of 2009 influenza A(H1N1) virus circulation [101]. The researchers reported a vaccine efficacy (VE) of 61.5% (CI, 15.5–82.5%) for 2009 H1N1 influenza vaccine against diagnosed 2009 influenza A(H1N1) infection during the study period among all mothers in the study cohort [101].

A separate population-based study of 117,347 pregnant women in Norway estimated that vaccination during the second or third trimester of pregnancy resulted in a 70% reduction in influenza diagnosis following vaccination with adjuvanted A(H1N1) vaccine (adjusted hazard ratio, 0.30; CI, 0.25–0.34) [53].

While there is significant heterogeneity among these eight clinical studies, presenting wide-ranging estimates of vaccine effectiveness in pregnant women (from −15 to 70%), the evidence of effectiveness data based on laboratory-confirmed influenza is mounting and compelling. The cumulative evidence to date provides three studies showing significant clinical effectiveness during seasonal influenza years, 35.8% against respiratory disease in a RCT [79], 50.4% protection against laboratory-confirmed influenza in a RCT [83], and one large data-base study documenting VE of 44–53% [84]. Two studies of vaccine effectiveness during the 2009 A(H1N1) pandemic estimated VE of 61.5% (unadjuvanted) and 70% (adjuvanted), suggesting that vaccination during a pandemic season may offer more benefit than during non-pandemic years.

These more recent estimates using laboratory-confirmed endpoints are well within the reported vaccine effectiveness for healthy, nonpregnant adults. When combined with the well-documented observation that the antibody response to influenza vaccine in pregnant women is similar to that of nonpregnant women, all current evidence suggests that efficacy of influenza vaccines in pregnant women is similar to the nonpregnant population.

5.2. Maternal vaccination to protect young infants

An important secondary benefit of maternal vaccination appears to be protection of infants from influenza infection during the first months of life, providing an important two-for-one benefit since no influenza vaccine is licensed or recommended for infants younger than 6 months of age.

Maternal vaccination has potential to protect newborns due to the transfer of maternal immunity. Transplacental transfer of antibodies occurs throughout pregnancy, with highest levels during the last 4–6 weeks of gestation [102, 103]. Antibodies (specifically IgG) cross the placenta from mother to fetus during the final weeks of pregnancy, while infants acquire additional immune protection during breastfeeding, when the main class of immunoglobulin transferred in breast milk is IgA [104].

Several studies have demonstrated transplacentally acquired antibodies after natural influenza infection in the mother. One study examined the cord sera of 26 infants who had culture-confirmed influenza when younger than 4 months of age. The authors found a direct correlation between the gestational age at the time of infection and the level of antibody in the cord serum ($p = 0.002$), suggesting a protective effect of transplacentally acquired antibody [105].

During the 1979 influenza epidemic, infants of mothers with serum antibody to influenza (seropositive) were compared to infants of mothers who were seronegative [106]. The infants of seropositive mothers had higher specific serum antibody (IgG) titers against the HA influenza protein than did infants of seronegative mothers. Good correlation was found between maternal antibody titers and titers in infants (correlation, 0.81). No such correlation was found for non-immune mothers and their infants (correlation, 0.24) [106]. However, this study showed no difference in incidence of influenza infection, although infants of immune mothers showed delayed onset of symptoms and shorter duration of illness, suggesting that passive maternal immunization may delay onset and severity.

5.2.1. Serological studies

When evaluating vaccination response to influenza, a serum antibody titer of ≥1:40 against the HA protein is considered to be clinically relevant, resulting in a 50% decrease in symptomatic infection and, therefore, serving as a correlate of protective immunity [107]. Recent analysis of published data indicates an even higher level of clinical protection, estimating that 70% of participants are protected at a titer of 1:40, with protection increasing gradually with higher titers [108].

In the absence of a widely accepted immune correlate of protection for influenza, the analysis of hemagglutinin inhibition (HAI) seroprotection rates is generally considered a useful indicator of protection in vaccinated persons. There are challenges associated with using this antibody titer as a correlate of protection in infants, however, particularly since this correlate was determined in healthy adults [41, 107]. In any event, the US Food and Drug Administration (FDA) uses this HAI antibody titer in evaluation of influenza vaccines, making the HAI antibody titer the standard used by most investigators [40], including those examining vaccine protection in neonates.

In a study examining transplacental transfer of antibody in response to vaccination, Englund et al. studied women during the last trimester of pregnancy who were vaccinated with IIV3 (A/Sichuan/H3N2, A/Taiwan/H1N1, B/Victoria). Maternal immunization resulted in the transfer of influenza-specific IgG to the infants. When measured at the time of delivery, the levels of antibody transferred were high, with between 87 and 99% of antibody detectable in the mother also detectable in the infant [78]. The antibody titers to at least two of the three influenza antigens (influenza H3N2 and influenza B) remained significantly elevated up to 2 months of age [78].

Sumaya and Gibbs vaccinated pregnant women and reported a similar correlation, finding that cord blood HAI antibody in infants correlated with titers of vaccine-stimulated HAI antibody in mothers, with HAI antibody detected in 54% of newborn serum and 73% of maternal serum [75]. This study did not examine infant influenza infection as an outcome, so the study was unable to correlate serum antibody levels with clinical outcome.

While these previous studies demonstrated that maternal antibody appears to be transferred to infants following both natural infection and vaccination, neither study discussed whether the level maternal antibody was high enough to confer protective immunity to the infant [41, 107]. Using HAI titer as a correlate of immunity, Steinhoff et al. did conduct an RCT of maternal influenza vaccine. Serum samples were obtained from 311 mothers before vaccination and at delivery and from 292 infants at birth at 10 weeks and 20–26 weeks later [109]. The proportion of mothers with a protective antibody titer (HAI ≥ 1:40) at the time of delivery was 88% for A/New Caledonia (H1N1), 98% for A/Fujian (H3N2), and 45% for B/Hong Kong. Similar proportions of infants had protective antibody titers at birth [109].

Yamaguchi et al. also examined the immune responses to influenza vaccination during pregnancy by measuring the effect of influenza vaccination (IIV3) in pregnancy, including maintenance of the specific antibody response, and the efficiency of transplacental transfer of the antibody to the fetus. The study included 125 pregnant women, 71 in their second trimester and 54 during the third trimester of pregnancy. The authors reported that vaccination at any time during pregnancy yielded protective levels of antibody in both maternal and fetal blood [110].

In a prospective study examining the immunogenicity and transplacental transmission of antibodies in pregnant women in Asia, Lin et al. enrolled 46 pregnant women who received a single dose of IIV3. Twenty-eight days after vaccination, the seroprotection rate in vaccinated women against H1N1, H3N2, and influenza B was 91.3, 84.8, and 56.5%, respectively [111].

Several additional studies have demonstrated transplacental antibody transfer following maternal vaccination with pandemic H1N1 vaccine. Three studies evaluated adjuvanted A(H1N1) vaccines, and two studied nonadjuvanted A(H1N1)vaccine. All five of the studies documented protective levels of antibody in significant percent of infants (79–95%).

Zuccotti et al. followed 69 mother-infant pairs. The women were vaccinated during their third trimester of pregnancy with MF59-adjuvanted influenza A(H1N1) vaccine. All of the mothers had HAI antibody titers at or above 1:40 at the time of delivery and throughout the 5 months of follow-up. Ninety-five percent of the infants had HAI antibody titers at or about 1:40 at both birth and 2 months of age. By 5 months of age, the proportion of infants with titers of 1:40 dropped to 81.2% [89], suggesting that passively acquired antibody at levels thought to be protective is transferred and persists for at least 5 months.

In a separate study performed at three sites in the UK, researchers followed infants born to mothers who were vaccinated with AS03-adjuvanted H1N1 vaccine during the second or third trimester of pregnancy. This study found that 79% of the infants of vaccinated mothers had serum antibody titers at or higher than 1:40 compared to a background immunity in 19% of infants of unvaccinated women ($p = 0.001$) [112].

Helmig et al. evaluated the serological response of a cohort of women immunized with adjuvanted A(H1N1) vaccine or by natural infection with A(H1N1)pdm09. The authors detected protective antibody levels (>1:40) in a significant number 17/19 (89.5%) of newborns born to vaccinated mothers ($p = 0.001$) [113]. Notably, while natural influenza infection conferred protective antibody levels in mothers, it did not contribute to protective levels in their infants; only 15.8% of infants born to women who had natural influenza infection during pregnancy developed protective levels of antibody at birth.

In a study of nonadjuvanted A(H1N1) vaccine, Tsatsaris et al. measured Ab titers in cord blood of 88 infants born to women vaccinated with a single dose of monovalent A(H1N1) vaccine. The researchers reported 95% (CI, 89–99%) of infants have protective levels of antibody (>1:40) at birth [114], and Fisher et al. also reported protective levels of Ab in cord blood of infants following maternal vaccination with 2009 monovalent A(H1N1) [115].

Taken together, these studies provide an important proof of concept for transplacentally acquired antibody, from either natural infection or vaccination of their mother, to potentially protect young infants from influenza infection and present maternal immunization as a promising strategy for reducing influenza infection in infants.

5.2.2. Clinical studies

Over the past 11 years, nine studies have been published evaluating the effect of maternal immunization on influenza in 97,656 infants across 15 influenza seasons. Six of these studies showed clinical protection; three studies did not (**Table 2**).

Study	Study period	Participants	Outcomes measured	Protection by maternal influenza vaccine
Black et al. [81]	1997–2002	49,585 pregnant women	Hospitalization for pneumonia and influenza	No difference in risk for hospitalization ($p = 0.235$) Adjusted hazard ratio: 0.956 (CI, 0.889–1.029) Clinical effectiveness: 4% (CI, –3 to 11%) No difference in risk including otitis media visit ($p = 0.506$) Adjusted hazard ratio: 0.938 (CI, 0.777 1.132) Clinical effectiveness: 6% (CI, –13 to 22%)
Munoz et al. [117]	1998–2003	225 infants of immunized mothers	Hospitalization or	No difference in hospitalization

http://dx.doi.org/10.5772/64368

Study	Study period	Participants	Outcomes measured	Protection by maternal influenza vaccine
		826 infants of nonimmunized mothers	clinic visits for respiratory conditions	During first month, infants of immunized moms had more clinic visits for bronchitis ($p = 0.04$) and fewer for respiratory distress ($p = 0.04$) No other differences
France et al. [116]	1995–2001	3160 infants of immunized mothers 37,969 infants of nonimmunized women	Medically attended acute respiratory illness (ARI)	No reduction in clinic visit rates Incident rate ratio: 0.96 (CI, 0.86–1.07)
Zaman et al. [79]	2004–2005	316 infant-mother pairs followed for 24 weeks	Clinic visits for respiratory illness Laboratory-confirmed influenza before 24 weeks of age (confirmation by rapid test)	63% effective at preventing laboratory-confirmed influenza in infants up to 6 months old (CI, 5–85%) 29% effective in preventing febrile illness (CI, 6.9–45.7%) 42% effective in preventing clinic visit (CI, 18.2–58.8%)
Benowitz et al. [118]	2000–2009	Infants less than 12 months old -220 cases -430 matched controls	Laboratory-confirmed influenza (confirmation by direct fluorescent antibody (DFA) test)	91.5% effective at preventing hospitalization of infants less than 6 months of age ($p = 0.001$; CI, 61.7–98.1%) No significant effect on infants older than 6 months
Eick et al. [120]	2002–2005	1169 infant-mother pairs	Laboratory-confirmed influenza (confirmation by viral culture, fourfold rise in HAI antibody in cord serum or rapid test)	Laboratory-confirmed influenza decreased among infants born to vaccinated women compared to controls Risk ratio 0.59 (CI, 0.37–0.93) Clinical effectiveness: 41% Hospitalization Risk ratio 0.61 (CI, 0.45–0.84) Clinical effectiveness: 39%
Poehling et al. [126]	2002–2009	Infants less than 6 months old hospitalized with fever or respiratory symptoms -151 cases -1359 controls	Laboratory-confirmed influenza (confirmation by viral culture or PCR)	Hospitalized infants whose mothers were immunized were 45–48% less likely to have laboratory-confirmed influenza Adjusted odds ratio (OR) 0.52 (CI, 0.30–0.91)
Sugimura et al. [127]	2010–2011	200 infants from birth to 6 months of age -106 infants of vaccinated mothers	Laboratory-confirmed influenza (confirmation by rapid test)	Significant difference in incidence of influenza between infants of vaccinated versus unvaccinated mothers ($p = 0.019$)

Study	Study period	Participants	Outcomes measured	Protection by maternal influenza vaccine
		-90 infants of unvaccinated mothers		
Madhi et al. [83]	2011–2012	2046 infants -1026 infants of vaccinated mothers - 1023 infants of placebo mothers	Laboratory-confirmed influenza RT-PCR	Vaccine efficacy of 48.8% (CI, 11.6–70.4%)

Table 2. Clinical effectiveness of maternal vaccination for protection of infants.

5.2.2.1. Studies finding no protective effect

In a retrospective cohort study of 48,639 infants, Black et al. found that infants born to vaccinated women had the same risk of hospitalization for influenza or pneumonia as infants of unvaccinated women (CI, 0.889–1.029). They also reported that maternal vaccination was not a significant determinant of risk for ILI or otitis media [81].

France et al. followed 3160 infants of immunized mothers and 37,969 infants of nonimmunized mothers from 1995–2001 and during four specific seasonal periods: peak influenza, respiratory syncytial virus predominant, periseasonal, and summer weeks [116]. They found no difference in medically attended ARI (incident rate ratio for peak influenza season 0.96, CI, 0.86–1.07), concluding "maternal influenza vaccination did not reduce visit rates during any of the four time periods and did not delay the onset of first respiratory illness" [116].

In a study that included an examination of data over five influenza seasons, Munoz et al. reported similar results, finding no difference in hospitalizations for respiratory illness during the peak of influenza season between infants of vaccinated mothers versus infants of non-vaccinated mothers [117].

5.2.2.2. Studies finding clinical protection

While the three earlier studies above found no benefit to infants from maternal vaccination, a more recent matched case-control study of infants less than 12 months old admitted to hospitals for seasonal influenza between 2000 and 2009 reported maternal vaccination to be 91.5% effective (CI, 61.7–98.1%, $p = 0.001$) in preventing hospitalization of infants younger than 6 months of age [118]. Maternal vaccination was not effective in preventing hospitalization for infants older than 6 months (−41.4% (CI, 0.153–0.918)). In this study, influenza cases from 2007 to 2009 were confirmed by direct fluorescent antibody (DFA) test, which was reported to be 96.2% sensitive and 99% specific for influenza [119]. A limitation to this study is that results from nine influenza seasons were combined, with no information regarding the strain match of vaccine to circulating strain for each influenza season. The researchers did not type the strain of influenza in infected infants, stating that they "did not have adequate power to assess the

http://dx.doi.org/10.5772/64368

vaccine's effectiveness by influenza season…and did not type strains to determine whether influenza infections were caused by strains included in the vaccine" [118].

Eick et al. conducted a study in the White Mountain and Navajo reservations over three influenza seasons, November 2002 to September of 2005. In this prospective cohort study, the effect of influenza vaccine during pregnancy on influenza infection in infants was compared between infants of vaccinated women and those born to non-vaccinated women. The authors analyzed 83 confirmed influenza cases. Of these cases, seven (86%) were confirmed by serology, ten (12%) by viral culture, and two (2%) by rapid influenza testing. Using these three measures of influenza infection, the authors reported a 41% reduction in the risk of laboratory-confirmed influenza for infants born to vaccinated women (RR 0.59, CI, 0.37–0.93) and a 39% reduction in the risk of ILI hospitalization (RR 0.61, CI, 0.45–0.84) [120].

The authors of this study pooled the results from three different assay methods, each with different sensitivities, to document influenza infection. Pooling assays with differing diagnostics represents a limitation of this study. Likewise, the use of serology to document influenza in most (86%) of cases represents a weakness of this study. The authors describe serological documentation of influenza infection as a fourfold or greater increase in HAI antibody in serum collected at 2–3 or 6 months compared with previous serum specimen [120]. Significant limitations have been reported regarding the use of serology in diagnosing influenza in adult patients that have been vaccinated with inactivated vaccines [121–123]. Using serology to document influenza infection in young infants presents additional complications.

Infants under 6 months of age have immature, immunologically inexperienced immune systems. Since their ability to produce antibody in response to infection is often delayed or completely absent, many of their serum antibodies are maternally derived. More than 50 years ago, the use of serology for diagnosis of influenza in infancy was questioned. During an influenza outbreak in Glasgow in 1953, fourfold increases in antibody were found in only 20% of infants admitted to pediatric pneumonia wards (as compared to 30% of adult cases) [124]. In two different outbreaks, antibody production was absent or considerably delayed in infected children under 18 months of age, even when virus could be isolated [125]. These observations illustrate the difficulties inherent in using serology to document influenza infection in young infants.

In the only randomized, blinded clinical study to assess infant protection, Zaman et al. reported a vaccine effectiveness of 63% (CI, 5–85%) against laboratory-confirmed influenza in infants up to 6 months of age [79]. Influenza was confirmed by rapid test (Z Stat Flu), which was reported to have a specificity of 80–90% and a sensitivity of 70–72% for type A and type B influenza. When respiratory illness and fever were used as measure of disease, the reported effectiveness was 29% (CI, 7–46%) [79].

A recent study sought to determine whether maternal vaccination during pregnancy was associated with a reduced risk or laboratory-confirmed influenza hospitalizations in 1510 infants over seven consecutive influenza seasons (2002–2003 through 2008–2009) and across three diverse geographic regions of the United States [126]. Of the 1510 infants hospitalized with fever or respiratory symptoms, 151 (10%) had laboratory-confirmed (by viral culture or

RT-PCR) influenza. The proportion of infants who were influenza positive varied significantly across influenza seasons, from 3% in 2006–2007 to 15% in 2003–2004. The percentage of women who were vaccinated also varied by season, from 10% in 2003–2004 to 38% in 2008–2009.

Among influenza-positive infants during all study years, 12% of their mothers reported being vaccinated during pregnancy, while 20% of mothers of influenza-negative infants reported receiving a vaccination [126], yielding an adjusted odds ratio of 0.52 (CI, 0.30–0.91) and suggesting that infants whose mothers received influenza vaccines during pregnancy were 48% less likely to have laboratory-confirmed influenza than infants of unvaccinated women [126].

In a randomized, placebo-controlled trial of influenza vaccination in South Africa, Madhi et al. followed 1026 infants born to women who received IIV3 and 1023 infants born to placebo recipients. The attack rate of influenza was lower among infants of vaccinated mothers (1.9%) than among those whose mothers received placebo vaccine (3.6%), yielding a vaccine effectiveness of 57.5% (CI, 7.6–70.4) in this population [83].

In a prospective study, Sugimura et al. assessed the incidence of fever and laboratory-confirmed influenza in newborns whose mothers were vaccinated during pregnancy with IIV3. Two hundred infants were followed from birth to 6 months of age. Fever was noted in 36 (34%) of the infants in the vaccinated group and 47 (52.2%) of infants born to unvaccinated mothers ($p < 0.007$). The incidence of influenza as diagnosed by rapid test was 0 (0%) and 5 (5.6%), respectively, ($p = 0.019$) [127].

The reviewed studies assessed hospitalization, clinic visits, ARI, or laboratory-confirmed influenza as primary outcomes. Rationale for influenza vaccination often includes additional secondary outcomes such as reduction of absenteeism for household contacts, secondary infections, acute otitis media, or community transmission of influenza. While these outcomes are important in measuring the broad impact of influenza, they do not provide accurate assessment of vaccine efficacy or effectiveness. Such an assessment is essential for evidence-based, reasoned development of public health policy and decision-making about influenza prevention.

In summary, the evidence for newborn protection through maternal vaccination is encouraging, but several studies exhibit methodological limitations. The results of studies measuring rates of ARI, clinic visit, or hospitalization range from no vaccine effect up to 42% effectiveness [81, 116, 117]. The six studies that used some form of laboratory-confirmed influenza (rapid tests, viral culture, or PCR) as the primary outcome are more encouraging, reporting vaccination effectiveness ranging from 41 to 91.5% [79, 83, 118, 120, 126, 127].

While outcomes and study designs differ, in general the data to date suggest that maternal vaccination has the potential to decrease influenza illness in newborns. As such, maternal immunization during pregnancy should continue to be recommended and encouraged for all women.

http://dx.doi.org/10.5772/64368

6. Current challenges

Influenza is a complex disease. For centuries it has eluded complete understanding or control. Constantly evolving and catching us by surprise, influenza is a perpetually emerging disease. The main tool for prevention of influenza is vaccination, the cornerstone for prevention of influenza disease. However, unlike many other vaccines, the effectiveness of influenza vaccines remains moderate to marginal across all populations [128], and in addition, the vaccines need to be administered every year. A universal influenza vaccine providing broad and long-lasting protection continues to be elusive.

These realities—difficult enough in the general population—are even more challenging to understand during pregnancy. Particularly complex is determining how, or if, the changing immune responses over pregnancy vis-a-vis influenza season and vaccination schedules impact vaccine effectiveness and disease outcomes in pregnant women.

A recent critique by Savitz et al. calls into question our most basic understanding of influenza infection during pregnancy, with a particular critique on the quality of the evidence for a benefit of maternal vaccination in prevention of harm from seasonal influenza [129]. Savitz et al. discuss the complications inherent in many current research practices, which serve to limit our understanding of the true picture of maternal influenza. Central to this critique is the notion that both pregnancy and influenza have temporal components; influenza typically is seasonal, with a 2–3-month period of circulation each year. But pregnancy has trimesters, each with distinct fetal developmental stages along with physiological and immunological changes in the expectant mother. To complicate this further, the risk of adverse outcomes from influenza infection is not equal across all trimesters of pregnancy. Therefore, optimizing risk and benefit of vaccination during pregnancy is complicated and likely requires reexamination of influenza risk and benefit across trimesters in association with months of influenza circulation [129].

A recent WHO review of influenza throughout pregnancy found insufficient data from comparable studies to discern which specific weeks, months, or trimesters influenza poses increased risk to pregnant women [130]. Savitz et al. assert that "As with all time dependent states, pregnancies must be followed longitudinally. There needs to be a week-by-week consideration of the pregnancy with regard to vaccination status and circulating influenza viruses" [129].

Aside from complications associated with potential differences in virus exposure across the trimesters of a pregnancy, risks posed to pregnant women also may differ according to the specific strain circulating during a given season, and, likewise, the immune response to vaccination also could differ based on strain [131].

Even when taking yearly strain differences into account, variation in immune responses across trimesters adds yet another complicating variable. It is widely accepted that the immune response to influenza vaccine in pregnant women is indistinguishable from that of nonpregnant women and that gestational age appears to have no effect on antibody response [75, 76, 132, 133].

Findings from more recent studies suggest that we may need to entertain a more nuanced approach to our understanding of the maternal immune response to influenza vaccination—precisely because immunogenicity and seroconversion may not tell the entire story.

In a 2011 study, Ohfuji et al. reported a lower seroprotective antibody response to pandemic A(H1N1) vaccine in pregnant women who had received prior seasonal influenza vaccine and suggested that the potential interference between pH1N1 and seasonal vaccination needed additional investigation [15]. Schlaudecker et al. directly compared immunogenicity of inactivated influenza vaccine in pregnant versus nonpregnant women and found that pregnancy modified antibody responses to the vaccine [134]. They demonstrated a significantly decreased postimmunization HAI geometric mean titer and a nonsignificantly decreased geometric mean ratio (fold increase) to influenza A antigens after influenza vaccine, even though overall seroconversion and seroprotection rates were comparable between the two groups of women. In a 2013 blinded randomized control study, Bischoff et al. found that the immune response to an adjuvanted pandemic A(H1N1) vaccine in pregnant women was decreased compared with nonpregnant women [133]. Sperling et al. examined HAI titers over pregnancy and found that timing of vaccination did not alter response, although there was a trend toward lower responses during the first trimester and six weeks postpartum [135].

A small study of 36 women during the 2012–2014 flu seasons suggests that T-follicular helper (Tfh) cell response to vaccination was highest during the first trimester of pregnancy. Tfh cells are required for the generation of high-quality antibody-producing B cells. Their expansion has been shown to be a predictor of response to influenza vaccination outside of pregnancy suggesting that immunologic changes during pregnancy may impact vaccine response. Notably, there was no significant expansion of Tfh after vaccination during either the second or third trimester [136].

In a study aimed to determine the optimal timing for vaccination within the second or third trimesters of pregnancy, Yamaguchi et al. reported that serum antibody levels in vaccinated women depended not on gestational stage but on the amount of time elapsed, since vaccination antibody titers decreased with time [110]. This observation is supported by other studies documenting that influenza-specific antibodies after vaccination are typically short lived [115].

Two separate studies of vaccine effectiveness in nonpregnant adults during the 2011–2012 influenza season also suggest that vaccine effectiveness wanes with time since vaccination [137, 138]. In both of these studies, vaccination effectiveness waned in people who were vaccinated 93 days—around 3 months—or more before presentation of symptoms. A similar observation was made by Fisher et al. who demonstrated a significant linear decline over time in HAI titers after pH1N1 infection or vaccination ($p = 0.04$ for infected and $p = 0.009$ for vaccinated) [115].

Taken together, these observations support a consensus that pregnant women are capable of mounting a robust immune response to influenza vaccination during the second and third trimester of pregnancy. Experimental evidence during the first trimester is less clear, due in part to a limited number of studies on influenza vaccination during the first trimester.

There is increasing evidence suggesting that—regardless of initial vaccine response—the level of vaccine-mediated anti-influenza-specific antibodies decreases with time. This waning of antibody implies that women vaccinated during the first trimester of pregnancy might be *less* well protected as their pregnancy progresses. It is well documented that serious influenza-related morbidity in healthy pregnant women most often occurs during the second and third trimester of pregnancy. So a reasonable goal appears to be ensuring the highest possible level of protection during the second and third trimesters. Studies on waning immunity suggest that this may be precisely opposite of what occurs in women who are vaccinated early in pregnancy; protection wanes as risk increases.

6.1. Timing maternal vaccination for protection of neonates

Cross-placental transfer of immunity occurs when antibodies cross the placenta via active transport, particularly in the final weeks of pregnancy. It is logical to assume that vaccine-induced maternal antibody transmitted to the fetus will provide protection to the infant during the first months of life, and several studies document increased antibody titers in infants of vaccinated mothers [120].

Comparable to studies of vaccinated mothers, researchers have demonstrated that the titers of influenza-specific antibodies in newborns, while not affected by trimester of maternal vaccination (within second or third trimester), do wane with time and are short lived [75]. Tsatsaris et al. also noted a trend toward lower cord blood antibody titer associated with longer intervals between maternal vaccination and delivery. A similar observation was made by Yamaguchi et al. who reported that transfer rate from the maternal blood to the fetal blood at time of delivery tended to be inversely correlated with duration of gestation postvaccination [110]. Some additional studies have hinted at lower cord blood titers among infants of women vaccinated in the first trimesters, but it is unclear if this is clinically significant [131].

Taken together, these studies serve to highlight the complicated nature of immunity particularly during pregnancy in response to vaccination and invite further virological and epidemiological studies to confirm and fully understand these observations and to correlate changes in antibody titer with clinical outcomes in both mothers and infants. As our understanding evolves, we may need to develop a more nuanced approach—one that takes into consideration the trimester of exposure to both circulating virus and vaccines—to optimize vaccine effectiveness during the period of highest risk of influenza disease.

The recommendation to vaccinate all pregnant women regardless of gestational age is motivated in part by operational concerns. Timing of the influenza vaccine campaigns occurs in the fall in temperate regions. Pregnancy, on the other hand, occurs throughout the year. Since pregnancy presents a period of regularly scheduled and repeat visits, a more tailored approach to influenza vaccine coverage may be appropriate in order to stack the odds in favor of the highest level of protection for both mother and infant.

7. Conclusions

The impact of influenza infection on pregnant women and newborns is well documented. The increased risk for morbidity and mortality has resulted in the universal recommendation that pregnant women be vaccinated for influenza at any stage of pregnancy [65]. Evidence to date suggests that influenza vaccination during pregnancy is similarly effective as in the nonpregnant population. Pregnant women mount robust immune response that correlates with clinical efficacy. This immunity then is transferred to the fetus during gestation, providing clinical benefit to infants less than 6 months of age. And while not a component of this review, there is substantial evidence that influenza vaccines are safe during all stages of pregnancy with no evidence of risk of adverse pregnancy outcome linked to influenza vaccines [3, 65, 131, 139, 140].

Gaps remain in our understanding of influenza risk over all seasons and trimesters, of maternal immunity, and of optimal timing of vaccination. To this end, in January of 2015, the Bill and Melinda Gates Foundation held a meeting of global stakeholders in the maternal influenza field. Participants identified a need for stronger evidence regarding, among other issues, the burden of disease and maternal immunization efficacy [141]. Expanding this evidence base will allow for a deeper understanding of influenza in this population and the development of more robust and efficacious public health approaches toward this disease.

Author details

Jill M. Manske

Address all correspondence to: jmmanske@stthomas.edu

University of St. Thomas, Saint Paul, MN, USA

References

[1] World Health Organization, WHO position paper on influenza vaccines. Wkly Epidemiol Record 2005; 33: 279–287)

[2] Tamma PD, Steinhoff MC, Omer SB. Influenza infection and vaccination in pregnant women. Expert Rev Respir Med 2010;4:321–8.

[3] Mak TK, Mangtani P, Leese J, Watson JM, Pfeifer D. Influenza vaccination in pregnancy: current evidence and selected national policies. Lancet Infect Dis 2008;8:44–52.

[4] Neuzil KM, Reed GW, Mitchel EF, Simonsen L, Griffin MR. Impact of influenza on acute cardiopulmonary hospitalizations in pregnant women. Am J Epidemiol 1998;148:1094–102.

[5] Schanzer DL, Langley JM, Tam TW. Influenza-attributed hospitalization rates among pregnant women in Canada 1994–2000. J Obstet Gynaecol Can 2007;29:622–9.

[6] Jamieson DJ, Theiler RN, Rasmussen SA. Emerging infections and pregnancy. Emerg Infect Dis 2006;12:1638–43.

[7] Skowronski DM, De Serres G. Is routine influenza immunization warranted in early pregnancy? Vaccine 2009;27:4754–70.

[8] Gaunt G, Ramin K. Immunological tolerance of the human fetus. Am J Perinatol 2001;18:299–312.

[9] Szekeres-Bartho J. Immunological relationship between the mother and the fetus. Int Rev Immunol 2002;21:471–95.

[10] Davies M, Browne CM. Pregnancy-associated nonspecific immunosuppression: kinetics of the generation and identification of the active factors. Am J Reprod Immunol Microbiol 1985;9:77–83.

[11] Saleeby E, Chapman J, Morse J, Bryant A. H1N1 influenza in pregnancy: cause for concern. Obstet Gynecol 2009;114:885–91.

[12] Laibl VR, Sheffield JS. Influenza and pneumonia in pregnancy. Clin Perinatol 2005;32:727–38.

[13] Griffiths PD, Ronalds CJ, Heath RB. A prospective study of influenza infections during pregnancy. J Epidemiol Community Health 1980;34:124–8.

[14] Lindsay L, Jackson LA, Savitz DA, Weber DJ, Koch GG, Kong L, et al. Community influenza activity and risk of acute influenza-like illness episodes among healthy unvaccinated pregnant and postpartum women. Am J Epidemiol 2006;163:838–48.

[15] Ohfuji S, Fukushima W, Deguchi M, Kawabata K, Yoshida H, Hatayama H, et al. Immunogenicity of a monovalent 2009 influenza A (H1N1) vaccine among pregnant women: lowered antibody response by prior seasonal vaccination. J Infect Dis 2011;203:1301–8.

[16] Dodds L, McNeil SA, Fell DB, Allen VM, Coombs A, Scott J, et al. Impact of influenza exposure on rates of hospital admissions and physician visits because of respiratory illness among pregnant women. CMAJ 2007;176:463–8.

[17] Cox S, Posner SF, McPheeters M, Jamieson DJ, Kourtis AP, Meikle S. Hospitalizations with respiratory illness among pregnant women during influenza season. Obstet Gynecol 2006;107:1315–22.

[18] Hartert TV, Neuzil KM, Shintani AK, Mitchel EF, Jr., Snowden MS, Wood LB, et al. Maternal morbidity and perinatal outcomes among pregnant women with respiratory hospitalizations during influenza season. Am J Obstet Gynecol 2003;189:1705–12.

[19] Kort BA, Cefalo RC, Baker VV. Fatal influenza A pneumonia in pregnancy. Am J Perinatol 1986;3:179–82.

[20] Housworth J, Langmuir AD. Excess mortality from epidemic influenza, 1957–1966. Am J Epidemiol 1974;100:40–8.

[21] Callaghan WM, Chu SY, Jamieson DJ. Deaths from seasonal influenza among pregnant women in the United States, 1998–2005. Obstet Gynecol 2010;115:919–23.

[22] Nuzum JW, Pilot I, Stangl FH, Bonar BE. 1918 pandemic influenza and pneumonia in a large civil hospital. IMJ Illinois Med J 1976;150:612–6.

[23] Freeman DW, Barno A. Deaths from Asian influenza associated with pregnancy. Am J Obstet Gynecol 1959;78:1172–5.

[24] Greenberg M, Jacobziner H, Pakter J, Weisl BA. Maternal mortality in the epidemic of Asian influenza, New York City, 1957. Am J Obstet Gynecol 1958;76:897–902.

[25] Harris JW. Influenza occurring in pregnant women: a statistical study of thirteen hundred and fifty cases. J Am Med Assoc 1919;72:978–80.

[26] Woolston, W.J., Conley D.O. Epidemic pneumonia (Spanish influenza) in pregnancy: effect in one hundred and one cases. J Am Med Assoc 1918;71:1898–9.

[27] CDC. Novel influenza A (H1N1) virus infection in three pregnant women—United States. MMWR Morb Mortal Wkly Rep 2009;58:497–500.

[28] Panda B, Panda A, Riley LE. Selected viral infections in pregnancy. Obstet Gynecol Clin North Am 2010;37:321–31.

[29] CDC. Hospitalized patients with novel influenza A (H1N1) virus infection-California. MMWR Morb Mortal Wkly Rep 2009;58:536–41.

[30] Jamieson DJ, Honein MA, Rasmussen SA, Williams JL, Swerdlow DL, Biggerstaff MS, et al. H1N1 2009 influenza virus infection during pregnancy in the USA. Lancet 2009;374:451–8.

[31] Louie JK, Acosta M, Jamieson DJ, Honein MA. Severe 2009 H1N1 influenza in pregnant and postpartum women in California. N Engl J Med 2010;362:27–35.

[32] Mosby LG, Rasmussen SA, Jamieson DJ. 2009 Pandemic influenza A (H1N1) in pregnancy: a systematic review of the literature. Am J Obstet Gynecol 2011.

[33] Callaghan WM, Creanga AA, Jamieson DJ. Pregnancy-related mortality resulting from influenza in the United States during the 2009–2010 pandemic. Obstet Gynecol 2015;126:486–90.

[34] Siston AM, Rasmussen SA, Honein MA, Fry AM, Seib K, Callaghan WM, et al. Pandemic 2009 influenza A(H1N1) virus illness among pregnant women in the United States. JAMA 2010;303:1517–25.

[35] Yates L, Pierce M, Stephens S, Mill AC, Spark P, Kurinczuk JJ, et al. Influenza A/H1N1v in pregnancy: an investigation of the characteristics and management of affected women and the relationship to pregnancy outcomes for mother and infant. Health Technol Assess 2010;14:109–82.

[36] Gerardin P, El Amrani R, Cyrille B, Gabriele M, Guillermin P, Boukerrou M, et al. Low clinical burden of 2009 pandemic influenza A (H1N1) infection during pregnancy on the island of La Reunion. PLoS One 2010;5:e10896.

[37] Zhang J, Troendle J, Reddy UM, Laughon SK, Branch DW, Burkman R, et al. Contemporary cesarean delivery practice in the United States. Am J Obstet Gynecol 2010;203:326e1–e10.

[38] Yawn DH, Pyeatte JC, Joseph JM, Eichler SL, Garcia-Bunuel R. Transplacental transfer of influenza virus. JAMA 1971;216:1022–3.

[39] Dulyachai W, Makkoch J, Rianthavorn P, Changpinyo M, Prayangprecha S, Payungporn S, et al. Perinatal pandemic (H1N1) 2009 infection, Thailand. Emerg Infect Dis 2010;16:343–4.

[40] Lieberman RW, Bagdasarian N, Thomas D, Van De Ven C. Seasonal influenza A (H1N1) infection in early pregnancy and second trimester fetal demise. Emerg Infect Dis 2011;17:107–9.

[41] Ortiz JR, Englund JA, Neuzil KM. Influenza vaccine for pregnant women in resource-constrained countries: a review of the evidence to inform policy decisions. Vaccine 2011;29:4439–52.

[42] Hewagama S, Walker SP, Stuart RL, Gordon C, Johnson PD, Friedman ND, et al. 2009 H1N1 influenza A and pregnancy outcomes in Victoria, Australia. Clin Infect Dis 2010;50:686–90.

[43] Uchide N, Ohyama K, Bessho T, Toyoda H. Induction of pro-inflammatory cytokine gene expression and apoptosis in human chorion cells of fetal membranes by influenza virus infection: possible implications for maintenance and interruption of pregnancy during infection. Med Sci Monit 2005;11:RA7–16.

[44] Shi L, Tu N, Patterson PH. Maternal influenza infection is likely to alter fetal brain development indirectly: the virus is not detected in the fetus. Int J Dev Neurosci 2005;23:299–305.

[45] McKinney WP, Volkert P, Kaufman J. Fatal swine influenza pneumonia during late pregnancy. Arch Intern Med 1990;150:213–5.

[46] Moretti ME, Bar-Oz B, Fried S, Koren G. Maternal hyperthermia and the risk for neural tube defects in offspring: systematic review and meta-analysis. Epidemiology 2005;16:216–9.

[47] Coffey VP, Jessop WJ. Maternal influenza and congenital deformities. A follow-up study. Lancet 1963;1:748–51.

[48] Hardy JM, Azarowicz EN, Mannini A, Medearis DN, Jr., Cooke RE. The effect of Asian influenza on the outcome of pregnancy, Baltimore, 1957–1958. Am J Public Health Nations Health 1961;51:1182–8.

[49] Saxen L, Hjelt L, Sjostedt JE, Hakosalo J, Hakosalo H. Asian influenza during pregnancy and congenital malformations. Acta Pathol Microbiol Scand 1960;49:114–26.

[50] Edwards MJ. Review: hyperthermia and fever during pregnancy. Birth Defects Res A Clin Mol Teratol 2006;76:507–16.

[51] Hansen C, Desai S, Bredfeldt C, Cheetham C, Gallagher M, Li D-K, et al. A large, population-based study of 2009 pandemic Influenza A virus subtype H1N1 infection diagnosis during pregnancy and outcomes for mothers and neonates. J Infect Dis 2012;206:1260–8.

[52] Luteijn JM, Brown MJ, Dolk H. Influenza and congenital anomalies: a systematic review and meta-analysis. Hum Reprod 2014;29:809–23.

[53] Haberg SE, Trogstad L, Gunnes N, Wilcox AJ, Gjessing HK, Samuelsen SO, et al. Risk of fetal death after pandemic influenza virus infection or vaccination. N Engl J Med 2013;368:333–40.

[54] Pierce M, Kurinczuk JJ, Spark P, Brocklehurst P, Knight M, Ukoss. Perinatal outcomes after maternal 2009/H1N1 infection: national cohort study. BMJ 2011;342:d3214.

[55] Moore DL, Vaudry W, Scheifele DW, Halperin SA, Dery P, Ford-Jones E, et al. Surveillance for influenza admissions among children hospitalized in Canadian immunization monitoring program active centers, 2003–2004. Pediatrics 2006;118:e610–9.

[56] Izurieta HS, Thompson WW, Kramarz P, Shay DK, Davis RL, DeStefano F, et al. Influenza and the rates of hospitalization for respiratory disease among infants and young children. N Engl J Med 2000;342:232–9.

[57] Neuzil KM, Mellen BG, Wright PF, Mitchel EF, Jr., Griffin MR. The effect of influenza on hospitalizations, outpatient visits, and courses of antibiotics in children. N Engl J Med 2000;342:225–31.

[58] Thompson WW, Shay DK, Weintraub E, Brammer L, Bridges CB, Cox NJ, et al. Influenza-associated hospitalizations in the United States. JAMA 2004;292:1333–40.

[59] Bhat N, Wright JG, Broder KR, Murray EL, Greenberg ME, Glover MJ, et al. Influenza-associated deaths among children in the United States, 2003–2004. N Engl J Med 2005;353:2559–67.

[60] Thompson WW, Weintraub, E., Shay, D.K., Brammer, L., Cox, N., Fukuda, K. Age-specific estimated of US influenza-associated deaths and hospitalizations. Int Congr Ser 2004;1263:316–20.

[61] Iwane MK, Edwards KM, Szilagyi PG, Walker FJ, Griffin MR, Weinberg GA, et al. Population-based surveillance for hospitalizations associated with respiratory syncytial virus, influenza virus, and parainfluenza viruses among young children. Pediatrics 2004;113:1758–64.

[62] Poehling KA, Edwards KM, Weinberg GA, Szilagyi P, Staat MA, Iwane MK, et al. The underrecognized burden of influenza in young children. N Engl J Med 2006;355:31–40.

[63] Centers for Disease Control. Surveillance for laboratory-confirmed, influenza-associated hospitalizations—Colorado, 2004–05 influenza season. MMWR Morb Mortal Wkly Rep 2005;54:535–7.

[64] Libster R, Bugna J, Coviello S, Hijano DR, Dunaiewsky M, Reynoso N, et al. Pediatric hospitalizations associated with 2009 pandemic influenza A (H1N1) in Argentina. N Engl J Med 2010;362:45–55.

[65] Fiore AE, Uyeki TM, Broder K, Finelli L, Euler GL, Singleton JA, et al. Prevention and control of influenza with vaccines: recommendations of the Advisory Committee on Immunization Practices (ACIP), 2010. MMWR Recomm Rep 2010;59:1–62.

[66] Centers For Disease Control. Key facts about 2009 H1N1 flu vaccine. http://www.cdc.gov/h1n1flu/vaccination/vaccine_keyfacts.htm. Published March, 2010. Accessed February 15, 2016.

[67] Ambrose CS, Luke C, Coelingh K. Current status of live attenuated influenza vaccine in the United States for seasonal and pandemic influenza. Influenza Other Respir Viruses 2008;2:193–202.

[68] Centers For Disease Control. General recommendations on immunization: recommendations of the Advisory Committee on Immunization Practices (ACIP). MMWR 2011; 60 (No. 2): 26.

[69] Yudin MH. Risk management of seasonal influenza during pregnancy: current perspectives. Int J Women's Health 2014;6:681–9.

[70] Fiore AE, Shay DK, Broder K, Iskander JK, Uyeki TM, Mootrey G, et al. Prevention and control of seasonal influenza with vaccines: recommendations of the Advisory Committee on Immunization Practices (ACIP), 2009. MMWR Recomm Rep 2009;58:1–52.

[71] Harper SA, Fukuda K, Uyeki TM, Cox NJ, Bridges CB. Prevention and control of influenza: recommendations of the Advisory Committee on Immunization Practices (ACIP). MMWR Recomm Rep 2004;53:1–40.

[72] Centers for Disease Control. Prevention and Control of Influenza: Recommendations of the Immunization Practices Advisory Committee (ACIP). MMWR Morb Mortal Wkly Rep 2013;62:10, 30.

[73] World Health Organization. WHO recommendations on pandemic (H1N1) 2009 vaccines. http://www.who.int/csr/disease/swineflu/notes/h1n1_vaccine_20090713/en/. July 2009. Accessed November 7, 2015.

[74] Centers For Disease Control. Updated interim recommendations for obstetric health care providers related to the use of antiviral medications in the treatment and prevention of influenza for the 2009–2010 season.http:// www.cdc.gov/h1n1flu/recommendations.htm. December 2009. Accessed January 12, 2016.

[75] Sumaya CV, Gibbs RS. Immunization of pregnant women with influenza A/New Jersey/76 virus vaccine: reactogenicity and immunogenicity in mother and infant. J Infect Dis 1979;140:141–6.

[76] Hulka JF. Effectiveness of polyvalent influenza vaccine in Pregnancy. Report of a Controlled Study during an Outbreak of Asian Influenza. Obstet Gynecol 1964;23:830–7.

[77] Deinard AS, Ogburn P, Jr. A/NJ/8/76 influenza vaccination program: effects on maternal health and pregnancy outcome. Am J Obstet Gynecol 1981;140:240–5.

[78] Englund JA, Mbawuike IN, Hammill H, Holleman MC, Baxter BD, Glezen WP. Maternal immunization with influenza or tetanus toxoid vaccine for passive antibody protection in young infants. J Infect Dis 1993;168:647–56.

[79] Zaman K, Roy E, Arifeen SE, Rahman M, Raqib R, Wilson E, et al. Effectiveness of maternal influenza immunization in mothers and infants. N Engl J Med 2008;359:1555–64.

[80] Manske JM. Efficacy and effectiveness of maternal influenza vaccination during pregnancy: a review of the evidence. Matern Child Health J 2013;18:1599–609.

[81] Black SB, Shinefield HR, France EK, Fireman BH, Platt ST, Shay D. Effectiveness of influenza vaccine during pregnancy in preventing hospitalizations and outpatient visits for respiratory illness in pregnant women and their infants. Am J Perinatol 2004;21:333–9.

[82] Munoz FM, Englund JA. A step ahead. Infant protection through maternal immunization. Pediatr Clin North Am 2000;47:449–63.

[83] Madhi SA, Cutland CL, Kuwanda L, Weinberg A, Hugo A, Jones S, et al. Influenza vaccination of pregnant women and protection of their infants. N Engl J Med 2014;371:918–31.

[84] Thompson MG, Li D-K, Shifflett P, Sokolow LZ, Ferber JR, Kurosky S, et al. Effectiveness of seasonal trivalent influenza vaccine for preventing influenza virus illness among pregnant women: a population-based case-control study during the 2010–2011 and 2011–2012 influenza seasons. Clin Infect Dis 2014;58:449–57.

[85] Centers for Disease Control. Use of Influenza A (H1N1) 2009 monovalent vaccine: recommendations of the Advisory Committee on Immunization Practices (ACIP). MMWR Morb Mortal Wkly Rep 2009;58:1–8.

[86] Centers for Disease Control. Seasonal Influenza and 2009 H1N1 influenza vaccination coverage among pregnant women–10 states, 2009–2010 influenza season. MMWR Morb Mortal Wkly Rep 2010;59:1541–5.

[87] Horiya M, Hisano M, Iwasaki Y, Hanaoka M, Watanabe N, Ito Y, et al. Efficacy of double vaccination with the 2009 pandemic influenza A (H1N1) vaccine during pregnancy. Obstet Gynecol 2011;118:887–94.

[88] Jackson LA, Patel SM, Swamy GK, Frey SE, Creech CB, Munoz FM, et al. Immunogenicity of an inactivated monovalent 2009 H1N1 influenza vaccine in pregnant women. J Infect Dis 2011;204:854–63.

[89] Zuccotti G, Pogliani L, Pariani E, Amendola A, Zanetti A. Transplacental antibody transfer following maternal immunization with a pandemic 2009 influenza A(H1N1) MF59-adjuvanted vaccine. JAMA 2010;304:2360–1.

[90] Abzug MJ, Nachman SA, Muresan P, Handelsman E, Watts DH, Fenton T, et al. Safety and immunogenicity of 2009 pH1N1 vaccination in HIV-infected pregnant women. Clin Infect Dis 2013;56:1488–97.

[91] Yung CF, Andrews N, Hoschler K, Miller E. Comparing the immunogenicity of AS03-adjuvanted 2009 pandemic H1N1 vaccine with clinical protection in priority risk groups in England. PLoS One 2013;8:e56844.

[92] Puleston R, Bugg G, Hoschler K, Konje J, Thornton J, Stephenson I, et al. Multi-centre observational study of transplacental transmission of influenza antibodies following vaccination with AS03(A)-adjuvanted H1N1 2009 vaccine. PLoS One 2013;8:e47448.

[93] Moro PL, Broder K, Zheteyeva Y, Walton K, Rohan P, Sutherland A, et al. Adverse events in pregnant women following administration of trivalent inactivated influenza vaccine and live attenuated influenza vaccine in the Vaccine Adverse Event Reporting System, 1990–2009. Am J Obstet Gynecol 2011;204:146e1–7.

[94] Kallen B, Olausson PO. Vaccination against H1N1 influenza with Pandemrix((R)) during pregnancy and delivery outcome: a Swedish register study. BJOG 2012;119:1583–90.

[95] Pasternak B, Svanstrom H, Molgaard-Nielsen D, Krause TG, Emborg HD, Melbye M, et al. Risk of adverse fetal outcomes following administration of a pandemic influenza A(H1N1) vaccine during pregnancy. JAMA 2012;308:165–74.

[96] Beau AB, Hurault-Delarue C, Vidal S, Guitard C, Vayssiere C, Petiot D, et al. Pandemic A/H1N1 influenza vaccination during pregnancy: a comparative study using the EFEMERIS database. Vaccine 2014;32:1254–8.

[97] Chambers CD, Johnson D, Xu R, Luo Y, Louik C, Mitchell AA, et al. Risks and safety of pandemic H1N1 influenza vaccine in pregnancy: birth defects, spontaneous abortion, preterm delivery, and small for gestational age infants. Vaccine 2013;31:5026–32.

[98] Heikkinen T, Young J, van Beek E, Franke H, Verstraeten T, Weil JG, et al. Safety of MF59-adjuvanted A/H1N1 influenza vaccine in pregnancy: a comparative cohort study. Am J Obstet Gynecol 2012;207:177.e1–8.

[99] Omon E, Damase-Michel C, Hurault-Delarue C, Lacroix I, Montastruc JL, Oustric S, et al. Non-adjuvanted 2009 influenza A (H1N1)v vaccine in pregnant women: the results of a French prospective descriptive study. Vaccine 2011;29:9649–54.

[100] Tavares F, Nazareth I, Monegal JS, Kolte I, Verstraeten T, Bauchau V. Pregnancy and safety outcomes in women vaccinated with an AS03-adjuvanted split virion H1N1 (2009) pandemic influenza vaccine during pregnancy: a prospective cohort study. Vaccine 2011;29:6358–65.

[101] Richards JL, Hansen C, Bredfeldt C, Bednarczyk RA, Steinhoff MC, Adjaye-Gbewonyo D, et al. Neonatal outcomes after antenatal influenza immunization during the 2009 H1N1 influenza pandemic: impact on preterm birth, birth weight, and small for gestational age birth. Clin Infect Dis 2013.

[102] Simister NE. Placental transport of immunoglobulin G. Vaccine 2003;21:3365–9.

[103] Munoz ET, Deem MW. Epitope analysis for influenza vaccine design. Vaccine 2005;23:1144–8.

[104] Van de Perre P. Transfer of antibody via mother's milk. Vaccine 2003;21:3374–6.

[105] Puck JM, Glezen WP, Frank AL, Six HR. Protection of infants from infection with influenza A virus by transplacentally acquired antibody. J Infect Dis 1980;142:844–9.

[106] Reuman PD, Ayoub EM, Small PA. Effect of passive maternal antibody on influenza illness in children: a prospective study of influenza A in mother-infant pairs. Pediatr Infect Dis J 1987;6:398–403.

[107] Plotkin SA. Correlates of protection induced by vaccination. Clin Vaccine Immunol 2010;17:1055–65.

[108] Coudeville L, Andre P, Bailleux F, Weber F, Plotkin S. A new approach to estimate vaccine efficacy based on immunogenicity data applied to influenza vaccines administered by the intradermal or intramuscular routes. Hum Vaccines 2010;6:841–8.

[109] Steinhoff MC, Omer SB, Roy E, Arifeen SE, Raqib R, Altaye M, et al. Influenza immunization in pregnancy—antibody responses in mothers and infants. N Engl J Med 2010;362:1644–6.

[110] Yamaguchi K, Hisano M, Isojima S, Irie S, Arata N, Watanabe N, et al. Relationship of Th1/Th2 cell balance with the immune response to influenza vaccine during pregnancy. J Med Virol 2009;81:1923–8.

[111] Lin S-Y, Wu E-T, Lin C-H, Shyu M-K, Lee C-N. The safety and immunogenicity of trivalent inactivated influenza vaccination: a study of maternal-cord blood pairs in Taiwan. PLoS One 2013;8:e62983.

[112] Puleston RL, Bugg G, Hoschler K, Konje J, Thornton J, Stephenson I, et al. Observational study to investigate vertically acquired passive immunity in babies of mothers vaccinated against H1N1v during pregnancy. Health Technol Assess 2010;14:1-82.

[113] Helmig RB, Maimburg RD, Erikstrup C, Nielsen HS, Petersen OB, Nielsen LP, et al. Antibody response to influenza A(H1N1)pdm09 in vaccinated, serologically infected and unaffected pregnant women and their newborns. Acta Obstet Gynecol Scand 2015;94:833–9.

[114] Tsatsaris V, Capitant C, Schmitz T, Chazallon C, Bulifon S, Riethmuller D, et al. Maternal immune response and neonatal seroprotection from a single dose of a monovalent nonadjuvanted 2009 influenza A(H1N1) vaccine: a single-group trial. Ann Intern Med 2011;155:733–41.

[115] Fisher BM, Van Bockern J, Hart J, Lynch AM, Winn VD, Gibbs RS, et al. Pandemic influenza A H1N1 2009 infection versus vaccination: a cohort study comparing immune responses in pregnancy. PLoS One 2012;7:e33048.

[116] France EK, Smith-Ray R, McClure D, Hambidge S, Xu S, Yamasaki K, et al. Impact of maternal influenza vaccination during pregnancy on the incidence of acute respiratory illness visits among infants. Arch Pediatr Adolesc Med 2006;160:1277–83.

[117] Munoz FM, Greisinger AJ, Wehmanen OA, Mouzoon ME, Hoyle JC, Smith FA, et al. Safety of influenza vaccination during pregnancy. Am J Obstet Gynecol 2005;192:1098–106.

[118] Benowitz I, Esposito DB, Gracey KD, Shapiro ED, Vazquez M. Influenza vaccine given to pregnant women reduces hospitalization due to influenza in their infants. Clin Infect Dis 2010;51:1355–61.

[119] Landry ML, Cohen S, Ferguson D. Real-time PCR compared to Binax NOW and cytospin-immunofluorescence for detection of influenza in hospitalized patients. J Clin Virol 2008;43:148–51.

[120] Eick AA, Uyeki TM, Klimov A, Hall H, Reid R, Santosham M, et al. Maternal influenza vaccination and effect on influenza virus infection in young infants. Arch Pediatr Adolesc Med 2011;165:104–11.

[121] McDonald JC, Andrews BE. Diagnostic methods in an influenza vaccine trial. Br Med J 1955;2:1232–5.

[122] Petrie JG, Ohmit SE, Johnson E, Cross RT, Monto AS. Efficacy studies of influenza vaccines: effect of end points used and characteristics of vaccine failures. J Infect Dis 2011;203:1309–15.

[123] Rapmund G, Johnson RT, Bankhead AS, Herman YF, Dandridge OW. The diagnosis of Asian influenza virus infection after recent immunization. U S Armed Forces Med J 1959;10:637–49.

[124] Grist NR, Landsman JB. Influenza in Glasgow, 1950–1953. Glasgow Med J 1955;36:69–75.

[125] Anderson SG, Donnelley M, French EL, Kalra SL, White J. Influenza in Victoria, 1950 and 1951. Med JAust 1953;2:44–7.

[126] Poehling KA, Szilagyi PG, Staat MA, Snively BM, Payne DC, Bridges CB, et al. Impact of maternal immunization on influenza hospitalizations in infants. Am J Obstet Gynecol 2011;204:S141–8.

[127] Sugimura T, Nagai T, Kobayashi H, Ozaki Y, Yamakawa R, Hirata R. Effectiveness of maternal influenza immunization in young infants in Japan. Pediatr Int 2015.

[128] Osterholm MT, Kelley NS, Sommer A, Belongia EA. Influenza vaccine efficacy and effectiveness: a new look at the evidence. Lancet Inf Dis, 2012;12:36–44.

[129] Savitz DA, Fell DB, Ortiz JR, Bhat N. Does influenza vaccination improve pregnancy outcome? Methodological issues and research needs. Vaccine 2015;33:6430–5.

[130] World Health Organization. WHO Influenza data taskforce –interim report.2015;1–24.

[131] Kay AW, Blish CA. Immunogenicity and Clinical Efficacy of Influenza Vaccination in Pregnancy. Front Immunol 2015;6:289.

[132] Murray DL, Imagawa DT, Okada DM, St Geme JW, Jr. Antibody response to monovalent A/New Jersey/8/76 influenza vaccine in pregnant women. J Clin Microbiol 1979;10:184–7.

[133] Bischoff AL, Folsgaard NV, Carson CG, Stokholm J, Pedersen L, Holmberg M, et al. Altered response to A(H1N1)pnd09 vaccination in pregnant women: a single blinded randomized controlled trial. PLoS One 2013;8:e56700.

[134] Schlaudecker EP, McNeal MM, Dodd CN, Ranz JB, Steinhoff MC. Pregnancy modifies the antibody response to trivalent influenza immunization. J Infect Dis 2012;206:1670–3.

[135] Sperling RS, Engel SM, Wallenstein S, Kraus TA, Garrido J, Singh T, et al. Immunogenicity of trivalent inactivated influenza vaccination received during pregnancy or postpartum. Obstet Gynecol 2012;119:631–9.

[136] Patel CG, Phillips Heine R, Staats J, Antczak B, Weaver K, Weinhold K, Swamy C. T-follicular helper (Tfh) cell expansion varies by trimester after influenza vaccination in pregnancy. AJOG,2016;214:S57–S58.

[137] Sullivan SG, Komadina N, Grant K, Jelley L, Papadakis G, Kelly H. Influenza vaccine effectiveness during the 2012 influenza season in Victoria, Australia: Influences of waning immunity and vaccine match. J Med Virol 2013;86:1017–1025.

[138] Kissling E, Valenciano M, Larrauri A, Oroszi B, Cohen JM, Nunes B, et al. Low and decreasing vaccine effectiveness against influenza A(H3) in 2011/12 among vaccination target groups in Europe: results from the I-MOVE multicentre case-control study. Euro Surveill 2013;18.

[139] Rasmussen SA, Watson AK, Kennedy ED, Broder KR, Jamieson DJ. Vaccines and pregnancy: past, present, and future. Semin Fetal Neonatal Med 2014;19:161–9.

[140] van der Maas N, Dijs-Elsinga J, Kemmeren J, van Lier A, Knol M, de Melker H. Safety of vaccination against influenza A (H1N1) during pregnancy in the Netherlands: results on pregnancy outcomes and infant's health: cross-sectional linkage study. BJOG 2015.

[141] Sobanjo-Ter Meulen A, Abramson J, Mason E, Rees H, Schwalbe N, Bergquist S, et al. Path to impact: A report from the Bill and Melinda Gates Foundation convening on maternal immunization in resource-limited settings; Berlin—January 29–30, 2015. Vaccine 2015;33:6388–95.

Chapter 10

Antibody Responses after Influenza Vaccination in Elderly People: Useful Information from a 27-Year Study (from 1988–1989 to 2014–2015)

Barbara Camilloni, Emilia Nunzi,
Michela Basileo and Anna Maria Iorio

Additional information is available at the end of the chapter

http://dx.doi.org/10.5772/104559

Abstract

Elderly people are more likely than younger people to get flu complications and respond suboptimally to influenza vaccination because of the presence of comorbidities and immunosenescence. In order to collect information about this issue, we evaluated data obtained in 27 winters of study, from 1988–1989 to 2014–2015, in frail elderly institutionalized people (≥60 years) vaccinated with commercially available seasonal trivalent inactivated influenza vaccines. The antibody response was examined comparing hemagglutination inhibition antibody titers in sera collected from 4461 volunteers before and 30 days after vaccination. Examining the results as crude mean responses, we evidenced the ability of influenza vaccines to induce significant increases in antibody titers against all the three vaccine antigens satisfying at least one of the three criteria of the Committee for Medical Products for Human Use (CHMP). Higher responses were found against A/H3N2 vaccine components and, examining different subgroups, in volunteers receiving 45 μg vaccine as compared with 30 μg and in female as compared with male subjects. Very elderly people (>75 years) gave better responses than younger elderly (≤75 years) at least against A/H1N1 strain and the last licensed potentiated vaccines (MF59-adjuvanted and intradermal) were more immunogenic than traditional vaccines (whole, subunit, and split).

Keywords: influenza vaccination, vaccine immunogenicity, HI antibody titers, CHMP criteria, elderly institutionalized people

1. Introduction

Influenza virus infections can affect all age groups, and older individuals are particularly at risk for influenza since, despite having no higher attack rate than younger adults, most influenza-related deaths and severe complications occur in this age group. Although influenza vaccination remains the mainstay in prevention, nonetheless, uncertainties regarding the effectiveness of the influenza vaccines in elderly adults are persistent [1, 2].

The higher rate of flu complications and the reduced vaccine efficacy are generally attributed to both concomitant comorbidities and immunosenescence, i.e., the age-related weakening of the immune system [3, 4].

As reported by Lambert et al. [5], the measurement of vaccine efficacy against influenza illness is a difficult task especially in older adults. Although influenza vaccine effectiveness depends not only on vaccine-induced immune response but also on annual variations in influenza incidence, circulating strain virulence, and the quality of the vaccine-to-circulating strain match [6], previous studies have established that a high serum antibody level can prevent infection at least in children and young adults [7–9], and serological studies based on the evaluation of influenza-specific antibody titers have been widely accepted and used as a surrogate marker for protection against influenza and vaccine efficacy.

Chronic underlying diseases, particularly cardiac and respiratory diseases, were shown to negatively influence the immune response after influenza vaccination in old people [10].

Three previous reviews on serological responses to inactivated seasonal vaccines in elderly people did not consider the possible role of chronic underlying illnesses, because there was not the possibility of controlling for the presence of serious illnesses [11] or because the elderly population was carefully selected to exclude any chronic diseases so that the results would reflect the effect of ageing on comparison with young people [12, 13].

In comparison with community-dwelling elderly people, residents of nursing homes are considered to be at a higher risk of serious influenza-related complications, because they are generally older, more debilitated, and more exposed to influenza infection once the virus is introduced because of the close environment in which they live [14]. However, evaluating vaccine immunogenicity, results reported in the review of Goodwin et al. [12] and results previously obtained in our laboratory [15] suggested that institutionalized elderly responded better when compared with community-dwelling elderly.

The aim of this chapter of the book is to examine the phenomenon of the decreased immunogenicity and efficacy of influenza vaccines in older persons from available data. We examined the data obtained by our research group in 27 winter seasons, from 1988–1989 to 2014–2015, of vaccine immunogenicity in a considerable number (4461) of elderly people (≥60 years of age), most of them with underlying medical conditions, vaccinated with commercially available seasonal trivalent inactivated influenza vaccines. Although some of the results obtained in the different winters were previously published, in the present report the results we obtained are cumulatively examined for the first time.

2. Materials and methods

2.1. Study design and vaccination

The volunteers initially enrolled in the prospective study of antibody response to influenza vaccination, conducted over a period of 27 consecutive winters, were 4461 elderly people, aged ≥60 years (mean age 80.5 year, range 60–106 years). Eighty-six percent of them were living in nursing homes in Central Italy.

After providing informed consent, all the subjects received one dose of trivalent inactivated influenza vaccine intramuscularly, in the deltoid, or intradermally. The vaccines used were commercially available inactivated trivalent vaccines for the winters from 1988–1989 to 2014–2015 produced by propagation of the virus in embryonated hens' eggs. Each dose of vaccine consisted of 10 μg (from 1988–1989 to 1991–1992) or 15 μg of hemagglutinin (HA) in a 0.5 ml dose (for vaccines administered intramuscularly) or in a 0.1 ml dose (for vaccines administered intradermally) for each of the three influenza strain antigens (A/H3N2, A/H1N1, and B influenza viruses). At the time of recruitment of this study, demographic data, health status, and history of influenza vaccination over the preceding year were obtained from each subject. Serum samples were obtained from the same subject before and 1 month after vaccination. Subjects were included in this study if they did not have a history of immediate hypersensitivity to eggs components. Subjects suffering from specific illnesses or chronic condition were not excluded. The study was conducted according to the Declaration of Helsinki and Good Clinical Practices. Since vaccines were assigned by local health authorities within the annual influenza campaign and sera were leftover sera from samples collected for clinical routine controls, the study did not need to be registered as a formal trial.

2.2. Determination of hemagglutination-inhibiting (HI) antibody titers and measurement results

HI antibody titers were determined using a standard microtiter method [16] with 0.5% chicken (from 1988–1989 to 1996–1997) or turkey erythrocytes (after 1996–1997). Antigens were prepared from the allantoic fluids of embryonated hens' eggs inoculated 3 days earlier with influenza virus. All sera were heat-inactivated at 56°C for 30 min and treated with potassium periodate and trypsin (from 1988 to 1994) or with receptor-destroying enzyme (RDE) of *Vibrio cholerae* (after 1994) to remove nonspecific inhibitors. The first dilution for antibody titration was 1:10. Pre- and postvaccination sera from each of the vaccines were frozen at −30°C until used and tested simultaneously for HI antibody titers using the same antigens as those in the vaccine. To eliminate any subjective bias, HI titers determinations were carried on in a blind fashion, i.e., with the tester unaware of which treatment the donor had received.

2.3. Criteria used for evaluating vaccines immunogenicity

HI antibody titers obtained by following the procedure indicated in the previous section were reported as protection rate (percentage of volunteers showing HI titers ≥40, considered to be associated with protection from influenza infection) [9], geometric mean titers (GMT;

any HI antibody titer <10 was considered equal to 5 for GMT calculation), ratio of postvaccination to prevaccination GMT values (GMTR), and seroconversion rate (percentage of subjects with a fourfold or greater increase in titer and with a postvaccination titer at least equal to 40 in seronegative volunteers). The antibody titers measured 1 month after vaccination were also evaluated according to the criteria of the Committee for Medicinal Products for Human Use (CHMP) for approval of influenza vaccines, which require that for individuals aged ≥60 years at least one of the following values must be met: seroprotection rate ≥60%, GMTR ≥2, or seroconversion rate ≥30% [17].

2.4. Statistical analyses

Statistical analyses and subanalyses considered in this work were applied to populations with a relatively large number of people, as a consequence both GMT and rate statistics were well approximated by a log normal and normal distributions, respectively. Moreover, since rates values were not close to 0 or 100%, thus significant differences between mean values of the groups were analyzed by Student's *t*-test. Both estimated mean values with their corresponding 95% confidence intervals (CI) the p-value of the *t*-statistic have been reported in the paper. In particular, *p*-values <0.01 were considered highly statistically significant, whereas *p*-values <0.05 were regarded as marginally statistically significant. Values of postvaccination GMT observed against different antigens and in different years were examined as such and also corrected for prevaccination status according to Beyer et al. [18] in order to verify that significant differences in the postvaccination status were independent on the prevaccination HI titers. Vaccine response was evaluated also according to the dosage of vaccine antigens (30 and 45 μg), gender, and age (≤75 and >75). For each antigen, significant differences between subpopulations means were evaluated and the corresponding statistical significance was indicated.

A multiple comparison test between groups of vaccine type and between antigens was executed by using one-way analysis of variance (ANOVA). Paired comparison values were presented only when one-way ANOVA comparison identified potentially significant differences. All statistical analyses were carried out using MATLAB® of MathWorks Inc. release 2014b.

3. Results

3.1. Study population and demographic characteristics

Table 1 reports the baseline characteristics of the 4461 elderly volunteers, aged ≥60 years (range 60–106) vaccinated with commercially available seasonal trivalent inactivated influenza vaccines for each year of the 27 consecutive winters (from 1988–1989 to 2014–2015) studied. The number of volunteers examined each year varied from 64 to 372. The mean age was lower in the first years studied (from 1988–1989 to 1998–1999) when a mixed population of community-dwelling and institutionalized elderly was examined (60–80 years) than in the other seasons when volunteers were totally recruited from nursing homes (82–86 years). The majority of elderly subjects has been previously vaccinated (61–100%). Although not reported in **Table 1**, percentage of volunteers, ≥80%, presented underlying diseases or risk factors for influenza and as a consequence used chronic drugs. The most frequent chronic diseases were cardiovascular, respiratory diseases, and diabetes. The most frequent drugs used were antihypertensive/inotropic drugs and benzodiazepines.

					Type of seasonal vaccine used[a]					
Season	**No. of subjects**	**Mean age (range)**	**Living situation[b]**	**Vaccination status prior to study[c]**	**Whole**	**Sub-u**	**Split**	**MF59**	**ID**	**Vaccine dosage**
1988–1989	282	73 (61–93)	M	na	232	50	–	–	–	30 μg
1989–1990	82	69 (60–83)	M	88%	–	59	23	–	–	30 μg
1990–1991	372	66 (60–87)	M	69%	159	213	–	–	–	30 μg
1991–1992	124	69 (60–93)	M	61%	108	–	16	–	–	30 μg
1992–1993	270	nd (>60)	M	96%	245	8	17	–	–	45 μg
1993–1994	298	76 (60–99)	M	na	51	–	247	–	–	45 μg
1994–1995	235	78 (60–100)	M	90%	32	–	203	–	–	45 μg
1995–1996	213	77 (60–100)	M	90%	–	213	–	–	–	45 μg
1996–1997	173	80 (60–99)	M	96%	–	173	–	–	–	45 μg
1997–1998	176	na (>60)	M	85%	36	140	–	–	–	45 μg
1998–1999	116	74 (60–102)	M	94%	–	110	6	–	–	45 μg
1999–2000	139	83 (60–103)	I	96%	–	46	78	15	–	45 μg
2000–2001	128	83 (60–103)	I	100%	–	82	46	–	–	45 μg
2001–2002	96	82 (60–104)	I	98%	–	–	96	–	–	45 μg
2002–2003	107	82 (60–105)	I	100%	–	–	107	–	–	45 μg
2003–2004	125	83 (60–101)	I	100%	–	–	33	92	–	45 μg
2004–2005	158	82 (60–99)	I	98%	–	–	36	122	–	45 μg
2005–2006	105	83 (60–99)	I	100%	–	–	40	65	–	45 μg
2006–2007	88	83 (60–98)	I	98%	–	–	21	67	–	45 μg
2007–2008	66	84 (61–102)	I	100%	–	–	–	66	–	45 μg
2008–2009	114	83 (60–103)	I	98%	–	–	–	114	–	45 μg

					Type of seasonal vaccine used[a]					
Season	No. of subjects	Mean age (range)	Living situation[b]	Vaccination status prior to study[c]	Whole	Sub-u	Split	MF59	ID	Vaccine dosage
2009–2010	64	83 (65–98)	I	100%	–	–	–	64	–	45 μg
2010–2011	112	85 (64–101)	I	100%	–	–	–	112	–	45 μg
2011–2012	151	84 (65–102)	I	98%	–	–	–	103	48	45 μg
2012–2013	252	85 (60–103)	I	100%	–	–	26	137	89	45 μg
2013–2014	204	86 (60–106)	I	100%	–	–	–	183	21	45 μg
2014–2015	211	84 (60–104)	I	100%	–	–	1	203	7	45 μg
Total	4461	85 (60–106)			863	1094	996	1343	165	

[a]Whole: whole-virus vaccine; Sub-u: sub-unit vaccine; Split: split-virus vaccine; MF59: subunit MF59-adjuvanted vaccine; ID: Intradermal subunit vaccine.
[b]I: Institutionalized elderly; M: mixed, both institutionalized and community living elderly.
[c]Percent of elderly having received influenza vaccination in the previous year.
na: not available

Table 1. Characteristics of studied population and type of influenza vaccines in the 27 winter seasons studied (from 1988/1989 to 2014/2015).

3.2. Vaccines

As reported in **Table 1**, different formulations such as whole, split (composed by viruses disrupted, by a detergent, and containing the internal and external component of the virus), and subunit (composed of just the purified surface glycoproteins of the virus, i.e., hemagglutinin (HA) and neuraminidase) of trivalent inactivated vaccines were used in the different years or in the same year. In the first four studied years (from 1988–1989 to 1991–1992), the HA concentration for each strain was lower (10 μg for each antigen) as compared with the concentration (15 μg for each antigen) of the vaccines used in all the years after the winter season 1991–1992. Whole and subunit formulations were administered respectively to 863 and 1094 volunteers in the first 13 years of the study (from 1988–1989 to 2001–2002). Nine hundred ninety-six elderly people were vaccinated with split vaccine in many years studied and, starting from the 1999–2000 season, 1343 volunteers received a subunit vaccine potentiated with MF59 adjuvant. In the last period of the study, a limited number of elderly people was vaccinated with vaccine administered intradermally (165 volunteers from 2011–2012 to 2014–2015). The percentages of previously influenza-vaccinated people were high and ranged from 88 to 100%, not considering 3 years (1990–1991, 69%; 1991–1992, 61%, and 1993–1994, data not available).

The antigenic composition of the vaccines used is reported in **Figure 1** and each year was formulated according to the recommendations of both "Ministero della Salute (Italy)" and

http://dx.doi.org/10.5772/104559

WHO (Northern Hemisphere) for the corresponding studied winter. During the 27-year period covered by our study (1988–2014), the WHO recommended 15 A/H3N2, 7 A/H1N1, and 12 B new influenza strains for inclusion in seasonal vaccines.

3.3. Overall response to influenza vaccination

The ability of licensed influenza vaccines to elicit an antibody response against vaccine antigens was examined comparing HI antibody titers in blood samples collected from the 4461 volunteers before and 1 month after vaccination with commercially available seasonal trivalent inactivated influenza vaccines in 27 consecutive winters (from 1988–1989 to 2014–2015).

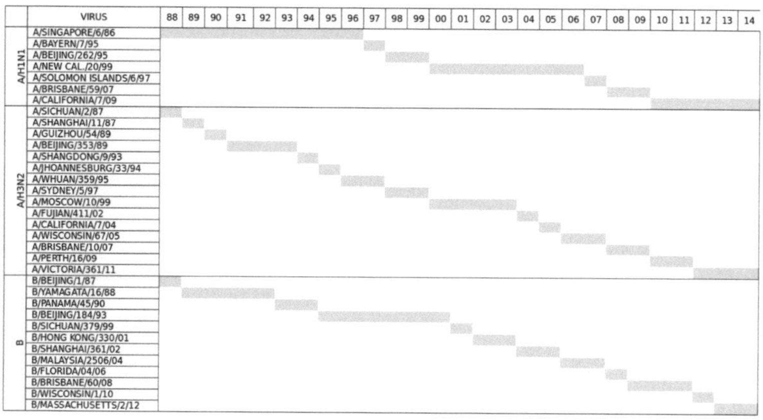

Figure 1. Recommended viruses for influenza vaccines by World Health Organization between 1988 and 2014.

Vaccine component (N = 4461)	Seroprotection rate (95% CI)		Seroconversion rate (95% CI)	GMT (95% CI)		Number of reached CHMP criteria/3
	Prevacc.	Postvacc.		Prevacc.	Postvacc. [GMTR]	
A/H3N2	35.1 [A,B]	65.7** [A,B]	30.0** [A,B]	20.9 [A,B]	54.6** [A,B] [2.6]	3/3
	(33.7–36.5)	(64.3–67.1)	(28.5–31.2)	(20.2–21.6)	(52.5–56.8)	
A/H1N1	23.5	52.6**	25.1	14.2	35.3 ** [2.5]	1/3
	(22.2–24.7)	(51.1–54.1)	(23.8–26.0)	(13.7–14.6)	(34.0–36.7)	
B	23.3	54.5**	25.6	14.5	35.7 ** [2.5]	1/3
	(22.1–24.5)	(53.0–55.9)	(24.3–27.1)	(14.1–14.9)	(34.5–37.0)	

**: p-value < 0.01 comparing pre- and postvaccination values.
A: p-value <0.01 comparing A/H3N2 and A/H1N1 antigens.
B: p-value <0.01 comparing A/H3N2 and B antigens.

Table 2. Mean values of the HI antibody responses observed in the 27-years study of the total population to the three influenza vaccine antigens and reachment CHMP criteria.

The HI antibody response after one dose of influenza vaccine was evaluated for each antigen (A/H1N1, A/H3N2, and B) and data obtained were processed in order to calculate, for each population considered in the paper, pre- and postvaccination seroprotection rate, seroconversion rate, pre- and postvaccination GMT, and GMTR together to their corresponding 95% confidence intervals. For each antigen, the values of these parameters referred to the overall population are reported in **Table 2**. One month after vaccination, statistically significant increases were found in the percentage of seroprotected volunteers and in the values of their corresponding GMT against all the three different vaccine antigens. The three CHMP requirements were satisfied 1 month after vaccination against the A/H3N2 vaccine component, whereas only the requested value of GMTR was reached against the A/H1N1 and B antigens.

Table 3 reports the results obtained examining the reachment of the CHMP criteria for each studied year against the three vaccine antigens. The seroprotection rate (HI titer ≥40) was higher than the requested 60% in 20 years against A/H3N2 (74%), 16 years against A/H1N1 (59%), and 14 years against B antigen (52%) of the 27 years studied. Values of GMTR satisfying the requested value ≥2 were found in 22 (81%), 25 (93%), and 21 (78%) years against A/H3N2, A/H1N1, and B vaccine components, respectively. The lower positive results were found for seroconversion requested to be ≥30%. This value was reached in 13 years against A/H3N2 (48%), 10 years against A/H1N1 (37%), and 8 years against B virus (30%). In some years none of the three CHMP criteria was satisfied, i.e., in 3 years against A/H3N2 (11%), 2 years against A/H1N1 (7%), and in 7 years against the B antigen (26%). Years with responses satisfying all the three CHMP criteria ranged between 22% (B antigen) and 48% (A/H3N2 antigen). Because the use of a vaccine featuring a novel antigen might affect the antibody response, considering data reported about vaccine antigenic composition in **Figure 1**, we identified the presence or absence of a novel vaccine component in each year studied, but we could not evidence any obvious association between vaccine HI antibody response and the presence of a new vaccine component.

Vaccine component	N. of years (%) [95% CI]			
	Seroprotection ≥60%	Seroconversion ≥30%	GMTR ≥2	Reachment of three CHMP criteria
A/H3N2	20 (74%) [55–93]	13 (48%) [29–67]	22 (81%) [67–96]	13 (48%)
A/H1N1	16 (59%) [41–78]	10 (37%) [18–56]	25 (93%) [78–107]	8 (30%)
B	14 (52%) [33–71]	8 (30%) [11–48]	21 (78%) [64–92]	6 (22%)

Table 3. Reachment of the CHMP criteria in the total population in the 27 years examined.

The data reported in **Table 2** evidenced differences in the values of the HI antibody titers against the three different vaccine antigens. HI antibody values against A/H3N2 antigen were in most instances significantly higher before and after vaccination as compared with those found both against A/H1N1 and B vaccine components.

Since the baseline serological status is considered to be important in evaluating immunogenicity of influenza vaccines and is regarded as capable of affecting the serological outcomes, in order to reduce the heterogeneity among the responses found against the three vaccine antigens, we examined the GMT values of the overall population correcting the postvaccination titers for the prevaccination status according to Beyer (**Figure 2**) [18].

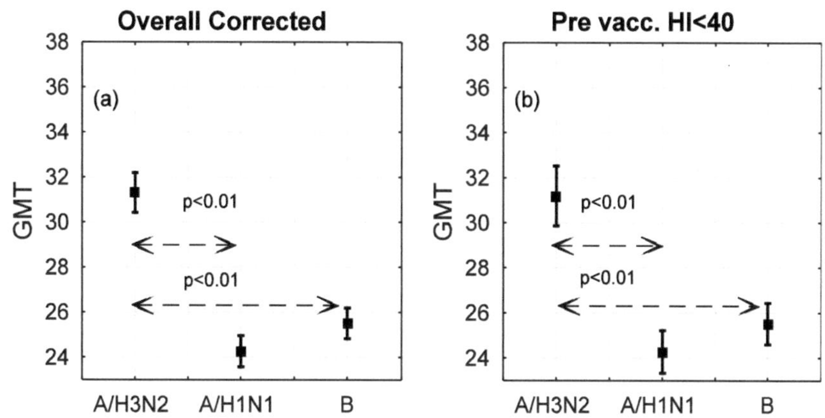

Figure 2. Postvaccination GMT values of: (a) the overall population corrected for the average prevaccination status according to Beyer; and (b) subjects unprotected before vaccination. Comparison of antigens is also shown when differences are significant. The bars indicate the ranges of the 95% confidence limits.

For comparison purposes, also the postvaccination GMT values of the prevaccination unprotected volunteers (HI < 40) are shown in **Figure 2** as indicated by the corresponding labels. The data reported confirmed that the responses against the A/H3N2 antigen were higher as compared with those against A/H1N1 and B antigens.

3.4. Factors associated with vaccine response

Since different factors may have an impact on vaccine response, we controlled for a number of variables for which we could obtain data. We did not consider the health status of the study participants, previous vaccination histories, and living situation, since a high percentage of the subjects had chronic underlying disease, was previously vaccinated, and was living in a nursing home.

3.4.1. Subanalysis according to different influenza vaccine dosages

In Italy, as in most European countries, seasonal trivalent influenza vaccines containing 10 μg HA for each antigen (30 μg) has been used until 1991. From 1992 onwards European influenza vaccines contain 15 μg HA per strain (45 μg), according to the European Harmonization of Requirements for Influenza Vaccines [17]. As a consequence, in the first 4 years of the 27-year period examined in our study, we used 30 μg and, after the winter 1991–1992, 45 μg vaccines.

Since previous observations suggested that increase in influenza vaccine dosage might be associated with an increase in antibody titers, at least against some of the vaccine strains [19, 20], we compared HI immune response following vaccination with 30 or 45 μg vaccines. As reported in **Table 1**, 860 (19%) and 3601 (81%) of the 4461 elderly subjects received respectively a 30 or a 45 μg trivalent influenza vaccine. **Table 4** reports the results obtained studying the induced HI antibody response. Significant increases were observed against all the three vaccine antigens comparing pre- and postvaccination data against all the three different vaccine antigens examining the percentages of seroprotected people and GMT values both after 30 and 45 μg vaccine administration.

Vaccine component	Vaccine dose (N)	Seroprotection rate		Seroconversion rate (95% CI)	GMT (95% CI)		
		Prevacc.	Postvacc.	(95% CI)	Prevacc.	Postvacc. [GMTR]	CHMP criteria satisfied
A/H3N2	30 μg	14.1 A	39.3**A	16.9 A	13.2 A	26.3**A [2.0]	1/3
	(860)	(11.7–16.4)	(36.0–42.6)	(14.5–19.4)	(12.4–14.0)	(24.6–28.0)	
	45 μg	40.1	72.0**	32.9	23.3	65.1** [2.8]	3/3
	(3601)	(38.5–41.7)	(70.5–73.5)	(31.4–34.4)	(22.4–24.3)	(62.3–68.0)	
A/H1N1	30 μg	10.2	35.7**A	20.8 A	9.5 A	22.5**A [2.4]	1/3
	(860)	(8.2–12.3)	(32.5–38.9)	(18.1–23.5)	(8.9–10.0)	(21.0–24.2)	
	45 μg	26.7	56.6**	26.1	15.6	39.4** [2.5]	1/3
	(3601)	(25.2–28.1)	(55.0–58.3)	(24.6–27.6)	(15.0–16.2)	(37.7–41.1)	
B	30 μg	5.1	30.0**A	21.2 A	8.1 A	19.9**A [2.5]	1/3
	(860)	(3.6–6.6)	(26.7–33.1)	(18.4–24.1)	(7.7–8.5)	(18.5–21.3)	
	45 μg	27.6	60.3**	26.6	16.6	41.1** [2.5]	2/3
	(3601)	(26.2–29.1)	(58.7–61.9)	(25.2–28.0)	(16.1–17.2)	(39.6–42.7)	

**: *p*-value <0.01 comparing pre- and postvaccination values.
A: *p*-value <0.01 comparing response between vaccine dosages (30 and 45 μg).

Table 4. HI antibody response in volunteers divided according to the vaccine dosage (30 or 45 μg).

At least one of the three CHMP requirements, i.e., the value of GMTR (≥2), was always reached using vaccine containing 30 μg of antigen but following 45 μg vaccine administration all the three parameters were satisfied against A/H3N2 antigen and two of them against the B antigen.

Postvaccination results observed after 45 μg vaccine administration were always significantly higher as compared with those after 30 μg vaccine.

However, comparing values found in the two groups of people before vaccination, we observed that the two groups were poorly comparable since there were differences in the prevaccination

http://dx.doi.org/10.5772/104559

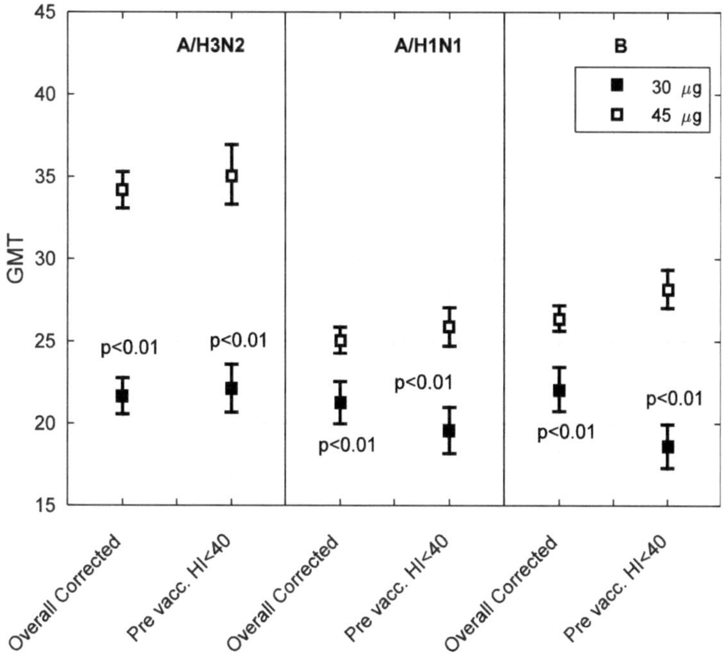

Figure 3. Postvaccination GMT values of populations divided according to the vaccine dosage (30 or 45 μg)), as indicated by legend labels. Postvaccination GMT values calculated on the overall population have been corrected for the average prevaccination status according to Beyer. For comparison purposes, post-GMT values of subjects unprotected before vaccination are also shown. The bars indicate the ranges of the 95% confidence limits.

status. Volunteers vaccinated with 45 μg vaccine showed prevaccination HI titers in most instances significantly higher as compared with the 30 μg volunteers. In order to have more homogeneous and comparable data, we examined vaccine immunogenicity both correcting the titers for prevaccination status of overall population [17], and considering only prevaccination unprotected volunteers (HI titers < 40). As shown in **Figure 3**, GMT corrected for prevaccination status confirmed that the increasing of the antigen dosage increments the response to the vaccine antigens. Postvaccination values found considering only people nonseroprotected before vaccination again evidenced a statistically significant higher response induced by 45 μg vaccine as compared with 30 μg.

3.4.2. Subanalysis of immunogenicity within the elderly groups, i.e., younger elderly (≤75 years) and very elderly (>75 years)

In a recent meta-analysis about the effect of age on the influenza vaccine–induced immune response based on studies from the past 20 years, Goodwin at al. [12] concluded that aged individual (>65 years) had a significantly reduced antibody response to vaccination. The studied elderly were categorized into two age groups, above or below 75 years. Antibody responses among the very elderly (≥75 years of age) were especially impaired with seroconversion levels at 32%, 46%, and 29% to A/H1N1, A/H3N2, and influenza B, respectively, compared with 42%, 51%, and 35% observed in people aged <75 to >65 years of age [12].

In order to have additive information we considered the immune responses found in volunteers of our study aged ≤75 or >75 years. The exact age was available for only 2712 people (61%) of the 4461 participants and 658 (24%) were aged ≤75 years and 2054 (76%) were >75 years. The results obtained are reported in **Table 5** and show that in both groups the vaccine administration induced significant increases in HI titers evaluated as percentage of seroprotected people (HI ≥ 40) and as GMT values. CHMP criteria were always satisfied for GMTR parameter (≥2) against all the three vaccine antigens. All the three requested values were reached in both groups against A/H3N2 antigen and only in >75 year group against A/H1N1 antigen. Against the B antigen, the requested value for seroconversion (≥30%) was not reached in both groups and the value for seroprotection (≥60%) was satisfied only in >75-year group.

Vaccine component	Group (*N*)	Seroprotection rate (95% CI)		Seroconversion rate (95% CI)	GMT (95% CI)		
		Prevacc.	Postvacc.		Prevacc.	Postvacc. [GMTR]	CHMP criteria satisfied
A/H3N2	≤75	28.5 [A]	60.7 ** [A]	31.8	16.5 [A]	46.9 ** [A] [2.8]	3/3
	(658)	(24.1–30.9)	(28.2–35.4)	(56.9–64.4)	(15.1–17.9)	(42.5–51.7)	
	Age >75	40.1	71.4 **	34.4	23.5	66.7 ** [2.8]	3/3
	(2054)	(37.9–42.2)	(69.4–73.3)	(32.4–36.4)	(22.3–24.8)	(62.7–70.9)	
A/H1N1	≤75	24.6	52.6 ** [A]	24.5 [A]	14.2 [a]	35.6 ** [A] [2.5]	1/3
	(658)	(21.3–27.9)	(48.7–56.4)	(21.2–27.8)	(13.0–15.4)	(32.3–39.3)	
	Age >75	26.9	60.3 **	29.8	15.7	42.5 ** [2.7]	3/3
	(2054)	(25.0–28.8)	(58.2–62.4)	(27.8–31.8)	(15.0–16.5)	(40.1–44.9)	
B	≤75	254.6 [A]	54.3 ** [A]	26.7	14.3 [A]	36.8 ** [A] [2.6]	1/3
	(658)	(21.3–27.9)	(50.4–58.0)	(23.4–30.0)	(13.2–15.5)	(33.4–40.5)	
	Age >75	30.6	62.8 **	26.4	18.0	42.6 ** [2.4]	2/3
	(2054)	(28.6–32.6)	(60.7–64.9)	(24.5–28.3)	(17.2–18.8)	(40.5–44.9)	

**: *p*-value <0.01 comparing pre- and post-vaccination values.
A: *p*-value <0.01 comparing response between age groups.
a: *p*-value <0.05 comparing response between age groups.

Table 5. HI antibody response of populations divided according to the age (younger elderly, ≤75 years, and very elderly, >75 years).

Comparing results obtained in the two groups, the responses observed in the oldest group (>75) were in most instances higher than those observed in the younger elderly (≤75). However, since the prevaccination status of these two groups were not fully comparable, we evaluated the values of GMT corrected for prevaccination status and GMT in people unprotected (HI < 40) before vaccination. Again the values were higher in the very elderly as compared with the younger against A/H1N1 for GMT corrected and against A/H1N1 and B for the GMT unprotected people (**Figure 4**).

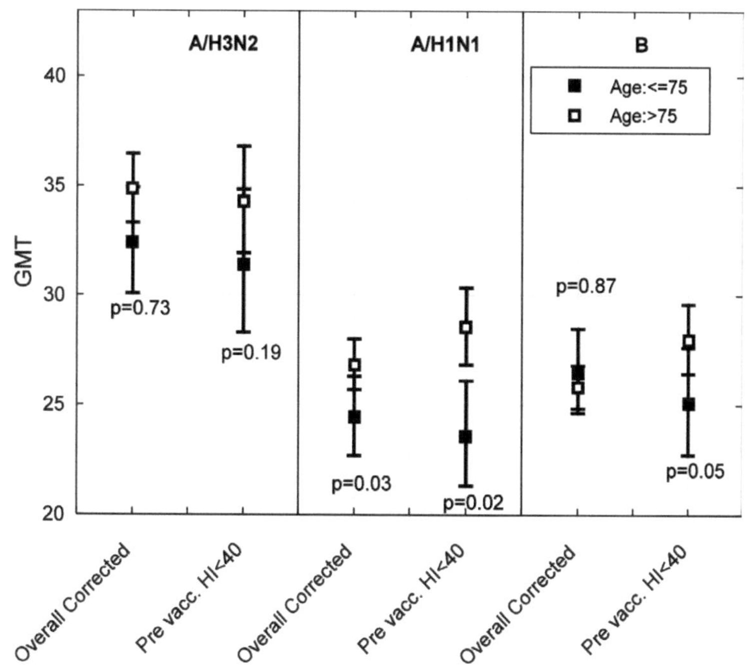

Figure 4. Postvaccination GMT values of populations divided according to the age class (younger elderly, ≤75 years, and very elderly, >75 years), as indicated in legend labels. Postvaccination GMT values calculated on the overall population have been corrected for the average prevaccination status according to Beyer. For comparison purposes, post-GMT values of subjects unprotected before vaccination are also shown. The bars indicate the ranges of the 95% confidence limits.

3.4.3. Subanalysis according to responses found in females and males

Previous data indicated that receipt of trivalent inactivated influenza vaccines results in significantly higher HI antibody titers among females than males, both in adults and elderly people [21].

In our study, sex data were available for about all the people studied (4457/4461) and the volunteers were prevalently females (70%). We examined the vaccine immunogenicity in females and males and the results are reported in **Table 6**. Postvaccination increases found against all the three vaccine antigens were statistically significant in both groups. All the three CHMP criteria were satisfied against A/H3N2 antigen in female subjects, whereas only the GMTR requirement was satisfied in males against A/H3N2 and both in males and females against A/H1N1 and B antigens. Comparison of postvaccination values evidenced statistically higher values in the female compared with male group. However, since differences were found also in the prevaccination values we compared the GMT corrected for the prevaccination status and examined the GMT found considering only volunteers not seroprotected before vaccination. The female responses were again higher than those of male against all the three vaccine antigens (**Figure 5**).

Vaccine components	Group (*N*)	Seroprotection rate (95% CI)		Seroconversion rate (95% CI)	GMT (95% CI)		EMA criteria satisfied
		Prevacc.	Postvacc.		Prevacc.	Postvacc. [GMTR]	
A/H3N2	F	36.9 ^{A}	68.7 ^{**A}	32.7 ^{A}	21.7 ^{A}	60.0 ^{**A} [2.8]	3/3
	(3142)	(35.2–38.5)	(67.1–70.3)	(31.0–34.4)	(20.8–22.6)	(57.3–62.9)	
	M	30.9	58.6 **	23.1	19.1	43.8 ** [2.3]	1/3
	(1315)	(28.4–33.4)	(55.9–61.3)	(20.8–25.4)	(17.9–20.4)	(40.9–46.9)	
A/H1N1	F	24.1	55.3 ^{**A}	27.7 A	14.4	38.0 ^{**A} [2.6]	1/3
	(3142)	(22.6–25.6)	(53.6–57.1)	(26.2–29.2)	(13.9–15.0)	(36.3–39.8)	
	M	22.1	46.2 **	18.7	13.6	29.8 ** [2.2]	1/3
	(1315)	(19.8–24.3)	(43.5–48.9)	(16.5–20.9)	(12.8–14.4)	(27.8–31.8)	
B	F	24.9 ^{A}	56.9 ^{**A}	26.7 ^{A}	15.2 ^{A}	38.2 ^{**A} [2.5]	1/3
	(3142)	(23.4–26.5)	(55.2–58.6)	(25.2–28.2)	(14.6–15.7)	(36.6–39.9)	
	M	19.3	48.6 **	22.7	13.0	30.5 ** [2.4]	1/3
	(1315)	(17.2–21.5)	(45.8–51.3)	(20.5–25.4)	(12.3–13.7)	(28.7–32.4)	

**: *p*-value <0.01 comparing pre- and post-vaccination values.
A: *p*-value <0.01 comparing response between M and F.

Table 6. HI antibody response of populations divided according to gender (male: M; female: F).

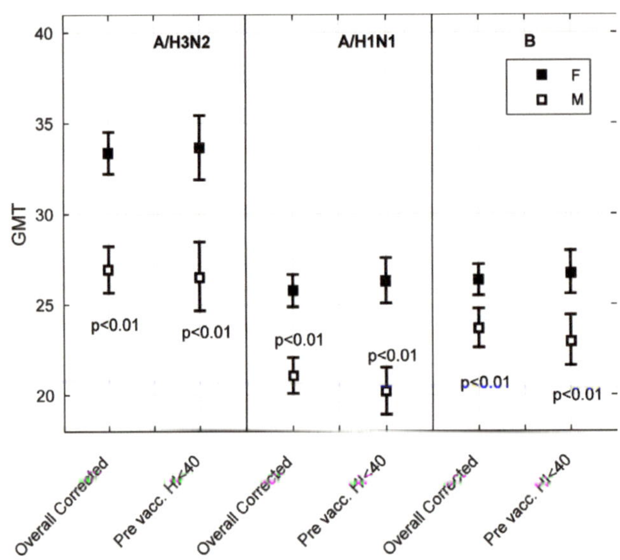

Figure 5. Postvaccination GMT values of populations divided according to gender (male: M and female: F) as indicated in legend labels. Postvaccination GMT values calculated on the overall population have been corrected for the average prevaccination status according to Beyer. For comparison purposes, post-GMT values of subjects unprotected before vaccination are also shown. The bars indicate the ranges of the 95% confidence limits.

3.4.4. *Evaluation of vaccine immunogenicity in "strong responder"*

Examining the antibody response after influenza vaccination, McElhaney et al. [22] considered as a vaccination efficiency-related parameter the HI antibody titer ratio between day 30 and day 0 and identified as weak/nonresponder people with a ratio 1– < 4 and as strong responders those with a ratio ≥4, i.e., people who seroconverted after vaccination. Using the same parameter we decided to evaluate in the groups identified as strong responders the induction of HI antibody response evaluated as GMT values against the three vaccine antigens.

The data obtained comparing results found in people who seroconverted after vaccination are reported in **Table 7**, and in most instances confirmed the results obtained examining the overall population of subgroups vaccinated with vaccine containing different dosages of antigens or subdivided in male and female. The responses induced by a 45 μg vaccine or in female were in most instances statistically higher than those induced by a 30 μg vaccine or in male volunteers, respectively. Moreover, the immune responses evaluated in volunteers with an age ≤ or >75 years were similar against A/H1N1 and B antigens and higher against the A/H3N2 antigen in people aged >75 years as compared with response in those ≤75 years.

Group	**A/H3N2**			**A/H1N1**			**B**		
	N **(total)**	**GMT post [GMTR] (95% CI)**	**Corrected GMT (95% CI)**	*N* **(total)**	**GMT post [GMTR] (95% CI)**	**Corrected GMT (95% CI)**	*N* **(total)**	**GMT post [GMTR] (95% CI)**	**Corrected GMT (95% CI)**
30 μg	146	84.0 ^{A} [7.6]	82.9 ^{A}	179	76.8 ^{A} [10.0]	86.81^{A}	182	83.8 ^{A} [9.7]	94.1 ^{A}
	(860)	(77.2–91.5)	(74.9–91.86)	(860)	(71.4–82.7)	(80.3–93.85)	(860)	(77.9–90.1)	(86.9–101.9)
45 μg	1185	164.7 [9.0]	133.6	940	127.4 [9.8]	126.1	959	110.2 [8.4]	118.9
	(3601)	(155.3–174.6)	(125.–142.7)	(3601)	(120.0–135.3)	(118.5–134.1)	(3601)	(104.3–116.4)	(112.1–126.3)
≤75	209	127.7 ^{A} [9.2]	112.9 ^{A}	161	123.0 [10.0]	121.6	176	113.4 [9.1]	122.7
	(658)	(111.4–146.4)	(99.3–128.3)	(658)	(106.1–142.6)	(104.7–141.2)	(658)	(98.6–130.4)	(105.3–143.1)
>75	707	183.3 [9.2]	146.2	612	127.6 [9.7]	128.35	543	112.8 [8.1]	117.3
	(2054)	(169.6–198.1)	(133.5–159.9)	(2054)	(118.7–137.2)	(119.3–138.2)	(2054)	(104.9–121.2)	(108.6–126.7)
F	1027	162.1 ^{A} [8.9]	130.3 ^{a}	872	120.3 [9.9]	121.6 ^{A}	842	113 ^{a} [8.9]	120.9 ^{A}
	(3142)	(152.2–172.5)	(121.7–139.6)	(3142)	(113.3–127.8)	(114.4–129.3)	(3142)	(106.7–119.6)	(113.8–128.4)
M	304	125.9 [8.4]	109.4	246	108.4 [9.3]	100.1	299	86.9 [7.8]	93.9
	(1315)	(113.4–139.7)	(97.1–123.1)	(1315)	(96.9–121.3)	(90.6–110.4)	(1315)	(79.9–94.4)	(86.3–102.2)

**: *p*-value <0.01 comparing pre- and postvaccination values.
A: *p*-value <0.01; a: *p*-value <0.05 comparing response between different groups.

Table 7. HI antibody response of strong responder population divided according to the vaccine dosage (30 or 45 μg), age class (younger elderly, μ75 years, and very elderly, >75 years), and gender (male: M; female: F).

3.4.5. Subanalysis according to the different types of vaccine used

Finally, since different vaccine formulations (whole, subunit, split, MF59-adjuvanted, and intradermally administered) were used in the 27 years studied, we compared the results obtained after administration of the different types of vaccine. Chi-square and one-way analysis of variance (ANOVA) were used for evaluating multiple comparisons among groups vaccinated with the different vaccine types. Estimates and comparison intervals are shown in **Figure 6**. Paired comparison *p*-values resulting from the multicomparison test are reported in **Tables 8** only when one-way ANOVA comparison identified potentially significant differences.

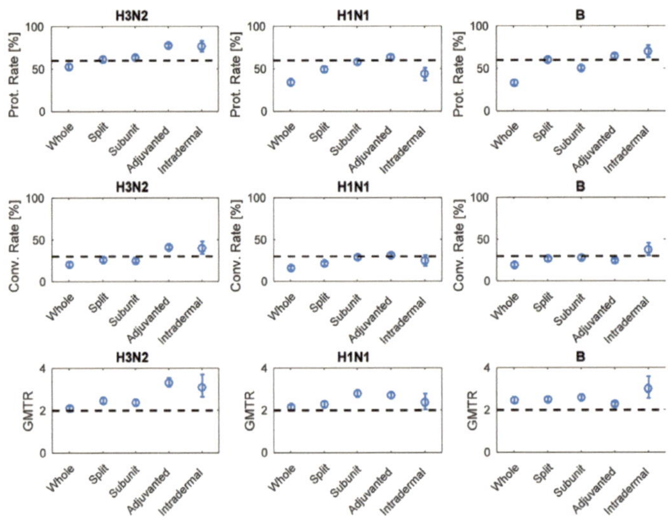

Figure 6. Values of CHMP parameters against the three vaccine antigens following vaccination with whole (N = 863), split (N = 996), subunit (N = 1094), MF-59 adjuvanted (N = 1343), and intradermally administered (N = 165) influenza vaccines. The black-dashed bold line in each figure represents the CHMP threshold value for the corresponding parameter. The bars indicate the ranges of the 95% confidence limits.

All vaccines used induced HI antibody responses satisfying at least one (prevalently GMTR value ≥2) of the three CHMP criteria. The antibody response induced by whole vaccine was in most instances lower as compared with responses induced by the others vaccines (**Table 8**). However, as reported in **Table 1**, many of the volunteers vaccinated with whole vaccine in the first years of the study received a vaccine with a low dose of antigen (30 μg). The responses induced by split and subunit vaccines against A/H3N2 and B antigens were similar; on the contrary against A/H1N1 antigen, the response induced by split vaccine was significantly lower as compared with subunit.

The two enhanced vaccines, MF59-adjuvanted and intradermal, induced similar and higher responses compared with conventional vaccines against A/H3N2 antigen.

Against A/H1N1, the response induced by MF59-adjuvanted vaccine was in most instances higher than conventional and intradermal vaccines.

http://dx.doi.org/10.5772/104559

Against B antigen, intradermal vaccine induced higher HI response than that induced by conventional and MF59-adjuvanted vaccines. In some cases the differences were statistically significant.

	p-Values (when <0.05)									
Parameter	**Whole /sub-u**	**Whole /split**	**Whole /MF59**	**Whole /ID**	**Split /sub-u**	**Split /MF59**	**Split /ID**	**Sub-u /MF59**	**Sub-u /ID**	**MF59 /ID**
A/H3N2 antigen										
Protection	<0.01	<0.01	<0.01	<0.01	–	<0.01	<0.01	<0.01	<0.01	–
Conversion	–	–	<0.01	<0.01	–	<0.01	<0.01	<0.01	<0.01	–
GMTR	<0.01	–	<0.01	<0.01	–	<0.01	<0.05	<0.01	<0.01	–
A/H1N1 antigen										
Protection	<0.01	<0.01	<0.01	–	<0.01	<0.01	–	<0.05	<0.01	<0.01
Conversion	–	<0.01	<0.01	–	<0.01	<0.01	–	–	–	–
GMTR	–	<0.01	<0.01	–	<0.01	<0.01	–	–	–	–
B antigen										
Protection	<0.01	<0.01	<0.01	<0.01	<0.01	–	–	<0.01	<0.01	–
Conversion	<0.01	<0.01	–	<0.01	–	–	<0.05	–	–	<0.01
GMTR	–	–	–	–	–	–	–	<0.01	–	<0.01

Whole: whole-virus vaccine; Sub-u: sub-unit vaccine; Split: split-virus vaccine; MF59: subunit MF59-adjuvanted vaccine; ID: Intradermal subunit vaccine.

Table 8. Paired comparison of results obtained in volunteers divided in groups according to the type of vaccine used for immunization. p-values resulting from the multicomparison test are reported only when one-way ANOVA comparison identified potentially significant differences.

4. Discussion

This study describes the humoral antibody response of 4461 elderly frail institutionalized volunteers prevalently vaccinated in the previous year after vaccination with influenza inactivated trivalent vaccines commercially available for the different years studied during a 27-year period (from winter season 1988–1989 to 2014–2015).

The first data were obtained by examining the results found in the 27-year period studied as crude mean responses and evidenced the ability of influenza vaccine administration to elicit antibody response in elderly volunteers (**Table 2**). One month after vaccination, significant increases were found against all the three vaccine antigens; however, vaccination induced significantly higher HI antibody titers against A/H3N2 antigen as compared with A/H1N1 and B strains. The higher responses against A/H3N2 strain were substantially confirmed considering the number of years in the 27-year period examined in which the CHMP criteria were fulfilled (**Table 3**) or comparing GMT values after correction for baseline titers or considering responses in prevaccination unprotected people (**Figure 2**).

In accordance with our results, higher titers after vaccination against A/H3N2 strain were previously found by Sasaki et al. [23] and Ohmit et al. [24], but it was not possible to discriminate between the possibility that A/H3N2 antigen is more immunogenic than A/H1N1 and B antigens or the possibility that the higher GMT and protection rate values might depend from earlier contact with the A/H3N2 virus due to vaccination or natural infection. Since all the volunteers were previously vaccinated, the possibility of the influence of a different circulation of A/H3N2 strains is more acceptable. The A/H3N2 viruses have the highest rate of evolution among the three influenza subtypes currently circulating, with antigenically distinct strains emerging on average 2–5 years and capable of a better diffusion among the population [25].

Further considerations about the results obtained derive from *post hoc* analyses conducted to determine whether vaccine dose, age, sex, and type of vaccine might influence the vaccine-induced humoral immune response.

Although the issue of increase in the antibody titers following increase in influenza vaccine dosage is not completely clarified [19, 20, 26], our data found using vaccines with 30 or 45 μg of antigens for vaccine dose, suggested that the increase in influenza vaccine dosage is generally associated with an increase in the induction of antibody titers. Significant antibody titers increases were observed both administering vaccines with 30 or 45 μg of antigens for vaccine dose against all the three vaccine antigens. However, postvaccination values following vaccination with 45 μg vaccine were in most instances statistically higher as compared with 30 μg both considering mean values for the overall population (**Table 4**) or GMT corrected for prevaccination status or calculated in prevaccination unprotected volunteers (**Figure 3**). In accordance with these observations, recently (December 2009) in the United States, a high-dose (60 μg HA per strain) trivalent inactivated influenza vaccine was licensed for people 65 years of age or older. The high dose vaccine was found to improve in people aged ≥65 years both antibody response and protection against laboratory-confirmed influenza illness [27, 28].

Considering vaccine immunogenicity in younger elderly (≤75 years) or in very elderly (>75 years), vaccine administration induced statistically significant increases in both groups. Comparing the two groups, the values were in many instances slightly higher in the very elderly as compared with younger elderly, and in some instances the differences were statistically significant. However, the differences persisted against A/H1N1 antigen both after correction for prevaccination status or calculation in unprotected volunteers before vaccination, and against B antigen only considering responses in unprotected people (**Figure 4**). The highest response of very elderly people as compared with younger elderly volunteers might be due to the fact that they probably represent a more selected group of elderly people capable of longer surviving and with a possible lower degree of age-associated alteration of the immune system [29].

However, since the differences were particularly evident against the A/H1N1 strain and are in accordance with previous data found in our laboratory showing in two different winter seasons a higher ability to give HI antibody response against A/H1N1 strains of people born between

1903 and 1919 as compared with volunteers born between 1920 and 1957, we cannot exclude the possibility that the differences might be due to cross-reactivity generated from exposure to the 1918 A/H1N1 virus or related A/H1N1 strains [30].

As far as sex could influence the immune response against influenza vaccines, our results confirmed previous data indicating that receipt of trivalent inactivated influenza vaccines results in significantly higher HI titers among females than males, both in adults and elderly people [21]. Significant rises in antibody titers were found after vaccination both in males and females, but the values observed in females were significantly higher as compared with males (**Table 6**) and the differences persisted also considering only GMT of volunteers unprotected before vaccination or GMT corrected for prevaccination status (**Figure 5**).

Sex hormones have been considered to be the most important mediators of sex differences and males with high level of testosterone have been found to have low antibody responses after influenza vaccination [31, 32].

However, since our data were obtained in elderly people, i.e., after the reproductive senescence, they support the hypothesis that the sex hormones are not the only mediator of sex differences in humoral response to influenza vaccination and there is the possibility that genetic differences also might underlie sex-based differences in adaptive immune response to viral vaccines [21, 33].

These results (vaccine dose, age, and sex) were, at least in part, confirmed also considering responses evaluated in strong responder, i.e., in volunteers showing a positive response after vaccination (**Table 7**).

Comparison of the different type of vaccines used in the 27-year period evidenced higher immunogenicity of the new "enhanced vaccines" specially licensed for elderly individuals, i.e., adjuvanted and intradermally administered vaccines, as compared with traditional whole, subunit, and split vaccines (**Table 7**, **Figure 6**) supporting previously published data [34, 35].

Our study had several limitations. The most important are that our observations may apply only to frail seniors living in care facilities and that the subanalysis groups were not fully comparable. However, since institutionalized people represent a significant target group for influenza vaccination, it is important to analyze their response to influenza vaccines. An additional limitation is the lack of data demonstrating clinical efficacy against influenza infection and illness. Although there is substantial evidence that HI antibody titers represent a good correlate of protection from severe illness in young adults, the predictive value of these measurements in older adults might be variable. Although the number of volunteers and of winter seasons we examined was considerable and comparable to the data reported in a review, differently from a review on influenza vaccine immunogenicity, the results obtained in each year were considered cumulatively not taking into account of the different characteristics of the vaccines used through the 27-year period. Indeed, the antigenic composition of influenza vaccines differ, even considerably, from one year to another, since it is updated each year to match the strains circulating in the community and inactivated influenza vaccines are available in different formulations (whole, split, and subunit with or without adjuvants), which are administered intramuscularly or intradermally. Moreover, a further aspect that should be carefully considered as compared with those of a review on HI antibody titers after influenza vaccine administration is the HI assay itself. HI test is not standardized across laboratory and was found to be highly variable and sensitive to factors such as reagents, erythrocyte source, and virus passage history. The results reported in the present report were all obtained in the same laboratory, although in different years and although, some changes were introduced in the HI test used during the 27-year period as reported in Section 2.

In conclusion, our data evidenced that the use of influenza vaccination appears to be an appropriate strategy to address the challenge of influenza infections of the elderly. However, they underline the need of studies for new improved influenza vaccines, since, as previously found, the vaccine-induced HI antibody responses against the three vaccine antigens were different and resulted not satisfactory against A/H1N1 and B antigen, since the postvaccination values of seroprotected volunteers were lower than the requested 60% (**Table 3**).

Moreover, they underline the necessity to expand researches and approaches to understand immunosenescence and its relationship to vaccine-induced immunity in order to have more valid vaccines. The vaccine-induced stimulation of HI antibody response following vaccination was found not only to be higher against one vaccine component as compared with the other two, but also to be influenced by different factors as vaccine dose, age, sex, and type of vaccine. It is therefore important, as suggested by Lambert et al. [5], both to understand the mechanisms that result in these differences and to use such information to devise more immunogenic influenza vaccine candidates.

Author details

Barbara Camilloni*, Emilia Nunzi, Michela Basileo and Anna Maria Iorio

*Address all correspondence to: barbara.camilloni@unipg.it

Department of Experimental Medicine, University of Perugia, Perugia, Italy

References

[1] Thompson WW, Shay DK, Weintraub E, Brammer L, Cox N, et al. Mortality associated with influenza and respiratory syncytial virus in the United States. JAMA. 2003;289(2): 179–186. DOI: 10.1001/jama.289.2.179

[2] Mullooly JP, Bridges CB, William W, Thompson WW, Chenb J, Weintraub E, et al. Influenza- and RSV-associated hospitalizations among adults. Vaccine. 2007;25(5):846–855. DOI: 10.1016/j.vaccine.2006.09.041

[3] Targonski PV, Jacobson RM, Poland GA. Immunosenescence: role and measurement in influenza vaccine response among elderly. Vaccine. 2007;25(16):3066–3069.

[4] Chen WH, Kozlovsky BF, Effros RB, Grubeck-Loebenstein B, Edelman R, et al. Vaccination in the elderly: an immunological perspective. Trends Immunol. 2009;30(7):351–359. DOI: 10.1007/978-3-0346-0219-8

[5] Lambert ND, Ovsyannikova IG, Pankratz VS, Jacobson RM, Poland GA. Understanding the immune response to seasonal influenza vaccination in older adults: a systems biology approach. Expert Rev Vaccines. 2012;11(8):985–994. DOI: 10.1586/erv.12.61

[6] Nichol KL. Challenger in evaluating influenza vaccine effectiveness and the mortality benefits controversy. Vaccine. 2009;27:6305–6311. DOI: 10.1016/j.vaccine.2009.07.006

[7] Hobson D, Curry RL, Beare AS, Ward-Gardner A. The role of serum haemagglutination-inhibiting antibody in protection against challenge infection with influenza A2 and B viruses. J Hyg (Lond). 1972;70(4):767–777.

[8] Potter CW. Determinants of immunity to influenza infection in man. Br Med Bull. Oxford JS. 1979;35(1):69–75.

[9] Katz JM, Hancock K, Xu X. Serologic assay for influenza surveillance, diagnosis and vaccine evaluation. Expert Rev Anti Infect Ther. 2011;9(6):669–683. DOI: 10.1586/eri.11.51

[10] McElhaney JE, Zhou X, Talbot HK, Soerhout E, Bleackley RC, et al. The unmet need in the elderly: how immunosenescence, CMV infection, co-morbidities and frailty are a challenge for the development of more effective influenza vaccines. Vaccine. 2012;30:2060–2067. DOI: 10.1016/j.vaccine.2012.01.015

[11] Beyer WE, Palache AM, Baljet M, Masurel N. Antibody induction by influenza vaccines in the elderly: a review of the literature. Vaccine. 1989;7(5):385–394. DOI: 10.1016/0264-410X(89)90150-3

[12] Goodwin K, Viboud C, Simonses L. Antibody response to influenza vaccination in the elderly: a quantitative review. Vaccine. 2006;24(8):1159–1169. DOI: 10.1016/j.vaccine.2005.08.105

[13] Seidman JC, Richard SA, Viboud C, Miller AM. Quantitative review of antibody response to inactivated seasonal influenza vaccines. Influenza Other Respirat Viruses. 2012;6(1):52–62. DOI: 10.1111/j.1750-2659.2011.00268.x

[14] Monto AS, Hornbuckle K, Ohmit SE. Influenza vaccine effectiveness among elderly nursing home residents: a cohort study. Am J Epidemiol. 2001;154:155–160. DOI: 10.1093/aje/154.2.155

[15] Iorio AM, Alatri A, Camilloni B, Neri M, Baglio G, et al. Antibody response to 1995–1996 influenza vaccine in institutionalized and non-institutionalized elderly women. Gerontology. 1999;45(1):31–38 . DOI: 10.1159/000022052

[16] Harmon MW, editor. Influenza viruses. Lennette EH (Ed.): Laboratory Diagnosis of Viral Infections. Second ed. New York: Marcel Dekker; 1992. pp. 515–534.

[17] Commission of the European Communities. Ad hoc working party on Biotechnology/Pharmacy. Harmonization of requirements for influenza vaccines. Biologicals. Document 111/3188/91-EN, Brussels; 1991.

[18] Beyer WE, Palache AM, Lüchters G, Nauta J, Osterhaus ADME. Seroprotection rate, mean fold increase, seroconversion rate: which parameter adequately expresses seroresponse to influenza vaccination?. Virus Res. 2004;103:125–132. DOI: 10.1016/j.virusres.2004.02.024

[19] Sullivan KM, Monto AS, Foster DA. Antibody response to inactivated influenza vaccines of various antigenic concentration. J Infect Dis. 1990;161(2):333–335. DOI: 10.1093/infdis/161.2.333

[20] Palache AM, Beyer WEP, Sprenger MJW, Masurel N, De Jonge S, et al. Antibody response after immunization with various vaccine doses: a double-blind, placebo-controlled, multi-centre, dose-response study in elderly nursing-home residents and young volunteers. Vaccine. 1993;11:3–7.

[21] Klein SL, Pekosz A. Sex-based biology and the rational design of influenza vaccination strategies. J Infect Dis. 2014;209(S3):S114–S119.

[22] McElhaney JE, Garmeau H, Camous X, Dupuis G, Pawelec G, et al. Predictors of the antibody response to influenza vaccination in older adults with type 2 diabetes. BMJ Open Diabetes Res Care. 2015;3(e000140). DOI: 10.1136/bmjdrc-2015-000140

[23] Sasaki S, He XS, Holmes TH, Dekker CL, Kemble GW, et al. Influence of prior influenza vaccination on antibody and B-cell responses. PLoS One. 2008;3(8). DOI: 10.1371/journal.pone.0002975

[24] Ohmit SE, Victor JV, Rotthoff JR, Teich ER, Truscon RK, et al. Prevention of antigenically drifted influenza by inactivated and live attenuated vaccines. N Engl J Med. 2006;355:2513–2522.

[25] Webster RG, Bean WJ, Gorman OT, Chambers TM, Kawaoka Y. Evolution and ecology of influenza A viruses. Microbiol Rev. 1992;56(1):152–179.

[26] Palache AM, Beyer WEP, Osterhaus ADME. Letter to the Editor Influenza vaccine dosages. Vaccine. 2008;26:2305–2306.

[27] Sullivan SJ, Jacobson R, Poland AG. Advances in the vaccination of the elderly against influenza: role of a high-dose vaccine. Expert Rev Vaccines. 2010;9(10):1127–1133. DOI: 10.1586/erv.10.117

[28] DiazGranados CA, Dunning AJ, Kimmel M, Kirby D, Treanor J, et al. Efficacy of high-dose versus standard-dose influenza vaccine in older adults. N Engl J Med. 2014;371:635–645. DOI: 10.1056/NEJMoa1315727

[29] Trzonkowski P, Mysliwska J, Pawelec G, Mysliwski A. From bench to bedside and back: the SENIEUR protocol and the efficacy of influenza vaccination in the elderly. Biogerontology. 2009;10:83–94. DOI: 10.1007/s10522-008-9155-5

[30] Iorio AM, Camilloni B, Lepri E, Neri M, Basileo M, Azzi A. Induction of cross-reactive antibodies to 2009 pandemic H1N1 influenza virus (pH1N1) after seasonal vaccination (Winters 2003/04 and 2007/08). Procedia Vaccinol. 2011;29:50–58. DOI: 10.1016/j.provac.2011.07.008

[31] Cook IF, Barr I, Hartel G, Pond D, Hampson AW. Reactogenicity and immunogenicity of an inactivated influenza vaccine administered by intramuscular or subcutaneous injection in elderly adults. Vaccine. 2006;24:2395–2402. DOI: 10.1016/j.vaccine.2005.11.057

[32] Furman D, Hejblum BP, Simon N, Jojic V, Dekker CL, et al. Systems analysis of sex differences reveals an immunosuppressive role for testosterone in the response to influenza vaccination. PNAS. 2013;111:869–874. DOI: 10.1073/pnas.1321060111

[33] Klein SL, Jedlicka A, Pekosz A. The Xs and Y of immune responses to viral vaccines. Lancet Infect Dis. 2015;5:338–349. DOI: 10.1016/S1473-3099(10)70049-9

[34] Basileo M, Iorio AM, Bartolini G, Bianchini C, Menculini G, et al. Comparative study of immunogenicity of split, intradermal and MF59-adjuvanted influenza vaccines in elderly institutionalized subjects. Procedia Vaccinol. 2014;8:18–23. DOI: 10.1016/j.provac.2014.07.004

[35] Camilloni B, Basileo M, Di Martino A, Donatelli I, Iorio AM. Antibody responses to intradermal or intramuscular MF59-adjuvanted influenza vaccines as evaluated in elderly institutionalized volunteers during a season of partial mismatching between vaccine and circulating A(H3N2) strains. Immunity Ageing. 2014; 11:10. DOI: 10.1186/1742-4933-11-10

Chapter 11

Chronic Obstructive Pulmonary Disease (COPD): Clinical and Immunological Effects of Mono-Vaccination Against Influenza Using an Immunoadjuvant Vaccine of a New Class Versus Combined Administration S. pneumoniae, H. influenzae, and Influenza Vaccines

Andrey Dmitrievich Protasov ,
Mikhail Petrovich Kostinov ,
Alexander Victorovich Zhestkov ,
Mikhail L'vovich Shteiner ,
Svetlana Vyacheslavovna Kazharova ,
Yuriy Vladimirovich Tezikov and
Igor Stanislavovich Lipatov

Additional information is available at the end of the chapter

http://dx.doi.org/10.5772/64292

Abstract

In Russian Federation, 27,300,000–41,200,000 acute upper and lower respiratory infections are reported annually. Patients with chronic obstructive pulmonary disease (COPD) are at higher risk of severe course, complications, and lethal outcomes of influenza. About 30% of COPD exacerbations are due to viral infections, and influenza A and B viruses are among the most common causes. The aim of our study was to assess exacerbation rate, number of courses of antibiotic chemotherapy, pulmonary function, and immunological effects of mono-vaccination with a new immunoadjuvant influenza vaccine vs. combined vaccination against pneumococcal infection, Hemophilus type b infection, and influenza in COPD patients. Both complex vaccination against Streptococcus pneumoniae, Haemophilus influenzae type b, and influenza and mono-vaccination with a new immunoadjuvant influenza vaccine led to statistically significant reduction in the number of COPD exacerbations and of antibiotic chemotherapy courses. Based on the obtained results, widespread implementation of mono-vaccina-

INTECH
open science | open minds

tion against influenza with a new immunoadjuvant influenza vaccine, as well as complex vaccination against bacterial respiratory infections and influenza can be recommended for COPD patients, as vaccination is beneficial for their functional status, that is, improves forced expiratory volume in 1 s (FEV1) and 6-minute walk test results. In our study, we evaluated immunogenicity of the new influenza immunoadjuvant vaccine administered as mono-vaccine to COPD patients in accordance with Committee for Proprietary Medicinal Products (CPMP) requirements.

Keywords: chronic obstructive pulmonary disease (COPD), vaccination, influenza, clinical effects, immunological effects

1. Introduction

In Russia, 27,300,000–41,200,000 acute upper and lower respiratory infections are reported annually. Patients with chronic obstructive pulmonary disease (COPD) are at higher risk of severe course, complications, and lethal outcomes of influenza. Therefore, influenza prevention in such patients is one of the most urgent tasks.

About 30% of COPD exacerbations are due to viral infections, and influenza A and B viruses are among the most common causes.

The best approach to prophylaxis is provided by vaccination because it combines the advantages of specificity, efficacy, safety, and cost-effectiveness. The GOLD guidelines (Global Initiative for Chronic Obstructive Lung Disease) recommend that influenza vaccination preferentially with split or subunit vaccines must be integrated into treatment strategies for all COPD patients regardless of the disease stage. However, further studies are needed to evaluate the efficacy and immunogenicity of modern adjuvant influenza vaccines [1].

It is not rarely that the risk of COPD exacerbation is associated not directly with the influenza virus as such, but rather with the development of bacterial superinfection, mainly caused by Streptococcus pneumoniae or Haemophilus influenzae type b [2–4].

In the Russian Federation, both inactivated and live vaccines against influenza have been licensed [5]. Antigenic composition of these vaccines is modified annually to adopt current epidemic situation and WHO guidelines. Recently, an innovative new class of immunoadjuvant influenza vaccines has evolved. The use of these vaccines in COPD patients will be outlined below.

According to CPMP criteria (Committee for Proprietary Medicinal Products), a vaccine is considered immunogenic, if at least one of the assessments meets the indicated requirements:

1. Seroconversion rate (at least fourfold increase in anti-hemagglutinin antibody titre): over 40% for individuals aging 18–60 years and over 30% among individuals above 60 years.
2. Seroprotection rate (number of individuals with protective titre of at least 1:40): over 70% for individuals aging 18–60 years and over 60% in individuals above 60 years.

3. Mean titre increase after vaccination: ≥2.5 in individuals aging 18–60 years and ≥2 in individuals above 60 years.

Vaccination against influenza for COPD patients is included into the National Immunization Calendar of the Russian Federation.

S. pneumoniae, H. influenzae, M. catarrhalis, and influenza virus are the most common causes of COPD infective exacerbations [6]. The standard of care for COPD patients includes vaccination against influenza and pneumococcal infection. Several serotypes of H. influenzae are known, and COPD exacerbation may be caused by each of them, including H. influenzae type b. Vaccine against H. influenzae type b is now available; therefore, it is of interest to evaluate a combined vaccination against S. pneumoniae, H. influenzae, and influenza in COPD patients and the effects of these vaccines on exacerbation rate and pulmonary function tests.

In adult COPD patients, the pioneer studies evaluating the therapeutic effect of PPV23 were performed in 2004. Elimination of S. pneumoniae from the sputum was observed in 52.9% cases, that is, at a lower rate compared to children. Other findings include increased levels of IgG against S. pneumoniae serotypes 3, 6B, 9N, 23F; decreased total IgE, and increased Wright's phagocytic index [7].

Immunization of COPD patients with PPV23 contributed to a 2.2-fold decrease in exacerbation rate by 18 months; at 12 months post vaccination, the duration of acute episodes decreased 1.8-fold compared to the control group [8].

Though disputable, the preliminary results regarding therapeutic effects of vaccination against respiratory infections were thus obtained. The common controversy is whether it is possible to improve the respiratory function tests in COPD patients through vaccination.

Study aim—to assess exacerbation rate, number of courses of antibiotic chemotherapy, pulmonary function, and immunological effects of mono-vaccination with a new immunoadjuvant influenza vaccine vs. combined vaccination against pneumococcal infection, Haemophilus type b infection, and influenza in COPD patients.

2. Material and methods

The study enrolled 170 patients with grade 1, 2, 3, 4 COPD (age 30–80 years) who had signed informed consent according to the study protocol approved by the ethics committee of the Samara State Medical University (Russian Federation) and Research Institute of Pulmonology (Moscow, Russian Federation). The diagnosis was determined according to GOLD guidelines (2012) [9].

Patients were divided into four groups. Group I enrolled 50 patients with COPD who continued to receive basic therapy for the main disease and were vaccinated with commercially available vaccines against pneumococcal infection (Pneumo 23, France), H. influenzae type b infection (Hiberix, Belgium), and influenza (new immunoadjuvant vaccine Grippol® plus,

Russian Federation). Vaccines were administered once intramuscularly into various parts of the body. Two patients from Group I did not complete the study per protocol (one patient died after a traffic accident, and one patient died from sudden massive pulmonary embolism). Therefore, the data from these patients were not included into final analysis, and it was based on 48 patients of Group I.

Group II (control for patients who received complex vaccination against pneumococcal infection, Haemophilus type b infection, and influenza) consisted of 80 patients with COPD of similar grade, who were not vaccinated and received only basic therapy.

Group III consisted of 20 COPD patients vaccinated against influenza with a new immunoadjuvant vaccine. Group IV (control for patients who received mono-vaccination against influenza with a new immunoadjuvant vaccine) enrolled 20 unvaccinated COPD patients. Groups II and IV were composed of patients who categorically rejected any vaccination, despite the information provided. Nevertheless, these patients gave their consent to participate in the study. All study patients were followed up for 1 year and subjected to function and immunological tests at baseline and at 12 months.

The use of two control groups was associated with enrollment of patients in two various study centers. Each study center enrolled subjects either to Group I (group of complex vaccination and control group) or to Group III (group of mono-vaccination against influenza and control group). Another reason for the use of two control groups was the probability that baseline characteristics of the patients in Group 1 and Group 3 will not be well balanced, and their comparison with the total control group will be incorrect. Our study is not a direct comparison between the groups of complex vaccination and mono-vaccination. We just compare each of these groups with its own control.

All study patients underwent a history taking (identification of risk factors for COPD, complaints for cough, sputum discharge, dyspnea of any grade worsened by physical exercise). To verify the diagnosis of COPD, all patients were subjected to pulmonary function tests and broncholytic test with 400 μg of salbutamol according to the standard techniques [8]. The study enrolled patients with Tiffeneau index forced expiratory volume in 1 s/forced vital capacity (FEV1/FVC) below 70%.

Inclusion criteria:

- Men and women above 30 years of age.
- Patients with mild/moderate/severe/extremely severe COPD.
- Patient's informed consent.

Exclusion criteria:

- Age below 30 years.
- Vaccination against pneumococcal infection within the previous 3 years.
- Previous vaccination against H. influenzae type b infection.

- Acute infectious diseases and tuberculosis.
- Active phase of chronic virus hepatitis.
- Mental disorders.
- Renal or hepatic failure.
- Malignancies.
- Exacerbation of chronic diseases.
- Hypersensitivity to vaccine components.
- Severe complications of previous vaccination.
- Pregnancy.
- Autoimmune disorders.

Patients were followed up by general practice physicians, pulmonologists, or allergologists-immunologists in the outpatient context or in hospitals, if hospitalization was required. In cases of COPD exacerbation, if necessary, patients were hospitalized to departments of pulmonology.

Patients meeting inclusion/exclusion criteria were divided into four groups. Groups II and IV enrolled patients who categorically rejected any vaccination. Other patients were first recruited to Group I to undergo complex vaccination and then to Group III to be vaccinated against influenza using a new immunoadjuvant vaccine. Sample size was determined by the number of vaccines.

All patients received basic bronchodilatory and anti-inflammatory therapies in accordance with the disease severity and GOLD guidelines (2012). At baseline, groups were well balanced for age, gender, disease severity, and scope of basic therapy, which remained unchanged throughout the study period. Vaccination was performed at remission in the outpatient context, follow-up period lasted for 12 months after vaccination.

PPV23 vaccine is a polyvalent pneumococcal vaccine manufactured by Sanofi aventis (France). It contains purified capsule S. pneumoniae polysaccharides of 23 serotypes. One dose of vaccine is 0.5 ml.

Hiberix is a conjugated vaccine to prevent infections caused by H. influenzae type b (GlaxoSmithKline Biologicals s.a., Belgium). One dose contains 10 μg of purified capsule polysaccharide isolated from str. H. influenzae type b conjugated with 30 μg of tetanus toxoid.

Grippol plus vaccine (NPO Petrovax Pharm, Russia) is a trivalent polymeric subunit immunoadjuvant vaccine (Petrovax, Russia) containing protective antigens isolated from purified influenza type A and B viruses grown in chicken embryos. One immunization dose (0.5 ml) contains at least 5 μg of hemagglutinin of epidemiologically relevant influenza subtype A (H1N1 and H3N2) and type B viruses, and polyoxidonium immunoadjuvant 500 μg in sodium phosphate buffer. Vaccine is free of preservatives.

Clinical efficacy of vaccination was assessed by the number of COPD exacerbations during the year before vaccination and after vaccination. COPD exacerbation was defined as increased dyspnea, cough, and sputum volume requiring medical advice and modification of current therapy documented by primary medical records.

Ventilation function was investigated using a Spiro S-100 spirometer (Russian Federation). The following parameters were measured: forced vital capacity (FVC), forced expiratory volume in 1 s (FEV1), and a calculated ratio of these two parameters (FEV1%/FVC), that is, modified Tiffeneau test. Exercise tolerance was assessed using the 6-minute walk test (6MWT) according to the standard protocol.

The levels of IgG antibodies against influenza virus strains were measured using standard HAI assay (hemagglutination inhibition assay) in accordance with the manufacturer's instructions to the kit.

The results were studied statistically using StatPlus 2009 Professional 5.8.4. Measures of central tendency and dispersion were chosen depending on the data distribution type. Continuous variables corresponding to normal distribution are presented as means (SD); variables differing from normal distribution as medians (interquartile distance). Categorical variables are presented as proportions (%) and absolute values.

The choice of statistical test depends on the data distribution type and evaluation of dispersion equality. The hypothesis of data distribution normality was tested (Shapiro-Wilks test). In cases of normal distribution of data in each sample, dispersion is to be compared between two distributions (Levene's test). If both criteria are met, Student's t test is selected, if no, its non-parametric alternative is used (Mann-Whitney test). The same is applicable to paired tests for comparisons of changing variables (pairwise Student's t test or Wilcoxon test for paired comparisons). Comparative analysis of categorical variables was performed using exact two-sided Fisher's test. Differences were statistically significant at $p < 0.05$ [10].

Prospective study design allows calculating the following statistics:

- Number of patients with exacerbations per year before and after vaccination.
- Absolute risk (AR) of exacerbation per year before and after vaccination.
- Relative risk (RR) of exacerbation per year before and after vaccination.
- Reduction of absolute risk (RAR) of exacerbation after vaccination.
- Reduction of relative risk (RRR) of exacerbation after vaccination.
- Chance of exacerbation.
- Odds ratio (OR) for exacerbation after vaccination compared to no vaccination.
- Number of patients needed to treat to prevent one additional bad outcome (NNTp).

About 95% CI of the difference of absolute risks (AR): the results are statistically significant, if 95% CI will not contain 0.

About 95% CI of the relative risk (RR): the results are statistically significant, if 95% CI will not contain 1.

About 95% CI for the odds ratio (OR): the results are statistically significant, if 95% CI will not contain 1.

3. Results and discussion

3.1. Clinical effects of vaccination in COPD patients

The clinical effects of vaccination (exacerbation rate) in COPD patients are characterized by groups in **Table 1**.

Parameter (formula)	**Before vaccination**				**After vaccination**			
	Group I Complex (n=48)	Group II Control I (n=80)	Group III Mono (n=20)	Group IV Control II (n=20)	Group I Complex (n=48)	Group II Control I (n=80)	Group III Mono (n=20)	Group IV Control II (n=20)
Number of COPD exacerbations over 12 months	2 [1,75; 3]	2 [1; 3]	2 [2; 3]	2 [1; 3]	0 [0; 1]***	2 [1; 3]	1 [0; 2]*	2 [1; 3]
Number of patients with exacerbations	44	67	16	17	18	71	10	18
Chance of exacerbation (no. patients with exacerbations /no. patients without exacerbations)	44/4 = 11	67/13 = 5.2	16/4 = 4	17/3 = 5.7	18/30 = 0.6	71/9 = 7.9	10/10 = 1	18/2 = 9
AP (no. patients with exacerbations /no. patients at risk of exacerbation)	44/48 = 0.92 = 92%	67/80 = 0.84 = 84%	16/20 = 0.8 = 80%	17/20 = 0.85 = 85%	18/48 = 0,38 = 38%	71/80 = 0.89 = 89%	10/20 = 0.5 = 50%	18/20 = 0.9 = 90%
	Flu+PPV23+ HIB (n=48)		**Control I (n=80)**		**Flu (n=20)**		**Control II (n=20)**	
OR (AR after vaccination/ AR without vaccination), 95% CI	0.38/0.92 = 0.41 = 41% (0.16; 1.08)		0.89/0.84 = 1.06 = 106% (0.49; 2.29)		0.5/0.8 = 0.63 = 63% (0.23; 1.69)		0.9/0.85 = 1.06 = 106% (0.19; 5.7)	
RAR (AR after vaccinations – AR without vaccination), 95% CI	0.38 – 0.92 = - 0.54 = - 54% (-1.53; 0.45)		0.89 – 0.84 = 0.05 = 5% (-0.76; 0.86)		0.5 – 0.8 = - 0.3 = - 30% (-1.29; 0.69)		0.9 – 0.85 = 0.05 = 5% (-1.63; 1.73)	
RRR (AR difference /AR without vaccination)	(92% - 38%)/92% = 0.59 = 59%		(84% - 89%)/84% = - 0.06 = -6%		(80% - 50%)/80% = 0.38 = 38%		(85% - 90%)/85% = - 0.06 = - 6%	
OR (chance with vaccination / chance without vaccination), 95% CI	0.6/11 = 0.05 = 5% (0.02; 0.17)#		7.9/5.2 = 1.52 = 152% (0.61; 3.78)		1/4 = 0.25 = 25% (0.06; 1.02)		9/5.7 = 1.58 = 158% (0.23; 10.8)	
NNTp (1/RAR)	1/0.54 = **1.9**		-		1/0.3 = **3.3**		-	

Notes: continuous variables are presented as medians and interquartile distances.
* p<0.05 vs. before vaccination in a given group (exact Fisher's test).
*** p<0.001 vs. before vaccination in a given group (exact Fisher's test).
# p<0.05.
Abbreviations: AR – absolute risk, RR – relative risk, RAR – reduction of absolute risk, RRR – reduction of relative risk, OR – odds ratio, NNTp – number of patients needed to treat to prevent unfavorable outcome.

Table 1. Number of exacerbations (calculated statistics) in COPD patients per year before and after vaccination.

Both complex and mono-vaccination resulted in a statistically significant reduction of the number of COPD exacerbations. The risk of COPD exacerbation was reduced by 54% after complex vaccination vs. 30% after mono-vaccination ($p > 0.05$ for all comparisons).

Parameter (formula)	Before vaccination				After vaccination			
	Group I Complex (n=48)	Group II Control I (n=80)	Group III Mono (n=20)	Group IV. Control II (n=20)	Group I Complex (n=48)	Group II Control I (n=80)	Group III Mono (n=20)	Group IV Control II (n=20)
Number of courses of antibiotic chemotherapy (ABC) over 12 months	2 [1; 3]	2 [1; 3]	2 [2; 3]	2 [1; 3]	0 [0; 1]***	2 [1; 3]	0 [0; 1]*	2 [1; 3]
Number of patients treated with ABC	41	62	17	15	15	63	11	18
Chance of ABC (no. patients treated with ABC/no. patients not treated with ABC)	41/7 = 5.9	62/18 = 3.4	17/3 = 5.7	15/5 = 3	15/33 = 0.5	63/17 = 3.7	11/9 = 1.2	18/2 = 9
AR (no. patients treated with ABC/no. patients not treated with ABC)	41/48 = 0.85 = 85%	62/80 = 0.78 = 78%	17/20 = 0.85 = 85%	15/20 = 0.75 = 75%	15/48 = 0.31 = 31%	63/80 = 0.79 = 79%	11/20 = 0.55 = 55%	18/20 = 0.9 = 90%
RR (AR with vaccination – AR without vaccination), 95% CI	**Combined (n=48)**		**Control I (n=80)**		**Mono (n=20)**		**Control II (n=20)**	
	0.31/0.85 = 0.36 = 36% (0.18; 0.73)#		0.79/0.78 = 1.01 = 101% (0.56; 1.82)		0.55/0.85 = 0.65 = 65% (0.21; 2.06)		0.9/0.75 = 1.2 = 120% (0.26; 5.48)	
RAR (AR with vaccination – AR without vaccination), 95% CI	0.31 – 0.85 = - 0.54 = - 54% (-1.25; 0.17)		0.79 – 0.78 = 0.01 = 1% (-0.58; 0.6)		0.55 – 0.85 = - 0.3 = - 30% (-1.45; 0.85)		0.9 – 0.75 = 0.15 = 15% (-1.37; 1.67)	
RRR (difference AR/AR without vaccination)	(85% - 31%)/85% = 0.64 = 64%		(78% - 79%)/78% = - 0.01 = -1%		(85% - 55%)/85% = 0.35 = 35%		(75% - 90%)/75% = - 0.2 = - 20%	
OR (chance with vaccination/chance without vaccination), 95% CI	0.5/5.9 = 0.08 = 8% (0.03; 0.22)#		3.7/3.4 = 1.09 = 109% (0.49; 2.41)		1.2/5.7 = 0.21 = 21% (0.05; 0.96)#		9/3 = 3 = 300% (0.49; 18.03)	
NNTp (1/RAR)	1/0.54 = **1.9**		-		1/0.3 = **3.3**		-	

Notes: continuous variables are presented as medians and interquartile distances.

* - $p<0.05$ vs. baseline value in a given group (exact Fisher's test).

*** - $p<0.001$ vs. baseline value in a given group (exact Fisher's test).

\# - $p<0.05$.

Abbreviations: AR – absolute risk, RR – relative risk, RAR – reduction of absolute risk, RRR – reduction of relative risk, OR – odds ratio, NNTp – number of patients needed to treat to prevent unfavorable outcome.

Table 2. Number of courses of antibiotic chemotherapy (calculated statistics) in COPD patients per year before and after vaccination in the groups considered.

As compared to unvaccinated patients, complex vaccination reduced the risk of COPD exacerbation by 59 vs. 38% reduction after mono-vaccination vs. increase by 6% in unvaccinated patients.

In the group of complex vaccination against pneumococcal, Haemophilus type b infection, and influenza, the chance of COPD exacerbation was 5% of that in unvaccinated patients ($p < 0.05$). In the group of mono-vaccination, the chance of COPD exacerbation was 25% of that without vaccination ($p > 0.05$).

Table 2 presents characteristics of the clinical effect of vaccination (i.e., number of courses of antibiotic chemotherapy) in different groups of COPD patients.

Both complex and mono-vaccination led to statistically significant reduction in the number of antibacterial chemotherapy courses.

The risk of antibiotic chemotherapy was reduced by 54% in the group of complex vaccination against pneumococcal, Hemophilus type b infection, and influenza vs. 30% in the group of mono-vaccination ($p > 0.05$ for all comparisons).

As compared to no vaccination, complex vaccination reduced the risk of antibiotic chemotherapy in patients with COPD by 64%, whereas mono-vaccination reduced it by 35%.

In the group of complex vaccination against pneumococcal, Hemophilus type b infection, and influenza, the chance of antibiotic chemotherapy was 8% of that in unvaccinated patients ($p < 0.05$). In the group of mono-vaccination, the chance of antibiotic chemotherapy was 21% of that in unvaccinated ($p < 0.05$).

3.2. The effect of vaccination on the pulmonary function tests in COPD patients

In COPD patients from Groups I and II, FVC changes did not undergo any statistically significant changes over 12 months (**Table 3**). In Group I (patients vaccinated against pneumococcal, Hemophilus type b infection, and influenza), forced expiratory volume in 1 s (FEV1) increased to 57.4% (2.0%) at 12 months vs. 53.9% (2.7%) at baseline ($p < 0.05$). In unvaccinated patients (Group II), these parameters remained unchanged: 54.1% (1.9%) at baseline vs. 50.4% (2.8%) at 12 months ($p > 0.05$), indicating that the rate of FEV1 decrease was lower in vaccinated COPD patients (Group I). Detailed characteristics of FEV1 changes in Groups I and II depending on the disease severity are given in **Table 4**, and **Table 5** outlines the same for Tiffeneau index.

COPD grade	At baseline		At 12 months	
	Abs., ml	%	Abs., ml	%
1 (n = 3/n = 24)	3611 (466)	100.7 (3)	3724 (489)	104 (0.4)
	3608 (206)	97.8 (3.2)	3572 (176)	95.6 (2.9)
2 (n = 23/n = 25)	2943 (180)	78.9 (3.3)	2867 (169)	79.3 (3.3)
	2936 (173)	77.9 (4.1)	2918 (167)	76.9 (3.5)
3 (n = 18/n = 25)	2301 (129)	55.2 (2.8)	2173 (208)	53.3 (3.5)
	2311 (128)	55.2 (2.7)	2086 (96.2)	51.2 (2.6)
4 (n = 4/n = 6)	1854 (116)	46.6 (5.6)	2158 (119)&	55.8 (3.8)&
	1845 (129)	45.2 (5.1)	1778 (106)	43.3 (2.2)
Total (n = 48/n = 80)	2653 (119)	68.7 (2.9)	2602 (131)	68.3 (2.9)
	2648 (122)	67.9 (2.5)	2562 (131)	64.8 (2.2)

Data are presented as means (standard deviation).
Group I patients in the numerator, Group II patients in the denominator.
& $p < 0.05$—differences between Groups I and II (Student's test).

Table 3. FVC changes in COPD patients from Groups I and II over 12 months.

COPD grade	At baseline		At 12 months	
	Abs., ml	%	Abs., ml	%
1 (n = 3/n = 24)	2412 (236)	86.7 (1.6)	2597 (337)	90.5 (1.1)$^{\&\&}$
	2399 (205)	85.8 (2.0)	2384 (136)	85.4 (1.2)
2 (n = 23/n = 25)	1954 (112)	66.1 (2.1)	1985 (109)	69.9 (2.6)$^{\&}$
	1959 (110)	66.4 (2.7)	1916 (102)	62.9 (1.4)
3 (n = 18/n = 25)	1274 (65.1)	39.1 (1.4)	1314 (101)	42.0 (2.2)
	1280 (69.3)	40.0 (1.3)	1204 (76.3)	37.2 (1.6)
4 (n = 4/n = 6)	876 (106.5)	26.9 (1.4)	951 (106.5)	28.6 (2.7)
	883 (115.5)	27.9 (1.2)	826 (97.2)	25.9 (1.0)
Total (n = 48/n = 80)	1638 (86.6)	53.9 (2.7)	1685 (95.4)	57.4 (2.0)$^{\&}$
	1642 (92.5)	54.1 (1.9)	1574 (94.4)	50.4 (2.8)

Data are presented as means (standard deviation).
Group I patients in the numerator, Group II patients in the denominator.
& $p < 0.05$; && $p < 0.01$—differences between Groups I and II (Student's test).

Table 4. FEV1 changes in COPD patients from Groups I and II over 12 months.

COPD grade	At baseline	At 12 months
	%	%
1 (n = 3/n = 24)	67.27 (1.95)	69.8 (0.1)
	66.34 (2.18)	68.4 (0.89)
2 (n = 23/n = 25)	67.14 (2.04)	69.9 (2.29)$^{\&}$
	66.85 (1.95)	64.24 (1.58)
3 (n = 18/n = 25)	56.68 (2.59)	62.39 (2.61)
	55.43 (2.12)	58.4 (2.53)
4 (n = 4/n = 6)	47.85 (6.69)	44.2 (4.95)
	47.38 (5.12)	45.84 (2.53)
Total (n = 48/n = 80)	61.62 (1.73)	64.93 (1.94)$^{\&}$
	60.98 (1.85)	59.13 (2.15)

Data are presented as means (standard deviation).
Group I patients in the numerator, Group II patients in the denominator.
& $p < 0.05$—differences between Groups I and II (Student's test).

Table 5. Tiffeneau index changes in COPD patients from Groups I and II over 12 months.

One year post vaccination, vaccinated COPD patients (Group I) showed 6MWT results that were 75.2% (2.8%) of the desired values vs. 60.4% (2.3%) in Group II patients ($p < 0.001$). Detail characteristics of the dynamics of the 6-minute walk test depending on the disease severity are given in **Table 6**.

COPD grade	At baseline		At 12 months	
	Abs., m	%	Abs., m	%
1 (n = 3/n = 24)	440 (49.0)	86.1 (8.6)	450 (54.5)	92.8 (4.3)
	434 (52.8)	84.7 (9.1)	429 (41.2)	83.5 (4.2)
2 (n = 23/n = 25)	355 (13.1)	71.8 (2.4)	401 (15.8)*,&&&	81.2 (3.1)*, &&&
	351 (10.2)	70.9 (2.6)	324 (8.7)#	64.1 (1.2)#
3 (n = 18/n = 25)	314 (21.1)	64.0 (3.8)	338 (26.4)	69.7 (4.3)&
	319 (20.3)	64.1 (3.6)	296 (17.1)	59.4 (1.7)
4 (n = 4/n = 6)	230 (45.2)	47.4 (13)	266 (37.3)	54 (12.3)
	235 (40.3)	48.6 (10.3)	213 (10.5)	44.2 (2.3)
Total (n = 48/n = 80)	335 (12.6)	67.8 (2.4)	369 (14.5)&&&	75.2 (2.8)*, &&&
	332 (18.4)	66.3 (2.6)	305 (10.5)	60.4 (2.3)

Data are presented as means (standard deviation).
Group I patients in the numerator, Group II patients in the denominator.
* $p < 0.05$ vs. baseline values in Group I (Student's test).
# $p < 0.05$ vs. baseline values in Group II (Student's test).
& $p < 0.05$; &&& $p < 0.001$—differences between Groups I and II (Student's test).

Table 6. Dynamics of 6MWT in COPD patients from Groups I and II over 12 months.

Detailed characteristics of spirometry data in COPD patients from Groups III and IV are presented in **Table 7**.

Parameter		Vaccinated against influenza (Group III, n = 20)		Unvaccinated (Group IV, n = 20)	
		At baseline	At 12 months	At baseline	At 12 months
FVC	Abs.	1.62 (0.18)	1.71 (0.13)	2.05 (0.12)	1.88 (0.16)
	%	37.69 (3.61)	42 (2.74)	47.06 (2.9)	41.94 (3.05)
FEV1	Abs.	1.13 (0.13)	1.17 (0.08)	1.48 (0.1)	1.38 (0.11)
	%	33.65 (3.43)	35.76 (2.16)	42.25 (2.76)	40.83 (3.46)
FEV1/FVC	%	52.7 (3.42)	46.46 (3.2)&	55.8 (2.18)	57.9 (2.66)

Data are presented as means (standard deviation).
& $p < 0.05$—differences between Groups III and IV at 12 months (Student's test).

Table 7. Spirometry values in COPD patients vaccinated against influenza (Group III) and in unvaccinated control patients (Group IV).

The analysis of the 6-minute walk test results showed a trend to distance increase by 13 m (+3.7%) 1 year after mono-vaccination ($p > 0.05$, Student's test).

Thus, the study demonstrated statistically significant increase in FEV1 [57.4% (2.0%)] at 12 months after complex vaccination when compared to unvaccinated COPD patients [50.4% (2.8%)]. This FEV1 increase was 3.5%, that is, not statistically significant vs. baseline value, although the positive trend was observed.

The group of mono-vaccination against influenza also demonstrated the positive trend of FEV1 increase, but the increase was only 2.11%, which is less than 3.5% in the group of complex vaccination.

In the group of complex vaccination, patients demonstrated significantly improved 6MWT results at 12 months vs. baseline distance. In Group I, the increase was 7.4% (+34 m), that is, statistically significant ($p < 0.05$). In patients vaccinated against influenza, 6MWT increase approached trend levels of significance.

3.3. Immunological effect of vaccination in patients with COPD

Previously, we have reported the dynamics of specific antibodies against influenza virus in COPD patients after complex vaccination against S. pneumoniae, H. influenzae type b, and influenza [11].

Combined vaccination against pneumococcal, H. influenzae type b and influenza is accompanied by production of antibodies to these infections, which persist during 1 year (observation period), regardless of disease severity. In patients with stage 4 COPD, the level of antibodies to influenza virus (strains A/H1N1, A/H3N2 and B) in post-vaccination period was lower than in patients with stages 1, 2, and 3. Probably, these patients should be vaccinated against influenza twice. Despite the fact that patients with COPD had lower levels of post-vaccination antibodies than control, they demonstrated apparent clinical effect throughout 12 months, which was recorded as reduction of both exacerbation number and the need in antibacterial medications. Combined vaccination against bacterial and viral infections contributes to the achievement of antibody levels leading to the development of significant clinical effect in patients with COPD.

Table 8 demonstrates lists immunogenicity parameter of the new immunoadjuvant vaccine against influenza after mono vaccination of COPD patients.

No statistically significant differences in immunogenicity were found between COPD patients and healthy participants vaccinated only against influenza, the latter, however, demonstrated a trend toward higher immune response to vaccination.

In the comparative analysis of COPD patients, in whom antibodies to all three influenza virus strains were detected at arbitrarily protective titres (≥1:40) at 6 months after vaccination, and patients, in whom, despite vaccination, antibody titres were <1:40, COPD patients at risk of low response to vaccination were identified. These patients had a long history of COPD with frequent respiratory infections and COPD exacerbations requiring hospitalization and systemic glucocorticosteroids or antibiotic chemotherapy.

Vaccine strains	Seroconversion, % (N ≥ 40%)		Seroprotection, % (N ≥ 70%)		Mean geometric antibody titre (N ≥ 40)		
	6 months	12 months	6 months	12 months	At baseline	6 months	12 months
A/H1N1/ Brisbane/ 59/07	60 ± 16	40 ± 16	58 ± 14	67 ± 14	20 ($\log_2$ 4.32 ± 0.36)	30.64 ($\log_2$ 4.94 ± 0.38)	33.64^p($\log_2$ 5.07 ± 0.28)
A/H3N2/ Uruguay/ 716/2007	70 ± 15	50 ± 16	75 ± 13	83.3 ± 11	24.75 ($\log_2$ 4.63 ± 0.63)	71.91 ($\log_2$ 6.17 ± 0.62)	59.93 ($\log_2$ 5.91 ± 0.38)
B/Florida/ 4/2006	30 [15; 45]	10 [1; 20]	100 ± 0	100 ± 0	46.94 ($\log_2$ 5.55 ± 0.30)	84.38 ($\log_2$ 6.4 ± 0.33)	59.9 ($\log_2$ 5.91 ± 0.38)

Marked values meet CPMP requirements.

Table 8. Immunogenicity parameters of the new immunoadjuvant vaccine against influenza after mono-vaccination of COPD patients (n = 15).

4. Conclusions

During post-vaccination period, treating physicians and patients as well focus their attention on the main disease course. The clinical course of the disease may be characterized by number of COPD exacerbations and the need for antibiotic chemotherapy. Both complex vaccination against S. pneumoniae, H. influenzae type b, and influenza and mono-vaccination with a new immunoadjuvant influenza vaccine led to statistically significant reduction in the number of COPD exacerbations and of antibiotic chemotherapy courses.

Our study had some limitations, that is, its pilot character, absence of randomization and blinding, and small sample size. As follows from the study results, complex vaccination of COPD patients against bacterial and viral respiratory infections have more expressed beneficial effects on their functional status when compared to mono-vaccination against influenza. Further well-designed multicenter clinical studies devoid of these limitations are needed to refine the hypothesis. Nevertheless, based on the obtained results, widespread implementation of mono-vaccination against influenza with a new immunoadjuvant influenza vaccine, as well as complex vaccination against bacterial respiratory infections and influenza can be recommended for COPD patients, as vaccination is beneficial for their functional status, that is, improves FEV1 and 6-minute walk test results.

Mono-vaccination of COPD patients using immunoadjuvant vaccines of a new class as well as combined vaccination against S. pneumoniae, H. influenzae, and influenza is associated with protective antibody titres. In our study, we evaluated immunogenicity of the new influenza immunoadjuvant vaccine administered as mono-vaccine to COPD patients in accordance with CPMP requirements. Immune response to vaccine strains of influenza virus was more intense and durable in initially seropositive patients compared to seronegative.

Combined vaccination against pneumococcal, H. influenzae type b and influenza is accompanied by production of antibodies to these infections. In patients with stage 4, COPD the level of antibodies to influenza virus (strains A/H1N1, A/H3N2 and B) in post-vaccination period was lower than in patients with stages 1, 2, and 3. Probably, these patients should be vaccinated against influenza twice. Combined vaccination against bacterial and viral infections contributes to the achievement of antibody levels leading to the development of significant clinical effect in patients with COPD.

Influenza prophylaxis in COPD patients implies annual influenza vaccination of all individuals having no contraindications regardless of the disease severity. Influenza vaccine prophylaxis must be included into patient's care plan and into the list of recommendations given by a pulmonologist at an outpatient visit or at discharge from hospital. If possible, simultaneous vaccination against S. pneumoniae, H. influenzae type b, and influenza is recommended as early as possible before the season of respiratory infections starts. Combined vaccination against respiratory infections has more significant effects on clinical characteristics and functional status of COPD patients and promotes production of specific antibodies not only against vaccine strains of influenza virus but also against S. pneumoniae and H. influenzae antigens contained in the corresponding vaccines.

Author details

Andrey Dmitrievich Protasov[1,2*], Mikhail Petrovich Kostinov[1,2], Alexander Victorovich Zhestkov[1,2], Mikhail L'vovich Shteiner[1,2], Svetlana Vyacheslavovna Kazharova[1,2], Yuriy Vladimirovich Tezikov[1,2] and Igor Stanislavovich Lipatov[1,2]

*Address all correspondence to: crosss82@mail.ru

1 Samara State Medical University, Samara, Russian Federation

2 Mechnikov Research Institute of Vaccines and Sera, Moscow, Russian Federation

References

[1] Chebykina A.V. Clinico-functional status and anti-influenza immune response in vaccinated patients with bronchial asthma and chronic obstructive pulmonary disease (COPD). [thesis]. Moscow:2012. 26 p. (In Russ.)

[2] Protasov A.D., Zhestkov A.V., Lavrenteva N.E., Kostinov M.P., Ryzhov A.A. Effect of complex vaccination against pneumococcal, Haemophilus type b infections and influenza in patients with chronic obstructive pulmonary disease. Journal of Microbiology, Epidemiology and Immunobiology. 2011;4:80–84. (In Russ.)

[3] Protasov A.D. Immunologic and clinical effects of combined use of pneumococcal vaccine, haemophilus influenzae type B vaccine and influenza vaccine in patients with COPD. [thesis]. Moscow: Right; 2012. 26 p. (In Russ.)

[4] Protasov A.D. The grounds for the development and introduction of the vaccine against M. catarrhalis for patients with chronic obstructive pulmonary disease. Medical Almanac. 2013;2(26):66–68. (In Russ.)

[5] Kostinov M.P., editor. Vaccination of adult subjects with bronchopulmonary pathology. A guide for physicians. Moscow: Art-studio "Constellation"; 2013. 112 p. (In Russ.)

[6] Protasov A.D., Zhestkov A.V., Kostinov M.P., Ryzhov A.A.. Changes in sputum bacterial landscape after vaccination against Streptococcus pneumoniae, Haemophilus influenzae type b and influenza in patients with chronic obstructive pulmonary disease. Pulmonology. 2012;5:23–27. (In Russ.)

[7] Dubinina V.V., Markelova E.V., Kostinov M.P. Immune response after "Pneumo-23" vaccination in persons of different age groups. Medical Immunology. 2005;7(2–3):259. (In Russ.)

[8] Chuchalin A.G, editor. Chronic obstructive pulmonary disease. Moscow: Atmosphere; 2008. 568 p. (In Russ.)

[9] Belevskii A.S., editor. Global strategy for the diagnosis, management, and prevention of chronic obstructive pulmonary disease. Moscow: Russian Respiratory Society; 2012. 80 p. (In Russ.)

[10] Lang T.A., Sesik M. How to describe statistical analysis in medicine. A manual for authors, editors and reviewers. Moscow: Applied medicine; 2011. 480 p. (In Russ.)

[11] Kostinov M.P., Protasov A.D., Zhestkov A.V., Pakhomov D.V., Chebykina A.V., Kostinova T.A. Post-vaccination immunity to pneumococcal, Haemophilus influenzae type B infection and influenza in patients with chronic obstructive pulmonary disease (COPD). J Vaccines Vaccin. 2014;5(2):1-5. doi:10.4172/2157-7560.1000221.